...a Pocket Dosing Guide 2010

Foreword

Welcome to the *PDR Pharmacopoeia Pocket Dosing Guide*, now in its 10th edition. This convenient little book is designed to be at your fingertips whenever you need to double-check dosage recommendations, review available forms and strengths, or confirm a pregnancy rating. The 2010 edition has been completely updated to include the newest drugs, forms, strengths, and indications.

To aid quick lookups and comparisons, PDR Pharmacopoeia is organized by major drug category and specific indication. Under each indication, you'll find applicable drugs sorted by class and listed alphabetically by generic name. For combination products, generic ingredients are listed alphabetically, with the strengths of the ingredients presented in the same order.

The book's major sections are listed on the Table of Contents page. The location of entries for specific brands, generics, and indications can be found in the index at the end of the book. For drugs with multiple uses, the index lists the page of each indication separately. Headings under a generic drug entry include listings for [illegible] single and combination forms of the generic product.

[illegible] *[illegible]opoeia* also offers [illegible]riety of quick- [illegible] [illegible]ently use[illegible] [illegible]as and compara- [illegible] [illegible]t location of these [illegible] end of the book.

The *PDR Pharmacopoeia* is drawn exclusively from FDA-approved drug labeling published in *Physicians' Desk Reference*® or supplied by the manufacturer. Although diligent efforts have been made to ensure the accuracy of this information, please remember that this book is sold without warranties, express or implied, and that the publisher and editors disclaim all liability in connection with its use.

Remember, too, that this book deals only with dosage for the typical patient, and includes little information on usage in special populations and circumstances. The need for dosage adjustments/warnings in the presence of hepatic or renal insufficiency is signaled in the Comments column of the entries. For details regarding these adjustments, as well as complete pediatric and geriatric dosage guidelines, consult the latest edition of *PDR*® or the manufacturer. Be sure to check these sources, too, whenever contraindications, warnings, or precautions may be an issue.

Throughout the book, you will find a drug's Controlled Substances Category (if any) immediately following its name. The drug's pregnancy rating and breastfeeding status appear in the Comments column of the entry. Keys to the symbols can be found below:

CII. High potential for abuse, leading to severe psychological or physical dependence. **CIII.** Abuse may lead to moderate or low physical dependence or high psychological dependence. **CIV.** Abuse may lead to limited physical dependence or psychological dependence. **CV.** Consequences of abuse are more limited than those of drugs in Category CIV.

USE-IN-PREGNANCY RATINGS

A. Controlled studies shown no risk. **B.** No evidence of risk in humans. **C.** Risk cannot be ruled out. **D.** Positive evidence of risk: Use only when no safer alternative exists for a serious problem. **X.** Contraindicated in pregnancy. **N.** Not rated.

Breastfeeding Safety

^ May be used in breastfeeding. > Caution advised or effect undetermined. v Contraindicated or not recommended.

H Dosage adjustment required for hepatic insufficiency.
R Dosage adjustment required for renal insufficiency.
W See Footnotes section.

DOSAGE FORMS

A key to the abbreviations may be found on page 4.

FOOTNOTES

A key to the footnotes begins on page 8.

PDR® PHARMACOPOEIA POCKET DOSING GUIDE 2010

PHYSICIANS' DESK REFERENCE

Director, Clinical Services: Sylvia Nashed, PharmD
Manager, Clinical Services: Nermin Shenouda, PharmD
Clinical Editors: Anila Patel, PharmD; Christine Sunwoo, PharmD
Manager, Production Purchasing: Thomas Westburgh
Manager, Art Department: Livio Udina
Associate Editor: Jennifer Reed
Project Manager: Don Pond

Executive Vice President, PDR: Thomas Rice
Vice President, Publishing & Operations: Valerie Berger
Vice President, Product & Solutions: Cy Caine
Senior Director, Editorial & Publishing: Bette Kennedy
Senior Product Manager: Richard Buchwald

Printed in USA 2010.1

ABBREVIATIONS

ABBREVIATIONS & DESCRIPTIONS	
CAP	community-acquired pneumonia
Cap	capsule
Cap,er	extended release capsule
CI	contraindicated
Cnt	concentrate
conc	concentration
Cre	cream
d	day
D/C	discontinue
Eli	elixir
Foa	foam
Gel	gel/jelly
gm	gram
h	hour
hs	at bedtime
IM	intramuscular
inj	injection
IU	international units
IV	intravenous

ABBREVIATIONS & DESCRIPTIONS	
ml	milliliter
mth	month
NTE	not to exceed
Oint	ointment
Pkt	packet
PO	by mouth
Pow	powder
prn	as needed
q	every
qd	once daily
qid	four times daily
qod	every other day
qow	every other week
SC	subcutaneous
Sl	sublingual
Sol	solution
Sol,Neb	solution, nebulized
Spr	spray(s)
Sup	suppository

kg	kilogram
Liq	liquid
Lot	lotion
Loz	lozenge
mcg	microgram
MDI	metered dose inhaler
mEq	milli-equivalent
mg	milligram
min	minute
miU	million international units
Susp	suspension
Syr	syrup
Tab	tablet
Tab,er	extended release tablet
tid	3 times daily
tiw	3 times weekly
U	units
w/a	while awake
wk	week
yo	years old

WEIGHTS & MEASURES; CONVERSIONS & FORMULAS

METRIC WEIGHT

1 kilogram (kg)	=	1,000 gram
1 gram (g)	=	1,000 mg
1 milligram (mg)	=	0.001 gm

METRIC WEIGHT

1 microgram (mcg)	=	0.001 mg
1 gamma	=	1 mcg

U.S. FLUID MEASURE

1 fluidrachm	=	60 minim (min)
1 fluidounce	=	8 fld drachm
	=	480 min

U.S. FLUID MEASURE

1 pint (pt)	=	16 fl oz
	=	7,680 min
1 quart (qt)	=	2 pt
	=	32 fl oz
1 gallon (gal)	=	4 qts
	=	128 fl oz

APOTHECARY WEIGHT

1 scruple	=	20 grains (gr)
1 drachm	=	3 scruples
	=	60 gr
1 ounce (oz)	=	8 drachms
	=	24 scruples
	=	480 gr
1 pound (lb)	=	12 oz
	=	96 drachms
	=	288 scruples
	=	5,760 gr

AVOIRDUPOIS WEIGHT

1 ounce	=	437.5 gr
1 pound	=	16 oz

CONVERSION FACTORS

1 gram	=	15.4 gr
1 grain	=	64.8 mg
1 ounce (AV)	=	28.35 gm
	=	437.5 gr
1 ounce (Ap)	=	31.1 gm
	=	480 gr
1 pound (Av)	=	453.6 gm
1 kilogram	=	2.68 pound Ap
	=	2.2 lbs Av
1 fluidounce	=	29.57 ml
1 fluidrachm	=	3.697 ml
1 minim	=	0.06 ml

COMMON MEASURES

1 teaspoonful	=	5 ml
	=	1/6 fl oz
1 tablespoonful	=	15 ml
	=	1/2 fl oz
1 wineglassful	=	60 ml
	=	2 fl oz
1 teacupful	=	120 ml
	=	4 fl oz

TEMPERATURE

For °F to °C, the formula is: 5/9 (°F minus 32) = °C
For °C to °F, the formula is: 9/5 °C plus 32 = °F
1 kelvin (K) = 9/5 °F

COCKCROFT/GAULT CREATININE CLEARANCE FORMULA

$$\text{ClCr (males* ml/min)} = \frac{(140 - \text{Age})(\text{Body Weight in kg})}{(\text{SrCr})(72\text{ kg})}$$

*For females multiply result by 0.85

BODY SURFACE AREA [BSA (M^2)]

BSA = ([Ht (cm) • Wt (kg)]/ 3600) 1⁄2

ANION GAP (AG)

AG = $(Na^+ + K^+) - (Cl^- + HCO_3^-)$ or AG = $Na^+ - (Cl^- + HCO_3^-)$

NEUTROPENIA CALCULATION

ANC = (% segs + % bands) X total WBC

FOOTNOTES

1 Potential neurotoxicity, ototoxicity & neuromuscular blockade. Avoid concurrent use w/ neurotoxic/nephrotoxic agents & diuretics.

2 Contraindicated in pregnant patients at term & nursing mothers.

3 Give only under supervision of a physician experienced w/ antineoplastics.

4 Contraindicated in pregnancy. Increased risk of endometrial carcinoma.

5 Proarrhythmic properties/drug should only be used in life-threatening arrhythmias.

6 Risk of paralysis by spinal/epidural hematoma w/ neuraxial anesthesia/lumbar puncture. Increased risk w/ concomitant anticoagulation, NSAIDs, or traumatic/repeated lumbar puncture.

7 ACE Inhibitors can cause injury & death to developing fetus in 2nd & 3rd trimesters.

8 Excess amounts may lead to water & electrolyte depletion.

9 When used in pregnancy, primarily during 2nd & 3rd trimesters, drugs acting directly on renin-angiotensin system may cause injury & even death to developing fetus. D/C if pregnancy detected.

10 Attempt to taper or d/c at 3-6 mth intervals.

11 Should only be used by physicians experienced w/ immunosuppression therapy.

12 Granulocytopenia. Anemia. Thrombocytopenia. Carcinogenic, teratogenic & aspermatogenic in animal studies.

13 May cause or aggravate neuropsychiatric, autoimmune, ischemic & infectious disorders; monitor closely.

14 INH associated w/ hepatitis. Avoid in acute hepatic diseases.

15 Neutropenia. Agranulocytosis. TTP. Aplastic anemia.

16 Tumorigenic in chronic toxicity studies. Avoid unnecessary use.

17 Abrupt cessation may induce arrhythmia or MI.

18 Abrupt cessation may exacerbate angina.

19 Monitor for bone marrow, lung, liver & kidney toxicities. Serious toxic reactions.

20 Risk of ocular damage, aging skin & skin cancer. Do not interchange w/ Oxsoralen-Ultra without retitration.

21 Risk of ocular damage, aging skin & skin cancer. Do not interchange w/ regular Oxsoralen or 8-Mop. Determine minimum phototoxic dose & phototoxic peak time.

22 Overdose in children can cause death.

23 Chromosomal aberrations. Severe bone marrow suppression.

24 Avoid if CrCl <30 ml/min.

25 CI during pregnancy. Thromboembolism, thrombotic & thrombophlebitic events reported. Peliosis hepatitis & benign hepatic carcinoma observed w/ long-term use. Associated w/ benign intracranial HTN.

26 Risk of agranulocytosis, seizures, myocarditis, other cardiovascular/respiratory effects. Increased mortality in elderly patients w/ dementia-related psychosis.

27 See Immunization chart for details.

28 Not for prevention of CV disease or dementia. Increased risks of MI, stroke, invasive breast cancer, pulmonary emboli, DVT & probable dementia in postmenopausal women. Prescribe at lowest effective doses for shortest duration.

29 May increase risk of suicidality in children, adolescents & young adults.

30 Increased risk of death in elderly patients w/ dementia-related psychosis.

31	Lactic acidosis & severe hepatomegaly w/ steatosis reported.
32	Severe acute exacerbations of hepatitis B reported in patients who have discontinued anti-hepatitis B therapy; monitor hepatic function closely.
33	Fatal hypersensitivity reactions reported.
34	Associated w/ hematologic toxicity. Prolonged use associated w/ myopathy.
35	Fatal & nonfatal pancreatitis reported.
36	May cause severe peripheral neuropathy.
37	Chronic administration may result in nephrotoxicity; monitor renal function w/, or if at risk of, renal dysfunction.
38	HIV resistance may emerge.
39	May cause severe hypersensitivity reactions including anaphylaxis. May cause severe hemolysis w/ G6PD deficiency. Use associated w/ methemoglobinemia. May interfere w/ uric acid measurements.
43	Serious GI adverse events reported; d/c if constipation or symptoms of ischemic colitis develop.
44	Caution w/ auditory or renal impairment. Avoid/caution w/ other ototoxic or nephrotoxic agents.
45	Intracranial hemorrhage, hepatitis & hepatic decompensation reported w/ ritonavir co-administration. Monitor closely w/ chronic hepatitis B or C co-infection.
46	Serious & sometimes fatal infections & bleeding occur very rarely.
47	NSAIDs may cause increased risk of serious CV thrombotic events, MI & stroke.
48	NSAIDs may cause increased risk of serious GI events.
49	High potential for abuse; avoid prolonged use. Misuse may cause sudden death & serious CV adverse events.

50 CI w/ phosphodiesterase type 5 (PDE5) inhibitors (eg, sildenafil, vardenafil, & tadalafil).

51 Swallow caps whole or sprinkle contents on applesauce. Do not crush, chew, or dissolve cap beads. Avoid alcohol or any alcohol-containing medications; may result in rapid absorption of potentially fatal dose of morphine.

52 Not for use by females who are or may become pregnant or breastfeeding. Birth defects documented. Approved for marketing only under iPLEDGE. Prescriber & patient must be registered w/ iPLEDGE.

53 Increased susceptibility to infection & possible development of lymphoma & other neoplasms may result from immunosuppression.

54 Sodium oxybate is a GHB (gamma hydroxybutyrate), a known drug of abuse. Do not use w/ alcohol or other CNS depressants. Only available through Xyrem Success Program.

55 Severe neurologic events reported.

56 Potential for human birth defects, hematologic toxicity (neutropenia & thrombocytopenia) & DVT/PE. Avoid fetal exposure. Only available under a restricted distribution program called "Revassist."

57 Highly concentrated. Check dose carefully.

58 Do not administer IV or by other parenteral routes. Deaths & serious, life-threatening adverse events have occurred when contents of capsules have been injected parenterally.

59 Renal impairment is major toxicity. CI w/ nephrotoxic agents. Neutropenia reported. Carcinogenic, teratogenic & hypospermatic in animal studies.

60 Extreme caution w/ renal dysfunction. Monitor hematologic, renal & hepatic status.

61 Risk of fatal hepatotoxicity. CI w/ terfenadine, astemizole, cisapride, oral triazolam.

62 Increased risk of severe neurotoxic reactions w/ renal dysfunction. Avoid neurotoxic & nephrotoxic drugs.

63 Hematologic toxicity & opportunistic infections reported. Gradually increase dose to avoid infusion reactions.

64 Severe myelosuppression, hypersensitivity reactions & hepatotoxicity reported.

65 Fatal infusion reactions, tumor lysis syndrome, severe mucocutaneous reactions & progressive multifocal leukoencephalopathy reported.

66 NSAIDs may cause an increased risk of serious CV thrombotic events, MI, stroke & serious GI adverse events including bleeding, ulceration & perforation of the stomach or intestines.

67 Contraindicated for treatment of peri-operative pain in CABG surgery.

68 CI w/ PUD, GI bleeding/perforation, advanced renal impairment, risk of renal failure due to volume depletion, CV bleeding, hemorrhagic diathesis, incomplete hemostasis, high-risk of bleeding, prophylactic analgesic before major surgery, intra-operatively when hemostasis is critical, intrathecal/epidural use, L&D, nursing & w/ ASA, NSAIDs, or probenecid.

69 Contains potent CII opioid agonist w/ high potential for abuse & risk of respiratory depression. HP formulation is highly concentrated; do not confuse w/ standard parenteral formulations.

70 Dermatologic toxicities & severe infusion reactions reported.

71 CI w/ myasthenia gravis.

72 Deaths, cardiac & respiratory, reported during initiation & conversion of pain patients to methadone treatment from treatment w/ other opioid agonists.

73 May cause fatal anaphylactic or anaphylactoid reactions.

74 Not for use as prn analgesic. May cause fatal respiratory depression if not already tolerant to high doses of opioids. Swallow caps whole, sprinkle contents on applesauce or dissolve in water & give thru 16 French G-tube. Do not crush, chew, or dissolve cap pellets.

75 Increased mortality, serious CV/thrombolembolic events & increased risk of tumor progression or recurrence. (Renal Failure) Studies have shown greater risks for death & serious CV events when ESAs given to higher target Hgb levels; individualize dosing to achieve/maintain Hgb of 10-12 gm/dL. (Cancer) Use lowest dose needed to avoid RBC transfusions, use only for anemia due to concomitant myelosuppressive chemo & d/c following completion of chemo. (Perisurgery) Increased rate of DVT w/o prophylactic anticoagulation; consider DVT prophylaxis.

76 Increased mortality, serious CV/thrombolembolic events & increased risk of tumor progression or recurrence. (Renal Failure) Studies have shown greater risks for death & serious CV events when ESAs given to higher target Hgb levels; individualize dosing to achieve/maintain Hgb of 10-12 gm/dL. (Cancer) Use lowest dose needed to avoid RBC transfusions, use only for anemia due to concomitant myelosuppressive chemo & d/c following completion of chemo.

77 Increases risk of meningococcal infections; vaccinate 2 wks prior to receiving 1st dose.

78 Potential liver injury. CI in pregnancy. Available only thru Letairis Education and Access Program.

79 Thiazolidinediones may cause or exacerbate CHF in some patients. Use not recommended in patients w/ symptomatic heart failure.

80 May lead to increased susceptibility to infection & possible development of lymphoma. Female users of childbearing potential must use contraception.

81 CI in combination w/ capecitabine if AST/ALT >2.5x ULN or bilirubin >1x ULN due to increased toxicity & neutropenia-related death.

82 Thiazolidinediones may cause or exacerbate CHF in some patients. Use not recommended w/ symptomatic heart failure. Studies have shown an increased risk of myocardial ischemic events.

83 Metronidazole has been shown to be carcinogenic in mice & rats. Unnecessary use should be avoided.

84 *C.difficile*-associated diarrhea reported.

85 Increases risk of progressive multifocal leukoencephalopathy (PML). Available only through special restricted distribution program called the TOUCH™ Prescribing Program.

86 Serious infections, including TB, bacterial sepsis & other opportunistic infections, reported. Evaluate for TB risk factors & test for latent TB infection prior to initiation.

87 Serious, sometimes fatal, dermatologic reactions, aplastic anemia & agranulocytosis reported.

88 Abnormal elevation of serum K+ levels (≥5.5 mEq/L) can occur w/ all K+-sparing agents, including triamterene; monitor serum K+ at frequent intervals.

89 May cause QT interval prolongation, complete AV block, or APL differentiation syndrome. Monitor ECG, electrolytes & creatinine before & during therapy.

90 May increase susceptibility to infection & development of neoplasia. Neoral® & Sandimmune® are not bioequivalent. Increased skin malignancy risk w/ certain psoriasis therapies. May cause HTN & nephotoxicity; monitor renal function.

91 Cardiomyopathy, infusion reactions & pulmonary toxicity reported.

92 Infections & progressive multifocal leukoencephalopathy may occur.

93 Myocardial damage, infusion-related reactions & myelosuppression may occur. Reduce dose w/ hepatic impairment. Avoid substitution w/ doxorubicin HCl.

94 May cause GI perforation, wound dehiscence & fatal pulmonary hemorrhage.

95 May cause negative inotropic effects. CI w/ cisapride, pimozide, quinidine, dofetilide, levacetylmethadol. Serious CV events reported w/ CYP3A4 inhibitors.

96 Life-threatening peripheral ischemia w/ concomitant potent CYP3A4 inhibitors.

97 Co-administration w/ certain nonsedating antihistamines, sedative hypnotics, antiarrhythmics, or ergot alkaloids may result in potentially serious/life-threatening adverse events.

98 Fluoroquinolones associated w/ increased risk of tendinitis & tendon rupture in all ages. Risk further increased if >60 yo, taking corticosteroids, or w/ kidney, heart or lung transplants.

99 Abuse liability similar to other opioid analgesics. Not intended as prn analgesic. 100 mg & 200 mg tabs for use in opioid-tolerant patients only. Swallow whole.

100 May cause increased risk of serious cardiovascular thrombotic events, MI, stroke & serious GI adverse events.

101 Fatal hepatoxicity reported (children <2 yo at higher risk); monitor closely & perform LFTs prior to therapy & then periodically. Teratogenic effects & life-threatening pancreatitis reported.

102 Give cautiously w/ history of drug dependence or alcoholism. Chronic abusive use may lead to marked tolerance & psychological dependence w/ varying degrees of abnormal behavior. Monitor closely during withdrawal.

ANALGESICS

Arthritis Therapy

SEE ALSO NSAIDS

NAME	FORM/STRENGTH	DOSAGE	COMMENTS
Abatacept (Orencia)	**Inj:** 250 mg	**Adults: Rheumatoid Arthritis: Initial: IV: <60 kg:** 500 mg. **60-100 kg:** 750 mg. **>100 kg:** 1 gm. Infuse over 30 min. **Maint:** Give at 2 & 4 wks after initial infusion, then q4wks thereafter. **Peds: 6-17 yo: Polyarticular Juvenile Idiopathic Arthritis: >75 kg:** Follow adult dosing. **Max:** 1000 mg. **<75 kg: Initial:** 10 mg/kg. Infuse over 30 min. **Maint:** Give at 2 & 4 wks after initial infusion, then q4wks thereafter.	C v
Adalimumab (Humira)	**Inj:** 40 mg/0.8 ml	**RA/Psoriatic Arthritis/Ankylosing Spondylitis: Adults:** 40 mg SC every other wk. Patients w/ RA not taking MTX may derive additional benefit by increasing to 40 mg qwk.	B v **W** 86
Anakinra (Kineret)	**Inj:** 100 mg/0.67 ml	**RA: Adults: ≥18 yo:** 100 mg SC qd.	B >
Auranofin (Ridaura)	**Cap:** 3 mg	**RA: Adults: Usual:** 3 mg bid or 6 mg qd. **Max:** 9 mg/d.	C v May cause gold toxicity.

Azathioprine (Azasan)	**Tab:** 25 mg, 50 mg, 75 mg, 100 mg	**RA: Adults: Initial:** 1 mg/kg/d given qd-bid. **Titrate:** May increase by 0.5 mg/kg/d after 6-8 wks, then q4wks. **Max:** 2.5 mg/kg/d. **Maint:** May decrease by 0.5 mg/kg/d or 25 mg/d q4wks until lowest effective dose. If no response by Week 12, consider refractory.	D v **R** Risk of neoplasia, mutagenesis & hematologic toxicities.
Azathioprine (Imuran)	**Tab:** 50 mg	**RA: Adults: Initial:** 1 mg/kg/d given qd-bid. **Titrate:** May increase by 0.5 mg/kg/d after 6-8 wks, then q4wks. **Max:** 2.5 mg/kg/d. **Maint:** May decrease by 0.5 mg/kg/d or 25 mg/d q4wks until lowest effective dose. If no response by Week 12, consider refractory.	D v **R** Risk of neoplasia, mutagenesis & hematologic toxicities.
Celecoxib (Celebrex)	**Cap:** 50 mg, 100 mg, 200 mg, 400 mg	**Adults: ≥18 yo: OA:** 200 mg qd or 100 mg bid. **RA:** 100-200 mg bid. **AS: Initial:** 200 mg qd or 100 mg bid. **Titrate:** May increase to 400 mg/d after 6 wks. **Peds: ≥2 yo: JRA: 10-25 kg:** 50 mg bid. **>25 kg:** 100 mg bid. **Poor Metabolizers of CYP2C9 Substrates:** Half lowest recommended dose.	C D (≥30 wks gestation) v **H W** [66, 67]
Certolizumab pegol (Cimzia)	**Inj:** 200 mg/ml	**RA: Adults: Initial:** 400 mg SC, and at Weeks 2 & 4, followed by 200 mg qow. **Maint:** 400 mg SC q4wks. **Concomitant w/ MTX:** 200 mg qow.	B v **W** [86]

NAME	FORM/STRENGTH	DOSAGE	COMMENTS
Cyclosporine (Neoral)	**Cap:** 25 mg, 100 mg; **Sol:** 100 mg/ml	**RA: Adults ≥18 yo: Initial:** 2.5 mg/kg/d, taken bid. **Titrate:** Increase by 0.5-0.75 mg/kg/d after 8 wks & again after 12 wks. **Max:** 4 mg/kg/d. Decrease by 25-50% to control adverse events. **Combo w/ MTX: Maint:** 3 mg/kg/d or less. **Max:** 15 mg/wk.	C v **W** 90
Etanercept (Enbrel)	**Inj:** 25 mg, 50 mg/ml	**RA/Psoriatic Arthritis/Ankylosing Spondylitis: Adults:** 50 mg/wk SC. **JRA: Peds: 2-17 yo:** 0.8 mg/kg/wk SC. **Max:** 50 mg/wk.	B v **W** 86
Flavocoxid (Limbrel)	**Cap:** 250 mg, 500 mg	**OA: Adults: ≥18 yo:** 250-500 mg q12h for total daily dose of 500-1000 mg/d. May increase to 2 or more caps q12h under physician supervision.	N v
Hydroxychloroquine Sulfate (Plaquenil)	**Tab:** 200 mg	**RA: Adults: Initial:** 400-600 mg/d w/ food or glass of milk. Increase dose in 5-10d until optimum response. **Maint:** After 4-12 wks, 200-400 mg/d.	N >
Infliximab (Remicade)	**Inj:** 100 mg	**Adults: RA (Combo w/ MTX):** 3 mg/kg IV infusion; repeat at 2 & 6 wks. **Maint:** 3 mg/kg q8wks thereafter. **Incomplete Response:** May increase to 10 mg/kg or give q4wks. **Ankylosing Spondylitis:** 5 mg/kg IV infusion; repeat at 2 & 6 wks. **Maint:** 5 mg/kg q6wks thereafter. **Psoriatic Arthritis:** 5 mg/kg IV infusion; repeat at 2 & 6 wks. **Maint:** 5 mg/kg q8wks thereafter.	B v **W** 86

Leflunomide (Arava)	**Tab:** 10 mg, 20 mg	**RA: Adults: LD:** 100 mg qd x 3d. **Maint:** 20 mg qd. **Max:** 20 mg/d. **If dose not tolerated or ALT elevations >2 but ≤3x ULN:** Reduce dose to 10 mg/d. If elevations persist or ALT >3x UNL, d/c.	X v **H** CI in pregnancy. Hepatotoxicity. Immunosuppression.
Meloxicam (Mobic)	**Susp:** 7.5 mg/5 ml; **Tab:** 7.5 mg, 15 mg	**OA/RA: Adults: ≥18 yo: Initial/Maint:** 7.5 mg qd. **Max:** 15 mg/d. **JRA: Peds: ≥2 yo:** 0.125 mg/kg qd. **Max:** 7.5 mg/d.	C v **W** [66, 67]
Methotrexate Sodium (Rheumatrex)	**Tab:** 2.5 mg, 5 mg, 7.5 mg, 15 mg	**RA: Adults: Initial:** 7.5 mg once wkly or 2.5 mg q12h x 3 doses once wkly. **Max:** 20 mg/wk. Reduce to lowest effective dose. **JRA: Peds 2-16 yo:** 10 mg/m^2 once wkly. Adjust dose to optimal response.	X v CI in pregnancy & nursing. **W** [19]
Penicillamine (Cuprimine)	**Cap:** 250 mg	**RA: Adults: Initial:** 125-250 mg/d. **Titrate:** May increase by 125-250 mg/d q1-3mths. If needed after 2-3 mths, may increase by 250 mg/d q2-3mths. D/C if no improvement after 3-4 mths at dose of 1-1.5 gm/d. **Maint:** 500-750 mg/d. **Max:** 1.5g/d.	D v CI in pregnancy, renal insufficiency & agranulocytosis.
Rituximab (Rituxan)	**Inj:** 10 mg/ml	**RA: Adults:** Give w/ MTX. Give two-1000 mg IV infusions separated by 2 wks. Give methylprednisolone 100 mg IV (or equivalent) 30 min prior to each infusion to reduce incidence & severity of infusion reactions.	C v **W** [65]

NAME	FORM/STRENGTH	DOSAGE	COMMENTS
Sulfasalazine (Azulfidine EN)	**Tab,Delay:** 500 mg	**RA: Adults: Initial:** 0.5-1 gm qd. **Usual:** 1 gm bid. **Max:** 3 gm/d. **JRA: Peds: 6-16 yo:** 30-50 mg/kg/d given bid. **Max:** 2 gm/d.	B >;

Narcotics

NAME	FORM/STRENGTH	DOSAGE	COMMENTS
Codeine Phosphate/ Acetaminophen CIII (Tylenol with Codeine)	**Eli:** 12-120 mg/5 ml; **Tab:** (#3) 30-300 mg, (#4) 60-300 mg	**Tab: Adults:** 15 mg-60 mg codeine/dose & 300 mg-1 gm APAP/dose up to q4h prn. **Max:** 360 mg codeine & 4 gm APAP per 24h. **Peds:** 0.5 mg/kg of codeine. **Eli: Adults:** 15 ml q4h prn. **Peds: 3-6 yo:** 5 ml tid-qid. **7-12 yo:** 10 ml tid-qid.	C >
Fentanyl CII (Duragesic)	**Patch:** 12.5 mcg/h, 25 mcg/h, 50 mcg/h, 75 mcg/h, 100 mcg/h	**Adults & Peds: ≥2 yo: Opioid Tolerant:** Individualize dose based on opioid tolerance. **Initial:** Base on daily oral morphine dose (see PI). **Titrate:** Adjust dose after 3d based on daily supplemental opioid analgesic dose; use ratio of 45 mg/24h of oral morphine to a 12.5 mcg/h increase in Duragesic dose. May take 6d to reach equilibrium after dose change.	C v
Fentanyl Citrate CII (Actiq)	**Loz:** 0.2 mg, 0.4 mg, 0.6 mg, 0.8 mg, 1.2 mg, 1.6 mg	**Breakthrough Pain: Adults & Peds: ≥16 yo: Initial:** 0.2 mg for pain (consume over 15 min). **Titrate:** Increase to next strength if pain episodes require >1 unit/pain episode. **Maint:** 1 unit/pain episode. **Max:** 2 units/pain episode or 4 units/d.	C v CI in acute or post-op pain, non-opioid tolerant patients.

Fentanyl Citrate CII (Fentora)	**Tab, Buccal:** 100 mcg, 200 mcg, 400 mcg, 600 mcg, 800 mcg	**Breakthough Pain Associated w/ Cancer: Adults: Initial:** 100 mcg. Repeat once (30 min after starting dose) during a single episode. **Titration Above 100 mcg:** Use two 100 mcg tabs (1 on each side of buccal cavity); if not controlled, use two 100 mcg tabs on each side (total four 100 mcg tabs). **Titration Above 400 mcg:** Use 200 mcg tab increments. **Max:** Not >4 tabs simultaneously. Do not chew, crush, swallow, or dissolve; consume over 14-25 min.	◙C ❁v CI in acute or post-op pain, non-opioid tolerant patients.
Hydrocodone Bitartrate/ Acetaminophen CIII (Lorcet, Lorcet 10/650, Lorcet HD, Lorcet Plus)	(Hydrocodone-APAP) **Cap:** (HD) 5 mg-500 mg; **Tab:** (Plus) 7.5 mg-650 mg, (10/650) 10 mg-650 mg	**Adults: Usual:** (Plus, 10/650) 1 cap/tab q4-6h prn pain. **Max:** 6 tabs/caps/d. (HD) 1-2 caps q4-6h prn pain. **Max:** 8 caps/d.	◙C ❁v
Hydrocodone Bitartrate/ Acetaminophen CIII (Vicodin, Vicodin ES, Vicodin HP)	**Sol:** (Vicodin) 5-500 mg, (Vicodin ES) 7.5-750 mg, (Vicodin HP) 10-660 mg	**Pain: Adults: Usual: Vicodin:** 1-2 tabs q4-6h prn. **Max:** 8 tabs/d. **Vicodin HP:** 1 tab q4-6h prn. **Max:** 6 tabs/d. **Vicodin ES:** 1 tab q4-6h prn. **Max:** 5 tabs/d.	◙C ❁v
Hydrocodone Bitartrate/ Ibuprofen CIII (Reprexain, Vicoprofen)	**Tab:** (Reprexain) 5-200 mg, 7.5 mg-200 mg; (Vicoprofen) 7.5-200 mg	**Adults & Peds: ≥16 yo: Usual:** 1 tab q4-6h prn. **Max:** 5 tabs/d.	◙C ❁v

NAME	FORM/STRENGTH	DOSAGE	COMMENTS
Hydrocodone/ Acetaminophen CIII (Lortab)	**Sol:** 7.5-500 mg/15 ml; **Tab:** 2.5-500 mg, 5-500 mg, 7.5-500 mg, 10-500 mg	**Pain: Adults: Tabs:** (2.5-500 mg, 5-500 mg) 1-2 tabs q4-6h prn. **Max:** 8 tabs/d. (7.5-500 mg, 10-500 mg) 1 tab q4-6h prn. **Max:** 6 tabs/d. **Sol:** 15 ml q4-6h prn. **Max:** 90 ml/d. **Peds: ≥2 yo: Lortab: Sol: 12-15 kg:** 3.75 ml. **16-22 kg:** 5 ml. **23-31 kg:** 7.5 ml. **32-45 kg:** 10 ml. **≥46 kg:** 15 ml. May repeat q4-6h prn.	C v
Hydromorphone HCl CII (Dilaudid, Dilaudid-HP)	**Inj:** 1 mg/ml, 2 mg/ml, 4 mg/ml, (HP) 10 mg/ml; **Sol:** 1 mg/ml; **Sup:** 3 mg; **Tab:** 2 mg, 4 mg, 8 mg	**Adults:** Individualize dose. **Initial:** 1-2 mg SC/IM/IV q4-6h prn. (HP) 1-14 mg IM/SC; adjust dose based on response. (Sol) 2.5-10 mg PO q3-6h prn. (Tab) 2-4 mg PO q4-6h prn. (Sup) Insert 1 PR q6-8h prn. **Titrate:** Increase dose as needed. **Elderly:** Start at lower end of dosing range.	C v **W** 69
Meperidine HCl CII (Demerol Oral)	**Syr:** 50 mg/5 ml; **Tab:** 50 mg, 100 mg	**Adults: Usual:** 50-150 mg PO q3-4h prn. **Peds: Usual:** 0.5 mg/lb-0.8 mg/lb PO, up to adult dose, q3-4h prn. Mix syrup in 1/2 glass of water to prevent topical anesthetic effect on mucous membranes.	N >**H R** CI with MAOI use within 14 days.
Methadone HCl CII (Dolophine)	**Tab:** 5 mg, 10 mg	**Pain: Adults: Usual**: 2.5-10 mg PO/IM/SC q3-4h prn. Special dosing for detox/maintenance treatment.	N > **W** 72
Morphine Sulfate CII	**Sol:** 10 mg/5 ml, 20 mg/5 ml; **Tab:** 15 mg, 30 mg	**Adults: Sol:** 10-20mg q4h. **Tab:** 15-30 mg q4h.	C v
Morphine Sulfate CII (Avinza)	**Cap,ER:** 30 mg, 60 mg, 90 mg, 120 mg	**Adults: ≥18 yo: Conversion from PO Morphine:** Give total daily morphine dose as a single dose q24h. **Conversion from Parenteral Morphine: Initial:** Give about 3x previous daily parenteral morphine requirement. **Conversion from Other Parenteral or PO Non-Morphine Opioids: Initial:**	C v **W** 51

		Give 1/2 of estimated daily morphine requirement q24h. May supplement w/ immediate-release morphine or short-acting analgesics. **Titrate:** Adjust as frequently as qod. **Non-Opioid Tolerant:** 30 mg q24h. **Titrate:** Increase by no more than 30 mg q4d. **Max:** 1600 mg/d. The 60, 90, & 120 mg caps are for opioid-tolerant patients.	
Morphine Sulfate CII (Kadian)	**Cap,ER:** 10 mg, 20 mg, 30 mg, 50 mg, 60 mg, 80 mg, 100 mg, 200 mg	**Adults: Conversion From Other PO Morphine:** Give 50% of daily PO morphine dose q12h or 100% q24h. **Conversion from Parenteral Morphine:** Give about 3x previous daily parenteral morphine requirement. **Conversion from Other Parenteral or PO Opioids: Initial:** Give 1/2 of estimated daily morphine requirement q24h or give 1/4 of estimated daily morphine requirement q12h. May supplement w/ immediate-release morphine or short-acting analgesics. **Titrate:** Adjust as frequently as qod. **Non-Opioid Tolerant:** 20 mg q24h. **Titrate:** Increase by no more than 20 mg qod. **Max:** No ceiling dose.	C v **W** [74]
Morphine Sulfate CII (MS Contin)	**Tab,ER:** 15 mg, 30 mg, 60 mg, 100 mg, 200 mg	**Adults: Conversion from Immediate-Release Oral Morphine:** Give 1/2 of patient's 24h requirement as MS Contin q12h or give 1/3 of daily requirement as MS Contin q8h. **Conversion from Parenteral Morphine: Initial:** If daily morphine dose ≤120 mg/d, give MS Contin 30mg. **Titrate:** Switch to 60 mg or 100 mg MS Contin. Taper dose; do not d/c abruptly. Swallow whole.	C v **W** [99]

NAME	FORM/STRENGTH	DOSAGE	COMMENTS
Morphine Sulfate CII (Roxanol, Roxanol-T)	**Sol,Concentrate:** 20 mg/ml	**Adults: Usual:** 10-30 mg q4h. During 1st effective pain relief, dose should be maintained for at least 3 days before any dose reduction, if respiratory activity & other vital signs are adequate.	C > **H R W** 57
Nalbuphine (Nubain)	**Inj:** 10 mg/ml, 20 mg/ml	**Adults: ≥18 yo: Pain: Initial:** 10 mg/70kg IV/IM/SQ q3-6h prn. Adjust according to severity, physical status & concomitant agents. **Max:** 20 mg/dose or 160 mg/day. **Anesthesia Adjunct: Induction:** 0.3-3 mg/kg IV over 10-15 minutes. **Maint:** 0.25-0.5 mg/kg IV.	B >
Oxycodone HCl CII (Oxycontin)	**Tab,ER:** 10 mg, 20 mg, 40 mg, 80 mg	**Adults: ≥18 yo: Opioid Naive:** 10 mg q12h. **Titrate:** Increase to 20 mg q12h, then increase total daily dose by 25-50% of current dose. Increase q1-2d. **Conversion from Oxycodone:** Divide 24h oxycodone dose by 50% to obtain q12h dose. Round down to appropriate strength. **Opioid Tolerant:** May use 80 mg tabs. D/C other around-the-clock opioids. **With CNS Depressants:** Reduce by 1/3 or 1/2.	B v For continuous analgesia. Abuse potential. 80 mg tabs only for opioid-tolerant patients. Swallow whole.
Oxycodone HCl CII (OxyIR)	**Cap:** 5 mg	**Pain: Adults: Usual:** 5 mg q6h prn.	B v

Oxycodone HCl/ Acetaminophen CII (Percocet)	**Tab:** 2.5-325 mg, 5-325 mg, 7.5-325 mg, 7.5-500 mg, 10-325 mg, 10-650 mg	**Pain: Adults:** (2.5-325 mg) 1-2 tabs q6h prn. **Max:** 12 tabs/d. (5-325 mg) 1 tab q6h prn. **Max:** 12 tabs/d. (7.5-500 mg) 1 tab q6h prn. **Max:** 8 tabs/d. (10-650 mg) 1 tab q6h prn. **Max:** 6 tabs/d. (7.5-325 mg) 1 tab q6h prn. **Max:** 8 tabs/d. (10-325 mg) 1 tab q6h prn. **Max:** 6 tabs/d. Do not exceed 4 gm APAP/d.	C >
Oxycodone HCl/Aspirin CII (Endodan, Percodan)	**Tab:** 4.5-0.38-325 mg	**Pain: Adults: Usual:** 1 tab q6h prn. **Max:** 12 tabs/d.	B (Oxycodone) D (ASA) v
Oxycodone HCl/Ibuprofen CII (Combunox)	**Tab:** 5-400 mg	**Pain: Adults:** 1 tab/dose. Do not exceed 4 tabs/d & 7 days.	C v **W** 66, 67
Oxymorphone HCl CII (Opana, Opana ER)	**Tab:** (Opana) 5 mg, 10 mg; **Tab, ER:** (Opana ER) 5 mg, 10 mg, 20 mg, 40 mg	**Adults:** Individualize dose. **Opana: Opioid-Naive: Initial:** 5-20 mg q4-6h. Titrate based on response. **Max:** 20 mg/dose. **Conversion from Parenteral Oxymorphone:** Give 10x total daily parenteral oxymorphone dose in 4 or 6 equally divided doses. **Conversion from Other Oral Opioids:** Give half of calculated total daily dose in 4-6 equally divided doses, q4-6h. **Opana ER:** Swallow whole; do not break, chew, crush, or dissolve. **Opioid-Naive: Initial:** 5 mg q12h. Titrate based on response. **Usual:** Increase dose by 5-10 mg q12h every 3-7d. **Conversion from Opana:** Divide 24h Opana dose in half to obtain q12h dose. **Conversion from Parenteral Oxymorphone:** Give	C > **H R** Abuse potential. Do not crush, chew, or break ER tabs.

Continued on Next Page

NAME	FORM/STRENGTH	DOSAGE	COMMENTS
Oxymorphone HCl CII (Opana, Opana ER) *Continued*		10x total daily parenteral oxymorphone dose in 2 equally divided doses. **Conversion from Other Oral Opioids:** Divide calculated 24h Opana dose (refer to PI for conversion ratios) in half to obtain q12h dose.	
Pentazocine/ Naloxone HCl CIV (Talwin NX)	**Tab:** 50-0.5 mg	**Pain: Adults & Peds: ≥12 yo: Initial:** 1 tab q3-4h. **Titrate:** Increase to 2 tabs prn. **Max:** 12 tabs/d.	C > Not for inj.
Propoxyphene Napsylate CIV (Darvon-N)	**Tab:** 100 mg	**Pain: Adults: Usual:** 100 mg q4h prn. **Max:** 600 mg/d.	N > **H R**
Propoxyphene Napsylate/ Acetaminophen CIV (Darvocet-N)	**Tab:** 50-325 mg, 100-650 mg	**Pain: Adults: Usual:** 100 mg propoxyphene & 650 mg APAP q4h prn. **Max:** 600 mg/d of propoxyphene.	N > **H R**

NSAIDs

NAME	FORM/STRENGTH	DOSAGE	COMMENTS
Celecoxib (Celebrex)	**Cap:** 50 mg, 100 mg, 200 mg, 400 mg	**Adults: ≥18 yo: Acute Pain/Primary Dysmenorrhea: Day 1:** 400 mg, then 200 mg if needed. **Maint:** 200 mg bid prn. **OA:** 200 mg qd or 100 mg bid. **RA:** 100-200 mg bid. **AS:** 200 mg qd or 100 mg bid. **Titrate:** May increase to 400 mg/d after 6 wks. **Peds: JRA: ≥2 yo: 10-25 kg:** 50 mg bid. **>25 kg:** 100 mg bid. **Poor Metabolizers of CYP2C9 Substrates:** Half lowest recommended dose.	C D (≥30 wks gestation) v **H W** [66, 67]
Diclofenac Epolamine (Flector)	**Patch:** 180 mg	**Adults:** Apply 1 patch to most painful area bid.	C v **W** [66, 67]

Diclofenac Sodium/ Misoprostol (Arthrotec)	**Tab,Delay:** 50-0.2 mg, 75-0.2 mg	**Adults: OA:** 50 mg tid. **RA:** 50 mg tid-qid. If intolerable, give 50-75 mg bid for OA or RA.	X v Misoprostol is an abortifacient. **W** 66, 67
Diclofenac Sodium (Voltaren Gel)	**Gel:** 1%	**Adults:** Measure onto enclosed dosing card to appropriate 2 gm or 4 gm line. **Lower Extremities:** Apply 4 gm to affected foot, knee, or ankle qid. **Max:** 4 gm/d to any single joint. **Upper Extremities:** Apply 2 gm to affected hand, elbow, or wrist qid. **Max:** 8 gm/d to any single joint. Total dose should not exceed 32 gm/d over all affected joints. Avoid showering or bathing for at least 1h after application. Avoid open wounds, eyes, mucous membranes, external heat, and/or occlusive dressings. Avoid wearing clothing or gloves for ≥10 min after application.	C v **W** 66, 67
Diclofenac Sodium (Voltaren)	**Tab,Delay:** 25 mg, 50 mg, 75 mg; **Tab,ER:** 100 mg	**Adults: OA: Voltaren:** 50 mg bid-tid or 75 mg bid. **Voltaren-XR:** 100 mg qd. **RA: Voltaren:** 50 mg tid-qid or 75 mg bid. **Voltaren-XR:** 100 mg qd-bid. **Max:** 225 mg/d.	C v **W** 66, 67
Ibuprofen (Motrin, Children's, Motrin, Infants, Motrin, Junior)	**Drops:** (Infants') 50 mg/1.25 ml; **Susp:** (Children's) 100 mg/5 ml; **Tab:** (Junior) 100 mg; **Tab, Chew:** (Children's) 50 mg, (Junior) 100 mg	**Infants: 12-23 mths (18-23 lbs):** 1.875 ml (75 mg) q6-8h prn. **6-11 mths (12-17 lbs):** 1.25 ml (50 mg) q6-8h prn. **Children's/Junior: 11 yo (72-95 lbs)**: 300 mg q6-8h prn. **9-10 yo (60-71 lbs):** 250 mg q6-8h prn. **6-8 yo (48-59 lbs):** 200 mg q6-8h prn. **4-5 yo (36-47 lbs):** 150 mg q6-8h prn. **2-3 yo (24-35 lbs):** 100 mg q6-8h prn. **Max: 6 mths-11 yo:** 4 doses/d.	N >

NAME	FORM/STRENGTH	DOSAGE	COMMENTS
Ibuprofen (Motrin IB)	**Tab:** 200 mg	**Adults/Pediatrics: ≥12 yo:** 200 mg q4-6h while symptoms persist, may increase to 400 mg q4-6h. **Max:** 1200 mg/24h.	N >
Ibuprofen (Motrin)	**Susp:** 100 mg/5 ml; **Tab:** 400 mg, 600 mg, 800 mg	**Adults: OA/RA:** 300 mg qid or 400-800 mg tid-qid. **Pain:** 400 mg q4-6h. **≥6 mths: JRA:** 30-40 mg/kg/d given tid-qid. 20 mg/kg/d w/ milder disease. **6 mths-12 yo: Pain:** 10 mg/kg q6-8h. **Max:** 40 mg/kg/d.	C v **R W** [66, 67]
Indomethacin (Indocin, Indocin SR)	(Indocin) **Susp:** 25 mg/5 ml; (Indocin SR) **Cap,ER:** 75 mg; (Generic) **Cap:** 25 mg, 50 mg; **Cap,ER:** 75 mg; **Susp:** 25 mg/5 ml	**Adults & Peds: ≥14 yo: Indocin: RA/OA: Initial:** 25 mg PO bid-tid. **Titrate:** Increase by 25-50 mg/d wkly. **Max:** 200 mg/d. **Bursitis/Tendinitis:** 75-150 mg/d given tid-qid x 7-14d. **Acute Gouty Arthritis:** 50 mg PO tid until tolerable, then d/c. **Indocin SR: RA/OA: Initial:** 75 mg qd. **Maint:** 75 mg bid. Take w/ food.	C v **W** [66, 67]
Ketorolac Tromethamine (Toradol)	(Generic) **Inj:** 15 mg/ml, 30 mg/ml; **Tab:** 10 mg; (Toradol) **Tab:** 10 mg	**Adults: 16 to <65 yo: Single Dose:** 60 mg IM or 30 mg IV. **Multiple Dose:** 30 mg IV/IM q6h. **Max:** 120 mg/d. **Transition from IV/IM to PO:** 20 mg PO, then 10 mg PO q4-6h. **Max:** 40 mg/24h. **≥65 yo or <50 kg: Single Dose:** 30 mg IM or 15 mg IV. **Multiple Dose:** 15 mg IV/IM q6h. **Max:** 60 mg/d. **Transition from IV/IM to PO:** 10 mg PO q4-6h. **Max:** 40 mg/24h. Max duration is 5d.	C v **R** Short-term use only (≤5d).
Meloxicam (Mobic)	**Susp:** 7.5 mg/5 ml; **Tab:** 7.5 mg, 15 mg	**OA/RA: Adults: ≥18 yo: Initial/Maint:** 7.5 mg qd. **Max:** 15 mg/d. **JRA: Peds: ≥2 yo:** 0.125 mg/kg qd. **Max:** 7.5 mg/d.	C v **W** [66, 67]

Naproxen Sodium (Anaprox, Anaprox DS)	**Tab:** (Anaprox) 275 mg, (Anaprox DS) 550 mg	**Adults: RA/OA/Ankylosing Spondylitis:** 275 mg-550 mg bid. **Pain/Tendinitis/Bursitis: Initial:** 550 mg, then 550 mg q12h or 275 mg q6-8h prn. **Max:** 1100 mg/d for maint. **Acute Gout:** 825 mg, then 275 mg q8h. **JRA: Peds: ≥2 yo: Tab:** 5 mg/kg of naproxen bid.	C v **W** [66, 67]
Naproxen (Naprosyn)	(Naprosyn) **Susp:** 25 mg/ml; **Tab:** 250 mg, 375 mg, 500 mg; (EC-Naprosyn) **Tab,Delay:** 375 mg, 500 mg	**Adults: RA/OA/Ankylosing Spondylitis: Naprosyn:** 250-500 mg bid. **EC-Naprosyn:** 375-500 mg bid. **Acute Gout: Naprosyn: Initial:** 750 mg, then 250 mg q8h. **JRA: Peds: ≥2 yo:** 5 mg/kg of naproxen bid.	C v **W** [66, 67]

Salicylates

Aspirin (Bayer Aspirin)	**Chewtab:** 81 mg; **Tab:** 81 mg, 325 mg, 500 mg; **Tab,Delay:** 81 mg, 325 mg	**Pain: Adults & Peds: ≥12 yo:** 325-1000 mg q4-6h prn. **Max:** 4 gm/d.	N v Avoid use during 3rd trimester. **H R**

Miscellaneous

Acetaminophen (Tylenol Children's)	**Susp:** 160 mg/5 ml; **Tab,Chew:** 80 mg	**Peds:** Give q4h prn. **Max:** 5 doses/d. **2-3 yo (24-35 lbs):** 160 mg. **4-5 yo (36-47 lbs):** 240 mg. **6-8 yo (48-59 lbs):** 320 mg. **9-10 yo (60-71 lbs):** 400 mg. **11 yo (72-95 lbs):** 480 mg.	N >

NAME	FORM/STRENGTH	DOSAGE	COMMENTS
Acetaminophen (Tylenol Regular Strength)	**Tab:** 325 mg	**Adults & Peds: ≥12 yo:** 650 mg q4-6h prn. **Max:** 3900 mg/d. **6-11 yo:** 325 mg q4-6h prn. **Max:** 1625 mg/d.	N >
Acetaminophen (Tylenol Extra Strength)	**Sol:** 500 mg/15 ml; **Tab:** 500 mg	**Adults & Peds: ≥12 yo:** 1000 mg (2 tabs) q4-6h prn. **Max:** 4 gm/d. Avoid use for ≥10 days.	N >
Duloxetine (Cymbalta)	**Cap,Delay:** 20 mg, 30 mg, 60 mg	**Adults: Diabetic Peripheral Neuropathic Pain: Usual:** 60 mg/d given once daily. **Max:** 120 mg/d. May lower starting dose if tolerability is a concern. **Fibromyalgia: Initial:** 30 mg qd x 1 wk to adjust before increasing to 60 mg qd. **Max:** 60 mg qd. Do not chew or crush.	C v **H R W** [29]
Gabapentin (Neurontin)	**Cap:** 100 mg, 300 mg, 400 mg; **Sol:** 250 mg/5 ml; **Tab:** 600 mg, 800 mg	**Postherpetic Neuralgia: Adults:** 300 mg single dose on Day 1, then 300 mg bid on Day 2, & 300 mg tid on Day 3. Increase further prn pain. **Max:** 600 mg tid.	C > **R**
Lidocaine/Tetracaine (Synera)	**Patch:** 70-70 mg	**Adults & Peds: ≥ 3 yo: Venipuncture or IV Cannulation:** Apply to intact skin for 20-30 min prior to procedure. **Superficial Dermatological Procedure:** Apply to intact skin for 30 min prior to procedure.	B >
Lidocaine (Lidoderm Patch)	**Patch:** 5%	**Postherpetic Neuralgia: Adults:** Apply to intact skin, cover most painful area. Apply up to 3 patches, once for up to 12 h within 24-h period. May cut patches into smaller sizes before removal of the release liner. **Debilitated/Impaired Elimination:** Treat smaller areas. Remove if irritation or burning occurs; may re-apply when irritation subsides.	B >

Milnacipran HCl (Savella)	**Tab:** 12.5 mg, 25 mg, 50 mg, 100 mg; 4-week Titration Pack.	**Fibromyalgia: Adults:** 100 mg qd (50 mg bid). **Titrate: Day 1:** 12.5 mg qd. **Days 2-3:** 25 mg/d (12.5 mg bid). **Days 4-7:** 50 mg/d (25 mg bid). **After Day 7:** 100 mg/d (50 mg bid). May increase dose to 200 mg/d (100 mg bid) based on individual response. **Max:** 200 mg/d.	C v **R W** [29]
Pregabalin CV (Lyrica)	**Cap:** 25 mg, 50 mg, 75 mg, 100 mg, 150 mg, 200 mg, 225 mg, 300 mg	**Adults: Neuropathic Pain: Initial:** 50 mg tid (150 mg/d). **Titrate:** May increase to 300 mg/d within 1 wk. **Max:** 100 mg tid (300 mg/d). **Post-Herpetic Neuralgia: Initial:** 150 mg/d divided bid or tid. **Max:** 600 mg/d divided bid or tid. **Fibromyalgia: Initial:** 75 mg bid (150 mg/d). **Titrate:** May increase to 150 mg bid (300 mg/d) within 1 wk based on efficacy & tolerability. May further increase to 225 mg bid (450 mg/d) if needed. **Max:** 450 mg/d.	C v **R**
Tramadol HCl/Acetaminophen (Ultracet)	**Tab:** 37.5-325 mg	**Acute Pain: Adults:** 2 tabs q4-6h, up to 5d. **Max:** 8 tabs/d.	C v**H R**
Tramadol HCl (Ryzolt)	**Tab,ER:** 100 mg, 200 mg, 300 mg	**Moderate to Moderately Severe Chronic Pain: Adults:** Individualize dose: **Initial:** 100 mg/d. **Titrate:** 100 mg q2-3d to achieve adequate pain control and tolerability. For patients requiring 300 mg/d, titration should take at least 4d. **Usual:** 200-300 mg/d. **Max:** 300 mg/d. **Patients Currently on Tramadol IR Products:** Calculate 24h IR dose and initiate on a total daily dose rounded down to next lowest 100 mg increment. **Max:** 300 mg/d. **Elderly:** Start at low end of dosing range. Swallow whole with liquid.	C > **H R**

NAME	FORM/STRENGTH	DOSAGE	COMMENTS
Tramadol HCl (Ultram, Ultram ER)	**Tab:** 50 mg; **Tab,ER:** 100 mg, 200 mg, 300 mg	**Moderate to Moderately Severe Pain: Adults: ≥17 yo: Tab: Initial:** 25 mg qam. **Titrate:** Increase by 25 mg/d q3d to 25 mg qid, then by 50 mg/d q3d to 50 mg qid. **Maint:** 50-100 mg q4-6h prn. **Max:** 400 mg/d. **Tab,ER: Adults: ≥18 yo: Initial:** 100 mg qd. **Titrate:** Increase by 100-mg increments q5d. **Max:** 300 mg/d.	C v **H R**

ANTI-INFECTIVES

AIDS Therapy

CCR5 CO-RECEPTOR ANTAGONIST

NAME	FORM/STRENGTH	DOSAGE	COMMENTS
Maraviroc (Selzentry)	**Tab:** 150 mg, 300 mg	**Adults: >16 yo:** Give in combo w/ other antiretroviral medications. **With Strong CYP3A Inhibitors (w/ or w/o CYP3A inducers) Including PIs (except tipranavir/ ritonavir), Delavirdine:** 150 mg bid. **With NRTIs, Tipranavir/Ritonavir, Nevirapine, Other Drugs That Are Not Strong CYP3A Inhibitors/Inducers:** 300 mg bid. **With CYP3A Inducers (w/o strong CYP3A inhibitor):** 600 mg bid.	B v Hepatotoxicity reported.

FUSION INHIBITOR

NAME	FORM/STRENGTH	DOSAGE	COMMENTS
Enfuvirtide (Fuzeon)	**Inj:** 90 mg/ml	**Adults:** 90 mg SC bid. **Peds: 6-16 yo:** 2 mg/kg SC bid. **Max:** 90 mg bid. Inject into upper arm, anterior thigh, or abdomen.	B v

HIV INTEGRASE STRAND TRANSFER INHIBITOR

Raltegravir Potassium (Isentress)	**Tab:** 400 mg	**Adults:** 400 mg bid. **Concomitant w/ Rifampin:** 800 mg bid.	C v

NON-NUCLEOSIDE REVERSE TRANSCRIPTASE INHIBITORS & COMBINATIONS

Delavirdine Mesylate (Rescriptor)	**Tab:** 100 mg, 200 mg	**Adults & Peds:** **≥16 yo:** 400 mg tid.	C v
Efavirenz/Emtricitabine/ Tenofovir Disoproxil (Atripla)	**Tab:** 600-200-300 mg	**Adults:** **≥18 yo:** 1 tab qd on empty stomach. HS dosing may improve tolerability of nervous system symptoms. Avoid w/ CrCl <50 ml/min.	D v R **W** [31, 32]
Efavirenz (Sustiva)	**Cap:** 50mg, 200mg; **Tab:** 600mg	**Adults:** 600 mg qd. **Peds:** **≥3 yo:** **10 to <15 kg:** 200 mg qd. **15 to <20 kg:** 250mg qd. **20 to <25 kg:** 300 mg qd. **25 to <32.5 kg:** 350 mg qd. **32.5 to <40 kg:** 400 mg qd. **≥40kg:** 600 mg qd. Take on empty stomach, preferably at bedtime.	D v
Etravirine (Intelence)	**Tab:** 100 mg	**Adults:** 200 mg bid following a meal.	B v
Nevirapine (Viramune)	**Tab:** 200 mg; **Susp:** 50 mg/5 ml	**Adults:** **Initial:** 200 mg qd x 14d. **Maint:** 200 mg bid. **Peds:** **≥15 days:** 150 mg/m^2 qd x 14d, followed by 150 mg/m^2 bid. **Max:** 400 mg/d.	B v **H** Severe hepatotoxicity & skin reactions reported.

NAME	FORM/STRENGTH	DOSAGE	COMMENTS
NUCLEOSIDE REVERSE TRANSCRIPTASE INHIBITORS & COMBINATIONS			
Abacavir Sulfate/Lamivudine (Epzicom)	**Tab:** 600-300 mg	**Adults: ≥18 yo: CrCl >50 ml/min:** 1 tab qd.	◉C ❋v **R W** [31,32,33]
Abacavir Sulfate/Lamivudine/ Zidovudine (Trizivir)	**Tab:** 300-150-300 mg	**Adults & Adolescents: >40 kg & CrCl >50 ml/min:** 1 tab bid.	◉C ❋v **R W** [31,32,33,34]
Abacavir Sulfate (Ziagen)	**Sol:** 20 mg/ml; **Tab:** 300 mg	**Adults:** 300 mg bid or 600 mg qd. **Peds: ≥3 mths:** 8 mg/kg bid. **Max:** 300 mg bid. **14-21 kg:** 150 mg bid. **Max:** 300 mg/d. **>21 to <30 kg:** 150 mg in AM, 300 mg in PM. **Max:** 450 mg/d. **≥30 kg:** 300 mg bid. **Max:** 600 mg/d.	◉C ❋v **H W** [31,33]
Didanosine (Videx, Videx EC)	**Cap,Delay:** (Videx EC) 125 mg, 200 mg, 250 mg, 400 mg; **Sol:** (Videx) 2 gm, 4 gm	**Adults: ≥60 kg: Cap,Delay:** (Videx EC) 400 mg qd. **<60 kg: Cap,Delay:** (Videx EC) 250 mg qd. **Peds: >8 mths: Sol:** (Videx) 120 mg/m^2 bid. **2 wks-8 mths: Sol:** (Videx) 100 mg/m^2 bid. Take on empty stomach.	◉B ❋v **R W** [31, 35]
Emtricitabine (Emtriva)	**Cap:** 200 mg; **Sol:** 10 mg/ml	**Adults: ≥18 yrs: Cap:** 200 mg qd. **Sol:** 240 mg (24 ml) qd. **Peds: 0-3 mths: Sol:** 3 mg/kg qd. **3 mths-17 yrs: >33 kg: Cap:** 200 mg qd. **Sol:** 6 mg/kg qd. **Max:** 240 mg (24 ml).	◉B ❋v **R W** [31, 32]
Lamivudine/Zidovudine (Combivir)	**Tab:** 150-300 mg	**Adults & Peds: ≥12 yo:** 1 tab bid. Avoid if CrCl ≤50 ml/min or w/ dose-limiting adverse events.	◉C ❋v **H R W** [31, 32, 34]

Lamivudine (Epivir)	**Sol:** 10 mg/ml; **Tab:** 150 mg, 300 mg	**Adults:** 150 mg bid or 300 mg qd. **Peds: 3 mths-16 yo:** 4 mg/kg bid. **Max:** 150 mg bid. **Scored Tab: 14-21 kg:** 1/2 tab (75 mg) in am & 1/2 tab (75 mg) in pm. **21-30 kg:** 1/2 tab (75 mg) in am & 1 tab (150 mg) in pm. ≥**30 kg:** 1 tab (150 mg) in am & 1 tab (150 mg) in pm.	B v **R W** [31, 32]
Stavudine (Zerit)	**Cap:** 15 mg, 20 mg, 30 mg, 40 mg; **Sol:** 1 mg/ml	**Adults:** ≥**60 kg:** 40 mg q12h. **<60 kg:** 30 mg q12h. **Peds: Birth-13d:** 0.5 mg/kg q12h. ≥**14d & <30 kg:** 1 mg/kg q12h. **>30 kg:** Adult dose. Adjust dose based on peripheral neuropathy.	C v **R W** [31, 35]
Tenofovir Disoproxil Fumarate/Emtricitabine (Truvada)	**Tab:** 300-200 mg	**Adults:** ≥**18 yo: CrCl:** ≥**50 ml/min:** 1 tab qd. **CrCl: 30-49 ml/min:** 1 tab q48h.	B v **R W** [31, 32]
Zidovudine (Retrovir)	**Cap:** 100 mg; **Inj:** 10 mg/ml; **Syr:** 50 mg/ 5 ml; **Tab:** 300 mg	**Adults:** (Tab) 600 mg/d in divided doses. (Inj) 1 mg/kg IV over 1h 5-6x/d. **Peds: 6 wks to <18 yo:** 480 $mg/m^2/d$ PO in divided doses (240 mg/m^2 bid or 160 mg/m^2 tid). **Max:** 480 $mg/m^2/d$. **4 to <9 kg:** 12 mg/kg bid or 8 mg/kg tid. **Max:** 24 mg/kg/d. ≥**9 to <30 kg:** 9 mg/kg bid or 6 mg/kg tid. **Max:** 18 mg/kg/d. ≥**30 kg:** 300 mg bid or 200 mg tid. **Max:** 600 mg/d. **Prevention of Maternal-Fetal HIV Transmission: Adults: >14 wks Pregnancy:** 100 mg PO 5x/d until start of labor. **During L&D:** 2 mg/kg IV over 1h followed by 1 mg/kg/h IV infusion until clamping of umbilical cord. **Neonates:** 2 mg/kg PO q6h (or 1.5 mg/kg IV over 30 min q6h) starting within 12h after birth & continue through 6 wks of age.	C v **H R W** [31, 34]

NAME	FORM/STRENGTH	DOSAGE	COMMENTS
NUCLEOTIDE REVERSE TRANSCRIPTASE INHIBITORS			
Tenofovir Disoproxil (Viread)	**Tab:** 300 mg	**Adults:** 300 mg qd w/ a meal.	◙B ❋v **W** 31, 32
PROTEASE INHIBITORS			
Atazanavir Sulfate (Reyataz)	**Cap:** 100 mg, 150 mg, 200 mg, 300 mg	**Adults: Therapy-Naive:** 300 mg w/ ritonavir 100 mg qd. If intolerant to ritonavir, give atazanavir 400 mg qd. **Concomitant Tenofovir:** Atazanavir 300 mg w/ ritonavir 100 mg. **Concomitant H2-Receptor Antagonist:** Give w/, and/or at least 10h after, atazanavir 300 mg w/ ritonavir 100 mg. **Max:** Famotidine 40 mg bid (or equivalent). If ritonavir intolerant, give atazanavir 400 mg qd at least 2h before or 10h after H_2-receptor antagonist. **Concomitant PPIs:** Give PPI 12h prior to atazanavir 300 mg w/ ritonavir 100 mg. **Max:** Omeprazole 20 mg (or equivalent). **Concomitant Efavirenz:** Atazanavir 400 mg & ritonavir 100 mg w/ efavirenz on empty stomach hs. **Concomitant Buffered Didanosine:** Give atazanavir 2h before or 1h after didanosine. **Therapy-Experienced:** 300 mg w/ ritonavir 100 mg qd. **Concomitant H2-Receptor Antagonist:** Atazanavir 300 mg w/ ritonavir 100 mg w/, and/or at least 10h after, H_2-receptor antagonist. **Max:** Famotidine 20 mg bid. **Both Tenofovir & H2-Receptor Antagonist:** Atazanavir 400 mg w/ ritonavir 100 mg qd. **Peds: Therapy-Naive:**	◙B ❋v **H R**

		≥13 yo & ≥39 kg/Ritonavir Intolerant: 400 mg qd w/o ritonavir. **Therapy-Naive: 6-<18 yo: 15-<25 kg:**150 mg w/ ritonavir 80 mg. **25-<32 kg:** 200 mg w/ ritonavir 100 mg. **32-<39 kg:** 250 mg w/ ritonavir 100 mg. ≥**39 kg:** 300 mg w/ ritonavir 100 mg. **Therapy-Experienced: 6-<18 yo: 25-<32 kg:** 200 mg w/ ritonavir 100 mg. **32-<39 kg:** 250 mg w/ ritonavir 100 mg. ≥**39 kg:** 300 mg w/ ritonavir 100 mg qd. Take w/ food.	
Darunavir (Prezista)	**Tab:** 75 mg, 300 mg, 400 mg, 600 mg	**Adults: Treatment-Naive:** 800 mg w/ ritonavir 100 mg qd. **Treatment-Experienced:** 600 mg w/ ritonavir 100 mg bid. **Peds: 6 to <18 yo:** ≥**20 to <30 kg:** 375 mg w/ ritonavir 50 mg bid. ≥**30 to <40 kg:** 450 mg w/ ritonavir 60 mg bid. ≥**40 kg:** 600 mg w/ ritonavir 100 mg bid. Take w/ food.	C v
Fosamprenavir Calcium (Lexiva)	**Tab:** 700 mg; **Sus:** 50 mg/ml	**Adults: Therapy-Naive:** 1400 mg bid OR 1400 mg qd + ritonavir 200 mg qd OR 700 mg bid + ritonavir 100 mg bid. **PI-Experienced:** 700 mg bid + ritonavir 100 mg bid. **Peds: Sus: Therapy-Naive: 2-5 yo:** 30 mg/kg bid, not to exceed 1400 mg bid. **>6 yo:** 30 mg/kg bid, not to exceed 1400 mg bid OR 18 mg/kg + ritonavir 3 mg/kg bid, not to exceed 700 mg + ritonavir 100 mg bid. **Therapy-Experienced:** ≥**6 yo:** 18 mg/kg + ritonavir 3 mg/kg, not to exceed 700 mg + ritonavir 100 mg bid. **>47 kg:** May use adult monotherapy dose. When given in combination w/ ritonavir, tabs may be used for peds ≥39 kg.	C v **H**

NAME	FORM/STRENGTH	DOSAGE	COMMENTS
Indinavir Sulfate (Crixivan)	**Cap:** 100 mg, 200 mg, 333 mg, 400 mg	**Adults:** 800 mg q8h w/ water. Hydrate to prevent nephrolithiasis/urolithiasis.	C v **H**
Lopinavir/Ritonavir (Kaletra)	**Tab** 100-25 mg, 200-50 mg; **Sol:** 80-20 mg/ml	**Adults & Peds: >12 yo: Therapy-Naive:** 400/100 mg (2 tabs or 5 ml) bid or 800/200 mg qd (4 tabs or 10 ml). **Therapy-Experienced:** 400/100 mg (2 tabs or 5 ml) bid. Once daily administration not recommended. **Concomitant Efavirenz/Nevirapine/Fosamprenavir/ Nelfinavir: Therapy-Naive:** (Tab) 400/100 mg (2 tabs) bid. **Concomitant Efavirenz/Nevirapine/Amprenavir/Nelfinavir:** (Sol) 533/133 mg (6.5 ml) bid. **Concomitant Efavirenz/ Nevirapine/ Fosamprenavir w/o Ritonavir/Nelfinavir: Treatment-Experienced w/ Decreased Susceptibility to Lopinavir:** 600/150 mg (3 tabs) bid. **6 mths-12 yo: >40 kg:** 400/100 mg (2 tabs or 5 ml) bid. **15-40 kg:** (Sol) 10/2.5 mg/kg bid. **7 to <15 kg:** (Sol) 12/3 mg/kg bid. **Concomitant Efavirenz/Nevirapine/Amprenavir: >45 kg:** 533/133 mg (2 tabs or 6.5 ml) bid. **15-45 kg:** (Sol) 11/2.75 mg/kg bid. **7 to <15 kg:** (Sol) 13/3.25 mg/kg bid. Tablets can be taken w/ or w/o food. Oral sol must be taken w/ food.	C v
Nelfinavir Mesylate (Viracept)	**Pow (Susp):** 50 mg/gm; **Tab:** 250 mg, 625 mg	**Adults:** 1250 mg bid or 750 mg tid. **Peds: 2-13 yo:** 20-30 mg/kg tid. Take w/ food.	B v

Ritonavir (Norvir)	**Cap:** 100 mg; **Sol:** 80 mg/ml	**Adults: Initial:** 300 mg bid & increase q2-3d by 100 mg bid. **Maint:** 600 mg bid. **Concomitant Saquinavir:** Better tolerated w/ 400 mg bid. **Peds: >1 mth: Initial:** 250 mg/m^2 po bid. **Titrate:** Increase by 50 mg/m^2 bid q2-3d. **Maint:** 350-400 mg/m^2 po bid or highest tolerated dose. **Max:** 600 mg bid.	◉B ❁v **W** [97]
Saquinavir Mesylate (Invirase)	**Cap:** 200 mg; **Tab:** 500 mg	**Adults: >16 yo:** 1000 mg bid w/ ritonavir 100 mg bid. Take within 2h after full meal.	◉B ❁v Invirase & Fortovase not bioequivalent.
Tipranavir (Aptivus)	**Cap:** 250 mg; **Sol:** 100 mg/ml	**Adults:** 500 mg, w/ ritonavir 200 mg, bid. Take w/ food. **Peds: 2-18 yo:** 14 mg/kg, w/ ritonavir 6 mg/kg (or 375 mg/m^2 w/ ritonavir 150 mg/m^2), bid. **Max:** 500 mg, w/ ritonavir 200 mg, bid.	◉C ❁v **H W** [45]

Antiviral Agents

ANTI-CYTOMEGALOVIRUS AGENTS

Cidofovir (Vistide)	**Inj:** 75 mg/ml	**CMV Retinitis: Adults & Peds: Induction:** 5 mg/kg qwk x 2wks. **Maint:** 5 mg/kg q2wks. Patients must receive hydration & probenecid w/ each dose.	◉C ❁v **R W** [59]

NAME	FORM/STRENGTH	DOSAGE	COMMENTS
Ganciclovir (Cytovene)	**Cap:** 250 mg; **Inj:** 500 mg	**Adults: CMV Retinitis Treatment: Initial:** 5 mg/kg IV q12h x 14-21d. **Maint:** 5 mg/kg IV qd x 7d or 6mg/kg IV qd x 5 days/wk or 1000 mg PO tid or 500 mg PO 6x/d q3h, while awake. **CMV Retinitis Prevention in HIV Patients:** 1000 mg PO tid. **CMV Retinitis Prevention in Transplant Patients: Initial:** 5 mg/kg IV q12h x 7-14d. **Maint:** 5 mg/kg IV qd x 7d or 6 mg/kg IV x 5d/wk or 1000 mg PO tid. Take caps w/ food.	⦿C ❈v **R W** [12]
Ganciclovir (Vitrasert)	**Implant:** 4.5 mg	**CMV Retinitis: Treatment: Adults & Peds: ≥9 yo:** Each implant releases the drug over 5-8 mths; may remove or replace after depletion.	⦿C ❈v
Valganciclovir (Valcyte)	**Tab:** 450 mg	**Adults: CMV Retinitis: Induction:** 900 mg bid x 21d. **Maint:** 900 mg qd. **Prevention of CMV Disease in High-Risk Kidney, Heart, & Kidney-Pancreas Transplant Patients:** 900 mg qd within 10 days of transplant until 100 days post-transplant. Take w/ food.	⦿C ❈v **R** Follow exact dosing guidelines. **W** [12]

HEPATITIS

NAME	FORM/STRENGTH	DOSAGE	COMMENTS
Adefovir Dipivoxil (Hepsera)	**Tab:** 10 mg	**HBV: Adults & Peds: ≥12 yo:** 10 mg qd.	⦿C ❈v **R W** [31, 32, 37, 38]
Entecavir (Baraclude)	**Sol:** 0.05 mg/ml; **Tab:** 0.5 mg, 1 mg	**HBV: Adults/Peds: ≥16 yo: Nucleoside-Treatment-Naive:** 0.5 mg qd. **Receiving Lamivudine or Known Lamivudine Resistance Mutation:** 1 mg qd. Take on empty stomach.	⦿C ❈v **R W** [31, 32]

Hepatitis B (Recombinant)/ Hepatitis A Vaccine (Inactivated) (Twinrix)	**Inj:** 720 U-20 mcg	**Adults: 3-Dose Schedule:** 1 ml IM at 0-, 1- & 6-mths. **Alternative 4-Dose Schedule:** 1 ml IM on Days 0, 7 & 21-30 followed by booster dose at 12 mths. Inject into deltoid region.	C >
Interferon alfacon-1 (Infergen)	**Inj:** 30 mcg/ml	**HCV: Adults: ≥18 yo:** 9 mcg SC TIW x 24 wks, then 15 mcg SC TIW x 6 mths if needed.	C >
Lamivudine (Epivir-HBV)	**Sol:** 5 mg/ml; **Tab:** 100 mg	**HBV: Adults:** 100 mg qd. **Peds: 2-17 yo:** 3 mg/kg qd. **Max:** 100 mg/d.	C v **R W** [31, 32]
Peginterferon alfa-2a (Pegasys)	**Inj:** 180 mcg/0.5 ml, 180 mcg/ml	**HCV & HCV/HIV: Adults: ≥18 yo: Monotherapy:** 180 mcg SC once wkly x 48 wks. Adjust dose by neutrophils, platelets, severity of depression & renal/hepatic function. **HCV: With Copegus: Adults: ≥18 yo:** 180 mcg SC once wkly x 48 wks for genotypes 1, 4; x 24 wks for genotypes 2, 3. **HCV/HIV: With Copegus: Adults: ≥18 yo:** 180 mcg SC once wkly x 48 wks regardless of genotype. **HBV: Monotherapy:** 180 mcg SC once wkly x 48 wks.	C (monotherapy) X (w/ ribavirin) v **H R W** [13]
Peginterferon alfa-2b (Peg-Intron)	**Inj:** 50 mcg/0.5 ml, 160 mcg/ml, 80 mcg/ 0.5 ml, 120 mcg/0.5 ml, 150 mcg/0.5 ml	**HCV: Adults: ≥18 yo:** Administer SC once wkly x 1 yr. **Monotherapy: 50 mcg/0.5 ml vial: ≤45 kg:** 40 mcg (0.4 ml); **46-56 kg:** 50 mcg (0.5 ml). **80 mcg/0.5 ml vial: 57-72 kg:** 64 mcg (0.4 ml); **73-88 kg:** 80 mcg (0.5 ml). **120 mcg/0.5 ml vial: 89-106 kg:** 96 mcg (0.4 ml); **107-136 kg:** 120 mcg (0.5 ml). **150 mcg/0.5 ml vial: 137-160 kg:** 150 mcg (0.5 ml). **With Rebetol (varying**	C v **W** [13]

Continued on Next Page

NAME	FORM/STRENGTH	DOSAGE	COMMENTS
Peginterferon alfa-2b (Peg-Intron) *Continued*		**doses): 50 mcg/0.5 ml vial: <40 kg:** 50 mcg (0.5 ml). **80 mcg/0.5 ml vial: 40-50 kg:** 64 mcg (0.4 ml); **51-60 kg:** 80 mcg (0.5 ml). **120 mcg/0.5 ml vial: 61-75 kg:** 96 mcg (0.4 ml); **76-85 kg:** 120 mcg (0.5 ml). **150 mcg/0.5 ml vial: >85 kg:** 150 mcg (0.5 ml). Adjust dose based on wt, WBC, platelets, neutrophils, and/or severity of depression. **Peds: 3-17 yo: Combination Therapy w/ Rebetol:** 60 mcg/m^2/wk SC plus Rebetol 15 mg/kg/d in 2 divided doses x 48 wks in genotype 1 or 24 wks in genotype 2 & 3. Adjust dose based on wt, WBC, platelets, neutrophils, and/or severity of depression.	
Ribavirin (Copegus)	**Tab:** 200 mg	**HCV: Adults: ≥18 yo w/ Pegasys: Genotypes 1,4: <75 kg:** 500 mg bid x 48 wks. **≥75 kg:** 600 mg bid x 48 wks. **Genotypes 2,3:** 400 mg bid x 24 wks. **HCV/HIV: Adults: ≥18 yo w/ Pegasys:** 800 mg qd x 48 wks. Dosage adjustment or d/c based on CV status, Hgb, renal function.	◙X ❋v **R** CI in pregnancy, male partners of pregnant females & significant cardiac disease. Hemolytic anemia.
Ribavirin (Rebetol)	**Cap:** 200 mg; **Sol:** 40 mg/ml	**HCV: Adults: With Intron A: ≤75 kg:** 400 mg qam & 600 mg qpm. **>75 kg:** 600 mg qam & 600 mg qpm. Treat x 24-48 wks if no prior interferon (IFN) therapy & x 24 wks if prior IFN therapy. **With PEG-Intron:** 400 mg bid, qam & qpm, w/ food. Dose based on Hgb & cardiac history. **Peds: ≥3 yrs:** 15 mg/kg/day in divided doses qam & qpm. Use	◙X ❋v **R** CI in pregnancy, male partners of pregnant females & significant

		sol if =25 kg or cannot swallow caps. **With Intron A: 25-36 kg:** 200 mg bid, qam & qpm. **37-49 kg:** 200 mg qam & 400 mg qpm. **50-61 kg:** 400 mg bid, qam & qpm. **>61 kg:** Dose as adult. **Genotype 1:** Treat x 48 wks. **Genotype 2/3:** Treat x 24 wks.	cardiac disease. Hemolytic anemia.
Telbivudine (Tyzeka)	**Tab:** 600 mg; **Sol:** 100 mg/5 ml	**HBV: Adults & Peds: ≥16 yo: CrCl ≥50 ml/min: Tab:** 600 mg qd. **Sol:** 30 ml qd. **CrCl 30-49 ml/min: Tab:** 600 mg q48h. **Sol:** 20 ml qd. **CrCl <30 ml/min (not requiring dialysis): Tab:** 600 mg q72h. **Sol:** 10 ml qd. **ESRD: Tab:** 600 mg q96h.	B v **R W** [31, 32]
Tenofovir Disoproxil (Viread)	**Tab:** 300 mg	**HBV: Adults:** 300 mg qd w/ a meal.	B v **W** [31, 32]

HERPES INFECTION

Acyclovir Sodium (Zovirax Injection)	**Inj:** 25 mg/ml, 50 mg/ml	**Herpes Simplex: Adults & Peds: >12 yo:** 5 mg/kg IV q8h x 7d. **<12 yo:** 10 mg/kg IV q8h x 7d. **Birth-3 mths:** 10 mg/kg q8h IV x 10d. **Genital Herpes: Adults & Peds: >12 yo:** 5 mg/kg IV q8h x 5d. **Encephalitis: Adults & Peds: >12 yo:** 10 mg/kg IV q8h x 10d. **<12 yo:** 20 mg/kg IV q8h x 10d. **Zoster: Adults & Peds: >12 yo:** 10 mg/kg IV q8h x 7d. **<12 yo:** 20 mg/kg IV q8h x 7d.	B > **R**

NAME	FORM/STRENGTH	DOSAGE	COMMENTS
Acyclovir (Zovirax Oral)	**Cap**: 200 mg; **Susp:** 200 mg/5 ml; **Tab:** 400 mg, 800 mg	**Zoster:** 800 mg 5x/d x 7-10d. **Genital Herpes: Initial:** 200 mg 5x/d x 10d. **Maint:** 400 mg bid x 1 yr or 200 mg 3-5x/d x 1 yr. **Recurrent:** 200 mg 5x/d x 5d. **Varicella: ≥2 yo: <40 kg:** 20 mg/kg qid x 5d. **>40 kg:** 800 mg qid x 5d.	B > R
Famciclovir (Famvir)	**Tab:** 125 mg, 250 mg, 500 mg	**Adults: ≥18 yo: Zoster:** 500 mg q8h x 7d. **Genital Herpes: Recurrent:** 1000 mg bid x 1d. **Recurrent Suppression:** 250 mg bid up to 1 yr. **Recurrent Orolabial or Genital Herpes in HIV Patients:** 500 mg bid x 7d. **Recurrent Herpes Labialis:** 1500 mg single dose.	B > R
Valacyclovir HCl (Valtrex)	**Tab:** 500 mg, 1 gm	**Adults: Herpes Zoster:** 1 gm q8h x 7d. Start within 48h after onset of rash. **Genital Herpes: Initial:** 1 gm q12h x 10d. Start within 48h after onset of symptoms. **Recurrent Episodes: Treatment:** 500 mg q12h x 3d. Start at 1st sign/symptom of episode. **Suppressive Therapy w/ Normal Immune Function:** 1 gm q24h. **Alternative:** (≤9 episodes/yr) 500 mg q24h. **Suppressive Therapy w/ HIV & CD4 ≥100 cells/mm^3:** 500 mg q12h. **Reduction of Transmission of Genital Herpes:** (≤9 episodes/yr) 500 mg qd for source partner. **Herpes Labialis: Adults & Peds: ≥12 yo:** 2 gm q12h x 1d. Start at earliest symptom of cold sore. **Chickenpox: Peds: 2 to <18 yo:** 20 mg/kg q8h x 5d. Max 1 gm q8h. Start at earliest sign/symptom of chickenpox.	B > R

Amantadine HCl (Symmetrel)	**Tab:** 100 mg; **Syr:** 50 mg/5 ml	**Influenza A Prophylaxis & Treatment: Adults:** 200 mg qd or 100 mg bid. **≥65 yo:** 100 mg qd. **Peds: 9-12 yo:** 100 mg bid. **1-9 yo:** 4.4-8.8 mg/kg/d. **Max:** 150 mg/d.	C v **R**
Oseltamivir Phosphate (Tamiflu)	**Cap:** 75 mg; **Susp:** 12 mg/ml	**Treatment: Adults & Peds: ≥13 yo: Cap/Susp:** 75 mg bid x 5d, begin within 2d of symptom onset. **≥1 yo: Susp: ≤15 kg:** 30 mg bid x 5d. **>15-23 kg:** 45 mg bid x 5d. **>23-40 kg:** 60 mg bid x 5d. **>40 kg:** 75 mg bid x 5d. **Prophylaxis: Adults & Peds: ≥13 yo: Cap/Susp:** Begin within 2d of exposure. 75 mg qd for at least 10d, up to 6 wks w/ community outbreak. **≥1 yo: Susp: ≤15 kg:** 30 mg qd x 10d. **>15-23 kg:** 45 mg qd x 10d. **>23-40 kg:** 60 mg qd x 10d. **>40 kg:** 75 mg qd x 10d.	C > **R**
Rimantadine HCl (Flumadine)	**Tab:** 100 mg; **Syr:** 50 mg/5 ml	**Influenza A: Prophylaxis: Adults & Peds: ≥10 yo:** 100 mg bid. **<10 yo:** 5 mg/kg qd. **Max:** 150 mg/d. **Treatment: Adults:** 100 mg bid; begin within 48h of symptom onset & treat x 7d from initial symptom onset.	C v **H R**
Zanamivir (Relenza)	**Disk:** 5 mg/inh	**Adults & Peds: ≥7 yo: Treatment:** 2 inh (10 mg) q12h x 5d. **≥5 yo: Prophylaxis: Household Setting:** 2 inh (10 mg) qd x 10d. **Community Setting:** 2 inh (10 mg) qd x 28d. Give at same time qd.	C >

Bone and Joint Infection

AMINOGLYCOSIDES

NAME	FORM/STRENGTH	DOSAGE	COMMENTS
Amikacin Sulfate	**Inj:** 50 mg/ml, 250 mg/ml	**IM/IV: Adults, Children & Older Infants:** 7.5 mg/kg q12h or 5 mg/kg IM/IV q8h. **Max:** 1.5 gm/d **Newborns: LD:** 10 mg/kg. **Maint:** 7.5 mg/kg q12h.	D v **R W** [1]
Gentamicin Sulfate	**Inj:** 40 mg/ml	**IM/IV: Adults:** 3 mg/kg/d given q8h. **Max:** 5 mg/kg/d in 3-4 doses. Reduce to 3 mg/kg/d as soon as clinically indicated. **Peds:** 2-2.5 mg/kg q8h. **Infants/Neonates:** 2.5 mg/kg q8h. **≤1 wk:** 2.5 mg/kg q12h.	N >**R W** [1]
Tobramycin Sulfate	**Inj:** 10 mg/ml, 40 mg/ml, 1.2 gm	**IM/IV: Adults:** 3 mg/kg/d given q8h. **Max:** 5 mg/kg/d in 3-4 doses. Reduce to 3 mg/kg/d as soon as clinically indicated. **Peds: >1 wk:** 2-2.5 mg/kg q8h or 1.5-1.89 mg/kg q6h. **≤1 wk:** Up to 2 mg/kg q12h.	D > **R W** [1]

CEPHALOSPORINS

NAME	FORM/STRENGTH	DOSAGE	COMMENTS
Cefazolin	**Inj:** 500 mg, 1 gm, 10 gm, 20 gm	**IM/IV: Adults: Usual:** 500 mg-1 gm q6-8h. **Peds: Usual:** 25-50 mg/kg/d given as tid-qid. **Max:** 100 mg/kg/d.	B > **R** Safety in prematures & neonates unknown.

Cefotaxime Sodium (Claforan)	**Inj:** 500 mg, 1 gm, 2 gm, 10 gm	**IM/IV: Adults & Peds: ≥ 50 kg:** 1-2 gm q8h. **Max:** 12 gm/d. **1 mth-12 yo: <50 kg:** 50-180 mg/kg/d divided into 4-6 doses. **1-4 wks:** 50 mg/kg IV q8h. **0-1 wk:** 50 mg/kg IV q12h.	B > **R**
Cefoxitin (Mefoxin)	**Inj:** (Generic) 1 gm, 1 gm/50 ml, 2 gm, 2 gm/ 50 ml, 10 gm, (Mefoxin) 1 gm/50 ml, 2 gm/ 50 ml	**IV: Adults:** 1 gm q4h or 2 gm q6-8h. **Peds: ≥3 mths:** 80-160 mg/kg/d given as q4-6h. **Max:** 12 gm/d.	B > **R**
Ceftazidime (Fortaz)	**Inj:** 500 mg, 1 gm, 1 gm/ 50 ml, 2 gm, 2 gm/ 50 ml, 6 gm	**Adults:** 2 gm IV q12h. **Peds: 1 mth-12 yo:** 30-50 mg/kg IV q8h, up to 6 gm/d. **Neonates: 0-4 wks:** 30 mg/kg IV q12h.	B > **R**
Ceftriaxone Sodium (Rocephin)	**Inj:** (Rocephin) 500 mg, 1 gm; (Generic) 250 mg, 500 mg, 1 gm, 2 gm, 10 gm, 1 gm/50 ml, 2 gm/50ml	**Adults: IM/IV: Usual:** 1-2 gm qd (or in equally divided doses bid.) **Max:** 4 gm/d.	B >
Cefuroxime (Zinacef)	**Inj:** 750 mg, 1.5 gm, 7.5 gm	**IM/IV: Adults:** 1.5 gm q8h. **Peds: >3 mths:** 50 mg/kg q8h. **Max:** 4.5 gm/d.	B > **R**
Cephalexin (Keflex)	(Keflex) **Cap:** 250 mg, 500 mg, 750 mg; (Generic) **Cap:** 250 mg, 500 mg; **Susp:** 125 mg/ 5 ml, 250 mg/5 ml	**Adults: Usual:** 250 mg q6h. **Max:** 4 gm/d. **Peds: Usual:** 25-50 mg/kg/d in divided doses.	B >

NAME	FORM/STRENGTH	DOSAGE	COMMENTS
PENICILLINS			
Ticarcillin Disodium/ Clavulanate Potassium (Timentin)	**Inj:** 3 gm-100 mg, 3 gm-100 mg/100 ml, 30 gm-1 gm	**IV: Adults: ≥60 kg:** 300 mg/kg/d ticarcillin given q4h. **<60 kg:** 200-300 mg/kg/d ticarcillin given q4-6h. **Peds: ≥3 mths & <60 kg:** 50 mg/kg/d ticarcillin given q4-6h. **≥3 mths & ≥60 kg:** 3.1 gm q4-6h.	◙B ❁> **R**
QUINOLONES			
Ciprofloxacin HCl (Cipro Oral)	**Susp:** 250 mg/5 ml, 500 mg/5 ml; **Tab:** 250 mg, 500 mg, 750 mg	**Adults: ≥18 yo: Mild/Moderate:** 500 mg PO q12h x ≥4-6 wks. **Severe/Complicated:** 750 mg PO q12h x ≥4-6 wks.	◙C ❁v **R W** [98]
Ciprofloxacin (Cipro IV)	**Inj:** 10 mg/ml, 200 mg/ 100 ml, 400 mg/200 ml	**Adults: ≥18 yo: Mild/Moderate:** 400 mg IV q12h x ≥4-6 wks. **Severe/Complicated:** 400 mg IV q8h x ≥4-6 wks.	◙C ❁v **R W** [98]
MISCELLANEOUS			
Clindamycin (Cleocin)	**Cap:** 75 mg, 150 mg, 300 mg; **Inj:** 150 mg/ml, 300 mg/50 ml, 600 mg/ 50 ml, 900 mg/50 ml; **Susp:** 75 mg/5 ml	**IM/IV: Adults:** 600-2700 mg/d in 2-4 doses. **Max:** 600 mg IM single dose. **Peds: 1 mth-16 yo:** 20-40 mg/kg/d in 3-4 doses. **<1 mth:** 15-20 mg/kg/d in 3-4 doses. **PO: Adults:** 150-450 mg q6h. **Peds:** 8-20 mg/kg/d given 3-4 doses.	◙B ❁v(IV) ❁> (PO) **W** [84]

Imipenem/Cilastatin (Primaxin I.V.)	**Inj:** 250-250 mg, 500-500 mg	**IV: Adults: ≥70 kg: Mild:** 250-500 mg q6h. **Moderate:** 500 mg q6-8h or 1 gm q8h. **Severe:** 500 mg q6h or 1 gm q6-8h. **Max:** 50 mg/kg/d or 4 gm/d, whichever is lower. **Peds: ≥3 mths:** 15-25 mg/kg q6h. **Max:** 4 gm/d. **4 wks-3 mths & ≥1500 gm:** 25 mg/kg q6h. **1-4 wks & ≥1500 gm:** 25 mg/kg q8h. **<1 wk & ≥1500 gm:** 25 mg/kg q12h.	C > **R**
Metronidazole (Flagyl IV)	**Inj:** 500 mg/100 ml	**Adults: IV: LD:** 15 mg/kg. **Maint:** After 6h, 7.5 mg/kg q6h. **Max:** 4 gm/d.	B v**H** CI in 1st trimester. **W** 83
Metronidazole (Flagyl)	**Cap:** 375 mg; **Tab:** 250 mg, 500 mg	**Adults: PO:** 7.5 mg/kg q6h. **Max:** 4 gm/d.	B v**H** CI in 1st trimester. **W** 83

Fungal Infection

Amphotericin B Lipid Complex (Abelcet)	**Inj:** 5 mg/ml	**Invasive Fungal Infections: Adults & Peds:** 5 mg/kg as a single IV infusion at 2.5 mg/kg/h. If infusion time >2h, mix contents by shaking infusion bag q2h.	B v **R**

NAME	FORM/STRENGTH	DOSAGE	COMMENTS
Amphotericin B Liposome (Ambisome)	**Inj:** 50 mg; **Susp:** 100 mg/ml	**Adult & Peds:** Give over 120 min & reduce to 60 min if well tolerated. **Emperic Therapy in Febrile, Neutropenic Patients:** 3 mg/kg/d IV. **Aspergillosis/*Candida*/*Cryptococcus*:** 3-5 mg/kg/d IV. **Visceral Leishmaniasis:** (Immunocompetent) 3 mg/kg/d IV for Days 1-5, 14, 21. (Immunocompromised) 4 mg/kg/d IV for Days 1-5, 10, 17, 24, 31, 38. **Cryptococcal Meningitis in HIV Patients:** 6 mg/kg/d IV.	B v
Amphotericin B (Amphotec)	**Inj:** 50 mg, 100 mg	**Adults & Peds: Test Dose:** Infuse small amount over 15-30 min. **Treatment:** 3-4 mg/kg/day IV at 1 mg/kg/hr.	B v **R**
Anidulafungin (Eraxis)	**Inj:** 50 mg	**Adults: Candidemia/*Candida* Infections (Intra-Abdominal Abscess & Peritonitis): LD:** 200 mg on Day 1. Follow w/ 100 mg qd thereafter. Continue therapy for at least 14d after last positive culture. **Esophageal Candidiasis: LD:** 100 mg on Day 1. Follow w/ 50 mg qd thereafter. Treat for minimum of 14d & for at least 7d after symptoms resolve.	C >
Caspofungin Acetate (Cancidas)	**Inj:** 50 mg, 70 mg	**Adults: Invasive Aspergillosis/Empirical Therapy: LD:** 70 mg IV on Day 1. **Maint:** 50 mg/d IV. **Esophageal Candidiasis:** 50 mg/d IV. **Candidemia/*Candida* Infections (intra-abdominal abscesses, peritonitis, & pleural space infection): LD:** 70 mg IV on Day 1. **Maint:** 50 mg/d IV. **Concomitant Rifampin:** 70 mg IV qd. **Concomitant Nevirapine/Efavirenz/Carbamazepine/Dexamethasone/**	C > **H**

		Phenytoin: May need to increase dose to 70 mg IV qd. **Peds: 3 mths-17 yo: LD:** 70 mg/m^2 IV on Day 1. **Maint:** 50 mg/m^2 IV qd. May increase to 70mg/m^2 based on response. **Max:** 70 mg/d. **Concomitant Rifampin/ Nevirapine/Efavirenz/Carbamazepine/Dexamethasone/ Phenytoin:** 70 mg/m^2 IV qd. **Max:** 70 mg/d.	
Fluconazole (Diflucan)	**Inj:** 200 mg/100 ml, 400 mg/200 ml; **Susp:** 50 mg/5 ml, 200 mg/ 5 ml; **Tab:** 50 mg, 100 mg, 150 mg, 200 mg	**Adults: PO: Vaginal Candidiasis:** 150 mg single dose. **IV/PO: Oropharyngeal Candidiasis:** 200 mg on Day 1, then 100 mg qd x min 2 wks. **Esophageal Candidiasis:** 200 mg on Day 1, then 100 mg qd x min 3 wks & 2 wks after symptoms resolve. **Max:** 400 mg/d. **Systemic *Candida* Infections:** 400 mg/d. **UTI & Peritonitis:** 50-200 mg/d. **Cryptococcal Meningitis:** 400 mg on Day 1, then 200 mg qd x 10-12 wks after negative CSF culture. **Relapse Suppression in AIDS:** 200 mg qd. **Prophylaxis in BMT:** 400 mg qd. **Peds: IV/PO: Oropharyngeal Candidiasis:** 6 mg/kg on Day 1, then 3 mg/kg/d x min 2 wks. **Esophageal Candidiasis:** 6 mg/kg on Day 1, then 3 mg/kg/d x min 3 wks & 2 wks after symptoms resolve. **Max:** 12 mg/kg/d. **Systemic *Candida* Infections:** 6-12 mg/kg/d. **Cryptococcal Meningitis:** 12 mg/kg on Day 1, then 6 mg/kg/d x 10-12 wks after negative CSF culture. **Relapse Suppression in AIDS:** 6 mg/kg/d.	◙C ❊v **R**

NAME	FORM/STRENGTH	DOSAGE	COMMENTS
Griseofulvin, Microcrystalline (Grifulvin V)	**Susp:** 125 mg/5 ml; **Tab:** 500 mg	**Adults: Tinea Corporis, Cruris & Capitis:** 500 mg qd; **Tinea Pedis, Unguium:** 1 gm qd. **Peds: 30-50 lbs:** 125-250 mg qd. **>50 lbs:** 250-500 mg qd. Treat capitis x 4-6 wks, corporis x 2-4 wks, pedis x 4-8 wks, unguium x min 4 mths (fingernails) or 6 mths (toenails).	N > CI in pregnancy.
Itraconazole (Sporanox)	**Cap:** 100 mg; **Inj:** 10 mg/mL; **Sol:** 10 mg/ml	**Adults: Cap:** Take w/ full meal. **Blastomycosis/ Histoplasmosis:** 200 mg qd. May increase by 100 mg increments if no improvement. **Max:** 400 mg/d. Give bid if dose >200 mg/d. **Aspergillosis:** 200-400 mg/d. **Life-Threatening Infections: LD:** 200 mg tid x 1st 3d. Continue x min 3 mths & until infection subsides. **Onychomycosis: Toenail:** 200 mg qd x 12 consecutive wks. **Fingernail:** 200 mg bid x 1 wk, skip x 3 wks, then repeat. **Sol:** Take on empty stomach. Swish 10 ml at a time for several sec, then swallow. **Candidiasis: Oropharyngeal:** 200 mg/d x 1-2 wks. If refractory to fluconazole, give 100 mg bid. **Esophageal:** 100-200 mg qd x min 3 wks. Continue x 2 wks after symptoms resolve. **Inj: Blastomycosis/ Histoplasmosis/Aspergillosis:** 200 mg IV bid x 4 doses, followed by 200 mg qd. **Empiric Therapy in Febrile, Neutropenia w/ Suspected Fungal Infections:** 200 mg IV bid x 4 doses, followed by 200 mg qd x up to 14 days. Continue w/ oral sol 200 mg bid until resolution of clinically significant neutropenia.	C v **W** [95]

Ketoconazole (Nizoral)	**Tab:** 200 mg	**Adults: Initial:** 200 mg qd. **Titrate:** May increase to 400 mg qd. **Peds: ≥2 yo:** 3.3-6.6 mg/kg qd. For topical, see under Dermatology Antifungals.	C v **W** [61]
Micafungin Sodium (Mycamine)	**Inj:** 50 mg	**Adults: Esophageal Candidiasis:** 150 mg/d IV. ***Candida* Infection Prophylaxis in Hematopoietic Stem Cell Transplantation:** 50 mg/d IV.	C >
Nystatin	**Susp:** 100,000 U/ml; **Tab:** 500,000 U	**Oral Candidiasis: Adults & Peds: Susp:** 4-6 ml qid. Continue x 48h after relief of symptoms. **Infants: Susp:** 2 ml qid. **GI Candidiasis: Tab:** 500,000-1,000,000 U tid. Continue x min 48h after cure.	C >
Posaconazole (Noxafil)	**Susp:** 40 mg/ml	**Adults & Peds: ≥13 yo: Prophylaxis of Invasive Fungal Infections:** 200 mg (5 ml) tid. Base duration of therapy on recovery from neutropenia or immunosuppression. **Oropharyngeal Candidiasis: LD:** 100 mg (2.5 ml) bid on Day 1, then 100 mg qd for 13d. **Oropharyngeal Candidiasis Refractory to Itraconazole and/or Fluconazole:** 400 mg (10 ml) bid. Base duration of therapy on severity of underlying disease & clinical response. Give each dose w/ full meal or nutritional supplement.	C v
Terbinafine HCl (Lamisil)	**Granules:** 125 mg/pkt, 187.5 mg/pkt; **Tab:** 250 mg	**Adults: Onychomycosis: Tab: Fingernail:** 250 mg qd x 6 wks. **Toenail:** 250 mg qd x 12 wks. **Adults & Peds: ≥4 yo: Tinea Capitis: Granules:** Take qd w/ food x 6 wks. **<25 kg:** 125 mg/d. **25-35kg:** 187.5 mg/d. **>35kg:** 250 mg/d.	B v

NAME	FORM/STRENGTH	DOSAGE	COMMENTS
Voriconazole (Vfend)	**Inj:** 200 mg/30 ml; **Susp:** 40 mg/ml; **Tab:** 50 mg, 200 mg	**Adults: Invasive Aspergillosis/Infections Due to *Fusarium* spp. & *Scedosporium apiospermum*: (Inj) LD:** 6 mg/kg IV q12h x 1st 24h. **Maint:** 4 mg/kg IV q12h; may reduce to 3 mg/kg if unable to tolerate. Switch to PO when appropriate. **(PO) Maint: ≥40 kg:** 200 mg q12h. **<40 kg:** 100 mg q12h. **Esophageal Candidiasis: (PO) ≥40kg:** 200 mg q12h. **<40 kg:** 100 mg q12h. Treat for min of 14d & at least 7d following resolution of symptoms. **Candidemia Non-Neutropenic Patients/Deep Tissue *Candida* Infections: (Inj) LD:** 6 mg/kg IV q12h x 1st 24h. **(Inj) Maint:** 3-4 mg/kg IV q12h. **(PO) Maint: ≥40 kg:** 200 mg q12h. **<40 kg:** 100 mg q12h. Treat for at least 14d following resolution of symptoms or following last positive culture, whichever is longer. For PO maint dosing, if inadequate response may increase from 200 mg q12h to 300 mg q12h for ≥40 kg or from 100 mg q12h to 150 mg q12h for <40 kg. If unable to tolerate higher PO maint doses, may reduce by 50 mg steps from 300 mg q12h to min of 200 mg q12h for ≥40 kg or from 150 mg q12h to min of 100 mg q12h for <40 kg. **Concomitant Phenytoin: Maint: IV:** 5 mg/kg q12h. **PO: ≥40 kg:** 400 mg q12h. **<40 kg:** 200 mg q12h. **Concomitant Efavirenz: Maint:** 400 mg q12h & efavirenz 300 mg q24h. **Mild to Moderate Hepatic Cirrhosis: Maint:** Use 1/2 of maint dose. **CrCl <50 ml/min:** Use PO. Take PO 1 hr before or 1	D v **H R**

hr after a meal. Base duration on severity of underlying disease, recovery from immunosuppression, & clinical response.

Lower Respiratory Tract Infection

AMINOGLYCOSIDES

Drug	Form	Dosage	Ratings
Amikacin Sulfate	**Inj:** 50 mg/ml, 250 mg/ml	**IV: Adults, Children & Older Infants:** 7.5 mg/kg q12h or 5 mg/kg IM/IV q8h. **Max:** 1.5 gm/d. **Newborns: LD:** 10 mg/kg. **Maint:** 7.5 mg/kg q12h.	D v **R W** [1]
Gentamicin Sulfate	**Inj:** 40 mg/ml	**IV: Adults:** 3 mg/kg/d given q8h. **Max:** 5 mg/kg/d in 3-4 doses. Reduce to 3 mg/kg/d as soon as clinically indicated. **Peds:** 2-2.5 mg/kg q8h. **Infants/Neonates:** 2.5 mg/kg q8h. **≤1 wk:** 2.5 mg/kg q12h.	N >**R W** [1]
Tobramycin Sulfate	**Inj:** 10 mg/ml, 40 mg/ml, 1.2 gm	**IV: Adults:** 3 mg/kg/d given q8h. **Max:** 5 mg/kg/d in 3-4 doses. Reduce to 3 mg/kg/d as soon as clinically indicated. **Peds: >1 wk:** 2-2.5 mg/kg q8h or 1.5-1.89 mg/kg q6h. **<1 wk:** Up to 2 mg/kg q12h.	D > **R W** [1]

CARBAPENEM

Drug	Form	Dosage	Ratings
Ertapenem Sodium (Invanz)	**Inj:** 1 gm	**CAP: Adults/Peds: ≥13 yo:** 1 gm IM/IV qd. **3 mths-12 yo:** 15 mg/kg IM/IV bid (not to exceed 1 gm/d) . **Duration:** 10-14d. May give IV up to 14d; IM up to 7d.	B > **R**

NAME	FORM/STRENGTH	DOSAGE	COMMENTS
CEPHALOSPORINS			
Cefaclor	**Cap:** 250 mg, 500 mg; **Susp:** 125 mg/5 ml, 187 mg/5 ml, 250 mg/5 ml, 375 mg/5 ml	**Adults: Cap/Susp: Usual:** 250 mg q8h. **Severe Infections/ Pneumonia:** 500 mg q8h. **Peds: ≥1 mth: Cap/Susp:** 20 mg/kg/d given q8h. **Serious Infections:** 40 mg/kg/d. **Max:** 1 gm/d.	B >
Cefdinir (Omnicef)	**Cap:** 300 mg	**Adults & Peds: ≥13 yo: CAP:** 300 mg q12h x 10d. **ABECB:** 300 mg q12h x 5-10d or 600 mg q24h x 10d.	B > **R**
Cefepime HCl (Maxipime)	**Inj:** 500 mg, 1 gm, 2 gm	**Adults: Moderate-Severe:** 1-2 gm IV q12h x 10d. **Peds: 2 mths-16 yo: ≤40 kg:** 50 mg/kg IV q12h. **Max:** Do not exceed adult dose.	B > **R**
Cefixime (Suprax)	**Susp:** 100 mg/5 ml	**Pharyngitis/Tonsillitis: Adults & Peds: >12 yo or >50 kg: Tab/Susp:** 400 mg qd or 200 mg bid. **≤50 kg or ≥6 mths: Susp:** 8 mg/kg qd or 4 mg/kg bid.	B v **R**
Cefpodoxime Proxetil (Vantin)	**Susp:** 50 mg/5 ml, 100 mg/5 ml; **Tab:** 100 mg, 200 mg	**Adults & Peds: ≥12 yo:** 200 mg q12h x 10-14d.	B v **R**
Cefprozil (Cefzil)	**Susp:** 125 mg/5 ml, 250 mg/5 ml; **Tab:** 250 mg, 500 mg	**Acute Bronchitis/ABECB: Adults & Peds: ≥13 yo:** 500 mg q12h x 10d.	B > **R**
Ceftazidime (Fortaz)	**Inj:** 500 mg, 1 gm, 1 gm/50 ml, 2 gm, 2 gm/50 ml, 6 gm	**Uncomplicated Pneumonia: Adults:** 500-1000 mg IM/IV q8h. **Peds: 1 mth-12 yo:** 30-50 mg/kg IV q8h, up to 6 gm/d. **Neonates: 0-4 wks:** 30 mg/kg IV q12h.	B > **R**

Ceftriaxone Sodium (Rocephin)	**Inj:** (Rocephin) 500 mg, 1 gm; (Generic) 250 mg, 500 mg, 1 gm, 2 gm, 10 gm, 1 gm/50 ml, 2 gm/50ml	**Adults: IM/IV: Usual:** 1-2 gm qd (or in equally divided doses bid). **Max:** 4 gm/d.	◉B ✽>
Cefuroxime Axetil (Ceftin)	**Tab:** 250 mg, 500 mg	**Adults & Peds: ≥13 yo:** 250-500 mg bid x 5-10d.	◉B ✽v **R**
Cephalexin (Keflex)	(Keflex) **Cap:** 250 mg, 500 mg, 750 mg; (Generic) **Cap:** 250 mg, 500 mg; **Susp:** 125 mg/5 ml, 250 mg/5 ml	**Adults: Usual:** 250 mg q6h. **Max:** 4 gm/d. **Peds: Usual:** 25-50 mg/kg/d in divided doses.	◉B ✽>

KETOLIDES

Telithromycin (Ketek)	**Tab:** 300 mg, 400 mg,	**Mild-to-Moderate CAP: Adults:** 800 mg qd x 7-10d.	◉C ✽> **H R W** [71]

MACROLIDES

Azithromycin (Zithromax)	**Inj:** 500 mg; **Susp:** 100 mg/5 ml, 200 mg/5 ml, 1 gm/pkt; **Tab:** 250 mg, 500 mg, 600 mg	**CAP: Adults: ≥16 yo: PO:** 500 mg on Day 1, then 250 mg qd on Days 2-5. **IV:** 500 mg qd x at least 2d, then 500 mg PO qd to complete 7-10 day course. **Peds: ≥6 mths: Susp:** 10 mg/kg on Day 1, then 5 mg/kg on Days 2-5. **COPD: Adults: PO:** 500 mg qd x 3d or 500 mg on Day 1, then 250 mg qd on Days 2-5.	◉B ✽>

NAME	FORM/STRENGTH	DOSAGE	COMMENTS
Azithromycin (Zmax)	**Susp,ER:** 2 gm (27 mg/ml)	**CAP: Adults:** 2 gm single dose. **Peds: ≥6 mths:** 60 mg/kg single dose. **Max:** 2 gm single dose. Patients weighing >34 kg should receive adult dose. See PI for specific pediatric dosage info. Take on empty stomach.	B >
Clarithromycin (Biaxin XL)	**Tab,ER:** 500 mg	**Adults: ABECB/CAP:** 1 gm qd x 7d.	C > **R**
Clarithromycin (Biaxin)	**Susp:** 125 mg/5 ml, 250 mg/5 ml; **Tab:** 250 mg, 500 mg	**Adults: ABECB:** 250-500 mg q12h x 7-14d. **CAP:** 250 mg q12h x 7-14d. **Peds: ≥6 mths: Usual:** 7.5 mg/kg q12h x 10d.	C > **R**
Erythromycin (Erythromycin Base)	**Tab:** 250 mg, 500 mg	**Adults: Usual:** 250 mg q6h or 500 mg q12h. **Peds: Usual:** 30-50 mg/kg/d in divided doses. **Max:** 4 gm/d.	B >
Erythromycin Ethylsuccinate (E.E.S.)	**Susp:** 200 mg/5 ml, 400 mg/5 ml; **Tab:** 400 mg	**Adults: Usual:** 1600 mg/d in divided doses given q6h, q8h, or q12h. **Max:** 4 gm/d. **Peds: Usual:** 30-50 mg/kg/d in divided doses given q6h, q8h, or q12h. May double dose for more severe infections.	B >
Erythromycin Ethylsuccinate (EryPed)	**Chewtab:** 200 mg; **Susp:** 100 mg/2.5 ml, 200 mg/5 ml, 400 mg/5 ml	**Adults: Usual:** 1600 mg/d in divided doses given q6h, q8h, or q12h. **Max:** 4 gm/d. **Peds: Usual:** 30-50 mg/kg/d in divided doses given q6h, q8h, or q12h. May double dose for more severe infections.	B >
Erythromycin Stearate (Erythrocin)	**Tab:** 250 mg, 500 mg	**Adults: Usual:** 250 mg q6h or 500 mg q12h. **Peds: Usual:** 30-50 mg/kg/d in divided doses. **Max:** 4 gm/d.	B >

Erythromycin (Ery-Tab)	**Tab,Delay:** 250 mg, 333 mg, 500 mg	**Adults: Usual:** 250 mg qid, 333 mg q8h, or 500 mg q12h. **Peds: Usual:** 30-50 mg/kg/d in divided doses. **Max:** 4 gm/d.	B >
Erythromycin (PCE)	**Tab,ER:** 333 mg, 500 mg	**Adults: Usual:** 333 mg q8h or 500 mg q12h. **Peds: Usual:** 30-50 mg/kg/d in divided doses. **Max:** 4 gm/d.	B >

OXAZOLIDINONE

Linezolid (Zyvox)	**Inj:** 2 mg/ml; **Susp:** 100 mg/5 ml; **Tab:** 600 mg	**CAP/Nosocomial Pneumonia:** Treat x 10-14d. **Adults & Peds: ≥12 yo:** 600 mg IV/PO q12h. **Birth-11 yo:** 10 mg/kg IV/PO q8h.	C >

PENICILLINS

Amoxicillin/Clavulanate (Augmentin XR)	**Tab,ER:** 1000-62.5 mg	**Adults & Peds: ≥16 yo:** 2 tabs q12h x 7-10d.	B >
Amoxicillin/Clavulanate (Augmentin)	**Chewtab:** 200-28.5 mg, 250-62.5 mg, 400-57 mg; **Susp:** (per 5 ml) 125-31.25 mg, 200-28.5 mg, 250-62.5 mg, 400-57 mg; **Tab:** 250-125 mg, 500-125 mg, 875-125 mg	Dose based on amoxicillin component. **Adults & Peds: ≥40 kg: Tab:** 875 mg q12h or 500 mg q8h. May use 125 mg/5 ml or 250 mg/5 ml susp in place of 500 mg tab & 200 mg/5 ml susp or 400 mg/5 ml susp in place of 875 mg tab. **Chewtab/Susp: ≥12 wks:** 45 mg/kg/d given q12h or 40 mg/kg/d given q8h. **<12 wks:** 15 mg/kg q12h (use 125 mg/5 ml susp).	B > 2-250 mg tabs are not equivalent to 1- 500 mg tab. Only use 250 mg tab if peds ≥40 kg. Chewtab & tab not interchangeable. **H R**

NAME	FORM/STRENGTH	DOSAGE	COMMENTS
Amoxicillin (Amoxil)	(Amoxil) **Cap:** 500 mg; **Sus:** 50 mg/ml, 250 mg/5 ml, 400 mg/5 ml. (Generic) **Cap:** 250 mg, 500 mg; **Sus:** 125 mg/5 ml, 200 mg/5 ml, 250 mg/5ml, 400 mg/5 ml; **Tab:** 500 mg, 875 mg; **Tab,Chew:** 125 mg, 200 mg, 250 mg, 400 mg	**Adults & Peds: >40 kg:** 875 mg q12h or 500 mg q8h. **>3 mths & <40 kg:** 45 mg/kg/d given q12h or 40 mg/kg/d given q8h. ≤**3 mths: Max:** 15 mg/kg q12h.	B > **R**
Ampicillin	**Cap:** 250 mg, 500 mg; **Susp:** 125 mg/5 ml, 250 mg/5 ml	**Adults & Peds: >20 kg:** 250 mg qid. ≤**20 kg:** 50 mg/kg/d given tid-qid.	B v
Penicillin V Potassium (Penicillin VK, Veetids)	**Susp:** 125 mg/5 ml, 250 mg/5 ml; **Tab:** 250 mg, 500 mg	**Adults & Peds:** ≥**12 yo: Pneumococcal:** 250-500 mg q6h until afebrile x 2d.	B >
Piperacillin Sodium/ Tazobactam (Zosyn)	**Inj:** 40-5 mg/ml, 60-7.5 mg/ml, 2-0.25 gm, 3-0.375 gm, 4-0.5 gm, 4-0.5 gm/100 ml, 36-4.5 gm	**Adults: Usual:** 3.375 gm IV q6h x 7-10d. **Nosocomial Pneumonia:** 4.5 gm IV q6h x 7-14d plus aminoglycoside.	B > **R**

Ciprofloxacin HCl (Cipro Oral)	**Susp:** 250 mg/5 ml, 500 mg/5 ml; **Tab:** 250 mg, 500 mg, 750 mg	**Adults: ≥18 yo: Mild/Moderate:** 500 mg PO q12h x 7-14d. **Severe/Complicated:** 750 mg PO q12h x 7-14d. **Inhalational Anthrax (Post-Exposure): Adults:** 500 mg PO q12h x 60d. **Peds:** 15 mg/kg PO q12h x 60d. **Max:** 500 mg PO per dose.	C v **R W** [98]
Ciprofloxacin (Cipro IV)	**Inj:** 10 mg/ml, 200 mg/ 100 ml, 400 mg/200 ml	**Adults: ≥18 yo: Mild/Moderate:** 400 mg IV q12h x 7-14d. **Severe/Complicated:** 400 mg IV q8h x 7-14d. **Nosocomial Pneumonia:** 400 mg IV q8h x 10-14d. **Inhalational Anthrax (Post-Exposure): Adults:** 400 mg IV q12h x 60d. **Peds:** 10 mg/kg IV q12h x 60d. **Max:** 400 mg IV per dose.	C v **R W** [98]
Gemifloxacin Mesylate (Factive)	**Tab:** 320 mg	**Adults: ≥18 yo: ABECB:** 320 mg qd x 5d. **CAP:** 320 mg qd x 5d (*S.pneumoniae, H.influenzae, M.pneumoniae, C.pneumoniae*) or 7d (multi-drug resistant *S.pneumoniae, K.pneumoniae, or M.catarrhalis*).	C v **R W** [98]
Levofloxacin (Levaquin)	**Inj:** 5 mg/ml, 25 mg/ml; **Sol:** 25 mg/ml; **Tab:** 250 mg, 500 mg, 750 mg	**Adults: ≥18 yo: CAP:** 500 mg IV/PO qd x 7-14d or 750 mg IV/PO qd x 5d. **Nosocomial Pneumonia:** 750mg IV/PO qd x 7-14d. **ABECB:** 500 mg IV/PO x 7d. **Inhalation Anthrax (Post-Exposure):** 500 mg IV/PO qd x 60d.	C v **R W** [98]
Lomefloxacin (Maxaquin)	**Tab:** 400 mg	**ABECB: Adults: ≥18 yo:** 400 mg qd x 10d.	C v **R W** [98]
Moxifloxacin HCl (Avelox)	**Inj:** 400 mg/250 ml; **Tab:** 400 mg	**Adults: ≥18 yo:** 400 mg IV/PO qd x 5d (ABECB) or 7-14d (CAP).	C v **W** [98]

NAME	FORM/STRENGTH	DOSAGE	COMMENTS
Ofloxacin (Floxin)	**Tab:** 200 mg, 300 mg, 400 mg	**ABECB/CAP: Adults: ≥18 yo:** 400 mg q12h x 10d.	C v **H R W** [98]
SULFONAMIDES AND COMBINATIONS			
Sulfamethoxazole/ Trimethoprim (Septra, Septra DS, Sulfatrim Pediatric)	**Susp:** 200-40 mg/5 ml; **Tab:** (SS) 400-80 mg, (DS) 800-160 mg	**Adults:** 800 mg SMX & 160 mg TMP (1 DS tab, 2 SS tabs, or 20 ml) q12h x 14d.	C v **R** CI in pregnancy & nursing.
TETRACYCLINES			
Doxycycline Hyclate (Doryx)	**Cap,Delay:** 75 mg, 100 mg	**Adults:** 100 mg q12h on Day 1, then 100 mg qd or 50 mg q12h. **Severe:** 100 mg q12h. **Peds: >8 yo & ≤100 lbs:** 1 mg/lb bid on Day 1, then 1 mg/lb qd or 0.5 mg/lb bid. **Severe:** 2 mg/lb. **>100 lbs:** Adult dose. **Inhalation Anthrax (Post-Exposure): Adults:** 100 mg bid x 60d. **Peds: >8 yo & <100 lbs:** 1 mg/lb bid x 60d. **≥100 lbs:** Adult dose.	D v
Doxycycline Monohydrate (Monodox)	**Cap:** 50 mg, 100 mg	**Adults:** 100 mg q12h or 50 mg q6h on Day 1, then 100 mg qd or 50 mg q12h. **Severe:** 100 mg q12h. **Peds: >8 yo & ≤100 lbs:** 1 mg/lb bid on Day 1, then 1 mg/lb qd or 0.5 mg/lb bid. **Severe:** 2 mg/lb. **>100 lbs:** Adult dose. **Inhalation Anthrax (Post-Exposure): Adults:** 100 mg bid x 60d. **Peds: >8 yo & <100 lbs:** 1 mg/lb bid x 60d. **≥100 lbs:** Adult dose.	D v

Doxycycline Monohydrate (Vibramycin)	**Cap:** (Vibramycin) 100 mg; **Tab:** (Vibra-Tabs) 100 mg	**Adults:** 100 mg q12h on Day 1, then 100 mg qd or 50 mg q12h. **Severe:** 100 mg q12h. **Peds: >8 yo & ≤100 lbs:** 1 mg/lb bid on Day 1, then 1 mg/lb qd or 0.5 mg/lb bid. **Severe:** 2 mg/lb. **>100 lbs:** Adult dose. **Inhalation Anthrax (Post-Exposure): Adults:** 100 mg bid x 60d. **Peds: >8 yo & <100 lbs:** 1 mg/lb bid x 60d. **≥100 lbs:** Adult dose.	D v
Doxycycline Monohydrate (Vibramycin)	**Susp:** 25 mg/5 ml	**Adults:** 100 mg q12h or 50 mg q6h on Day 1, then 100 mg qd or 50 mg q12h. **Severe:** 100 mg q12h. **Peds: >8 yo & ≤100 lbs:** 1 mg/lb bid on Day 1, then 1 mg/lb qd or 0.5 mg/lb bid. **Severe:** 2 mg/lb. **>100 lbs:** Adult dose. **Inhalation Anthrax (Post-Exposure): Adults:** 100 mg bid x 60d. **Peds: >8 yo & <100 lbs:** 1 mg/lb bid x 60d. **≥100 lbs:** Adult dose.	D v
Minocycline HCl (Dynacin)	**Tab:** 50 mg, 75 mg, 100 mg	**Adults:** 200 mg PO, then 100 mg q12h or 50 mg qid. **Peds: >8 yo:** 4 mg/kg PO, then 2 mg/kg q12h.	D v **R**
Minocycline HCl (Minocin)	**Cap:** 50 mg, 100 mg; **Inj:** 100 mg	**Adults:** 200 mg PO/IV, then 100 mg q12h or 50 mg qid. **Peds: >8 yo:** 4 mg/kg PO/IV, then 2 mg/kg q12h.	D v **R**
Tetracycline HCl (Sumycin)	**Cap:** 250 mg, 500 mg; **Susp:** 125 mg/5 ml	**Adults:** 250 mg qid or 500 mg bid. **Peds: >8 yo:** 25-50 mg/kg divided bid-qid.	D v **R**

MISCELLANEOUS

NAME	FORM/STRENGTH	DOSAGE	COMMENTS
Clindamycin (Cleocin)	**Cap:** 75 mg, 150 mg, 300 mg; **Inj:** 150 mg/ml, 300 mg/50 ml, 600 mg/ 50 ml, 900 mg/50 ml; **Susp:** 75 mg/5 ml	**IM/IV: Adults:** 600-2700 mg/d in 2-4 doses. **Max:** 600 mg IM single dose. **Peds: 1 mth-16 yo:** 20-40 mg/kg/d in 3-4 doses. **<1 mth:** 15-20 mg/kg/d in 3-4 doses. **PO: Adults:** 150-450 mg q6h. **Peds:** 8-20 mg/kg/d given 3-4 doses.	◙B ❊v(IV) ❊> (PO) **W** [84]

Meningitis, Bacterial

AMINOGLYCOSIDES

NAME	FORM/STRENGTH	DOSAGE	COMMENTS
Amikacin Sulfate	**Inj:** 50 mg/ml, 250 mg/ml	**IV: Adults, Children & Older Infants:** 7.5 mg/kg q12h or 5 mg/kg IM/IV q8h. **Max:** 1.5 gm/d. **Newborns: LD:** 10 mg/kg. **Maint:** 7.5 mg/kg q12h.	◙D ❊v **R W** [1]
Gentamicin Sulfate	**Inj:** 40 mg/ml	**IV: Adults:** 3 mg/kg/d given q8h. **Max:** 5 mg/kg/d in 3-4 doses. Reduce to 3 mg/kg/d as soon as clinically indicated. **Peds:** 2-2.5 mg/kg q8h. **Infants/Neonates:** 2.5 mg/kg q8h. **≤1 wk:** 2.5 mg/kg q12h.	◙N ❊>**R W** [1]
Tobramycin Sulfate	**Inj:** 10 mg/ml, 40 mg/ml, 1.2 gm	**IV: Adults:** 3 mg/kg/d given q8h. **Max:** 5 mg/kg/d in 3-4 doses. Reduce to 3 mg/kg/d as soon as clinically indicated. **Peds: >1 wk:** 2-2.5 mg/kg q8h or 1.5-1.89 mg/kg q6h. **<1 wk:** Up to 2 mg/kg q12h.	◙D ❊> **R W** [1]

CARBAPENEM

Meropenem (Merrem)	**Inj:** 500 mg, 1 gm	**IV: Adults & Peds: ≥3 mths: >50 kg:** 1 gm q8h. **≤50 kg:** 40 mg/kg q8h. **Max:** 2 gm q8h.	B > **R**

CEPHALOSPORINS

Cefotaxime Sodium (Claforan)	**Inj:** 500 mg, 1 gm, 2 gm, 10 gm	**IV: Adults or >50 kg:** 2 gm q6-8h. **Max:** 12 gm/d. **1 mth-12 yo: <50 kg:** 50-180 mg/kg/d divided into 4-6 doses. **1-4 wks:** 50 mg/kg IV q8h. **0-1 wk:** 50 mg/kg IV q12h.	B > **R**
Ceftazidime (Fortaz)	**Inj:** 500 mg, 1 gm, 1 gm/ 50 ml, 2 gm, 2 gm/ 50 ml, 6 gm	**Adults:** 2 gm IV q8h. **Peds: 1 mth-12 yo:** 30-50 mg/kg IV q8h, up to 6 gm/d. **Neonates: 0-4 wks:** 30 mg/kg IV q12h.	B > **R**
Ceftriaxone Sodium (Rocephin)	**Inj:** (Rocephin) 500 mg, 1 gm; (Generic) 250 mg, 500 mg, 1 gm, 2 gm, 10 gm, 1 gm/50 ml, 2 gm/50ml	**IV: Adults:** 1-2 gm qd (or in equally divided doses bid). **Max:** 4 gm/d. **Peds:** Initial of 100 mg/kg (NTE 4 gm), then 100 mg/kg qd or (in equally divided doses q12h) x 7-14d. **Max:** 4 gm/d.	B >
Cefuroxime (Zinacef)	**Inj:** 750 mg, 1.5 gm, 7.5 gm	**IV: Adults:** 1.5 gm q6h. **Max:** 3 gm q8h. **Peds: >3 mths:** 200-240 mg/kg/d divided q6-8h.	B > **R**

PENICILLINS

Ampicillin Sodium	**Inj:** 250 mg, 500 mg, 1 gm, 2 gm	**IV: Adults & Peds:** 150-200 mg/kg/day given q3-4h.	B >

NAME	FORM/STRENGTH	DOSAGE	COMMENTS
Penicillin G Potassium (Pfizerpen)	**Inj:** 5 MU, 20 MU	**IV: Adults: *Listeria*:** 15-20 MU/d x 2 wks. ***Pasteurella*:** 4-6 MU/d x 2 wks. ***Meningococcus*:** 1-2 MU IM q2h or 20-30 MU/d continuous IV.	B >

Mycobacterium Avium Complex

NAME	FORM/STRENGTH	DOSAGE	COMMENTS
Azithromycin (Zithromax)	**Susp:** 100 mg/5 ml, 200 mg/5 ml, 1 gm/pkt; **Tab:** 600 mg	**Adults: Prevention:** 1200 mg qwk. **Treatment:** 600 mg qd w/ ethambutol 15 mg/kg/d.	B >
Clarithromycin (Biaxin)	**Susp:** 125 mg/5 ml, 250 mg/5 ml; **Tab:** 250 mg, 500 mg	**Prevention & Treatment: Adults:** 500 mg bid. **Peds: ≥20 mths:** 7.5 mg/kg bid. **Max:** 500 mg bid.	C > **R**
Rifabutin (Mycobutin)	**Cap:** 150 mg	**Adults:** 300 mg qd or 150 mg bid w/ food. Reduce dose w/ nelfinavir or indinavir.	B v **R**

Otitis Media, Acute

CEPHALOSPORINS

NAME	FORM/STRENGTH	DOSAGE	COMMENTS
Cefaclor	**Cap:** 250 mg, 500 mg; **Susp:** 125 mg/5 ml, 187 mg/5 ml, 250 mg/5 ml, 375 mg/5 ml	**Peds: ≥1 mth:** 40 mg/kg/d given in divided doses. **Max:** 1 gm/d.	B >
Cefdinir (Omnicef)	**Susp:** 125 mg/5 ml; 250 mg/5 ml	**Peds: 6 mths-12 yo:** 7 mg/kg q12h x 5-10d or 14 mg/kg q24h x 10d.	B > **R**

Cefixime (Suprax)	**Susp:** 100 mg/5 ml	**Adults & Peds: >12 yo or >50 kg: Tab/Susp:** 400 mg qd or 200 mg bid. **≤50 kg or >6 mths: Susp:** 8 mg/kg qd or 4 mg/kg bid.	◉B ❀v **R**
Cefpodoxime Proxetil (Vantin)	**Susp:** 50 mg/5 ml, 100 mg/5 ml; **Tab:** 100 mg, 200 mg	**Peds: 2 mths-11 yo:** 5 mg/kg q12h x 5d.	◉B ❀v **R**
Cefprozil (Cefzil)	**Susp:** 125 mg/5 ml, 250 mg/5 ml; **Tab:** 250 mg, 500 mg	**Peds: 6 mths-12 yo:** 15 mg/kg q12h x 10d.	◉B ❀> **R**
Ceftriaxone Sodium (Rocephin)	**Inj:** (Rocephin) 500 mg, 1 gm; (Generic) 250 mg, 500 mg, 1 gm, 2 gm, 10 gm, 1 gm/50 ml, 2 gm/50ml	**Peds:** 50 mg/kg IM single dose. **Max:** 1 gm/dose.	◉B ❀>
Cefuroxime Axetil (Ceftin)	**Susp:** 125 mg/5 ml, 250 mg/5 ml; **Tab:** 250 mg, 500 mg	**Peds: 3 mths-12 yo: Susp:** 15 mg/kg bid x 10d. **Max:** 1 gm/d. **Tab:** 250 mg bid x 10d.	◉B ❀> Tabs & susp not bioequivalent. **R**
Cephalexin (Keflex)	(Keflex) **Cap:** 250 mg, 500 mg, 750 mg; (Generic) **Cap:** 250 mg, 500 mg; **Susp:** 125 mg/5 ml, 250 mg/5 ml	**Peds:** 75-100 mg/kg/d in divided doses.	◉B ❀>

NAME	FORM/STRENGTH	DOSAGE	COMMENTS
MACROLIDES			
Azithromycin (Zithromax)	**Susp:** 100 mg/5 ml, 200 mg/5 ml; 1 gm/pkt	**Peds: ≥6 mths:** 30 mg/kg x 1 dose; 10 mg/kg qd x 3d; or 10 mg/kg qd x 1d, then 5 mg/kg qd on Days 2-5.	◙B ❀>
Clarithromycin (Biaxin)	**Susp:** 125 mg/5 ml, 250 mg/5 ml; **Tab:** 250 mg, 500 mg	**Peds: ≥6 mths:** 7.5 mg/kg q12h x 10d.	◙C ❀> **R**
MACROLIDES AND COMBINATIONS			
Erythromycin Ethylsuccinate/ Sulfisoxazole Acetyl (Pediazole)	**Susp:** 200-600 mg/5 ml	**Peds: ≥2 mths:** Dose based on 50 mg/kg/d erythromycin or 150 mg/kg/d sulfisoxazole given tid-qid x 10d. **Max:** 6 gm/d sulfisoxazole.	◙C ❀v
PENICILLINS			
Amoxicillin/Clavulanate (Augmentin ES-600)	**Susp:** 600-42.9 mg/5 ml	**Peds: 3 mths-12 yo: <40 kg:** 45 mg/kg q12h based on amoxicillin component x 10d. Not interchangeable w/ other Augmentin susp.	◙B ❀> **H R**
Amoxicillin/Clavulanate (Augmentin)	**Chewtab:** 200-28.5 mg, 250-62.5 mg, 400-57 mg; **Susp:** (per 5 ml) 125-31.25 mg, 200-28.5 mg, 250-62.5 mg, 400-57 mg; **Tab:**	Dose based on amoxicillin component. **Peds: ≥40 kg: Tab:** 500 mg q12h or 250 mg q8h. May use 125 mg/5 ml or 250 mg/5 ml susp in place of 500 mg tab & 200 mg/5 ml or 400 mg/5 ml susp in place of 875 mg tab. **≥12 wks: Susp/Chewtab:** 45 mg/kg/d given q12h or 40 mg/kg/d given q8h. **<12 wks: Susp:** 15 mg/kg q12h (use 125 mg/5 ml susp).	◙B ❀> 2- 250 mg tabs are not equivalent to 1- 500 mg tab. Only use 250 mg tab if peds ≥40 kg.

	250-125 mg, 500-125 mg, 875-125 mg		Chewtab & tab not interchangeable. **H R**
Amoxicillin (Amoxil)	(Amoxil) **Cap:** 500 mg; **Sus:** 50 mg/ml, 250 mg/5 ml, 400 mg/5 ml. (Generic) **Cap:** 250 mg, 500 mg; **Sus:** 125 mg/5 ml, 200 mg/5 ml, 250 mg/5ml, 400 mg/5 ml; **Tab:** 500 mg, 875 mg; **Tab,Chew:** 125 mg, 200 mg, 250 mg, 400 mg	**Peds: >40 kg:** 500-875 mg q12h or 250-500 mg q8h, depending on severity. **>3 mths:** 25-45 mg/kg/d divided q12h or 20-40 mg/kg/d divided q8h, depending on severity. **≤3 mths: Max:** 15 mg/kg q12h.	◙B ❃> **R**

SULFONAMIDES AND COMBINATIONS

Sulfamethoxazole/ Trimethoprim (Septra, Septra DS, Sulfatrim Pediatric)	**Susp:** 200-40 mg/5 ml; **Tab:** (SS) 400-80 mg, (DS) 800-160 mg	**Peds: ≥2 mths:** 4 mg/kg TMP & 20 mg/kg SMX q12h x 10d.	◙C ❃v **R** CI in pregnancy & nursing.

Pneumocystis Carinii Pneumonia

Atovaquone (Mepron)	**Susp:** 750 mg/5 ml	**Adults & Peds: ≥13 yo:** Take w/ food. **Prevention:** 1500 mg qd. **Treatment:** 750 mg bid x 21d.	◙C ❃>

NAME	FORM/STRENGTH	DOSAGE	COMMENTS
Sulfamethoxazole/ Trimethoprim (Septra, Septra DS, Sulfatrim Pediatric)	**Susp:** 200-40 mg/5 ml; **Tab:** (SS) 400-80 mg, (DS) 800-160 mg	**Treatment: Adults & Peds:** 15-20 mg/kg TMP & 75-100 mg/kg SMZ divided q6h x 14-21d. **Prophylaxis: Adults:** 1 DS tab qd. **Peds:** 150 mg/m^2/d TMP & 750 mg/m^2 SMZ divided bid x 3 consecutive days/wk. **Max:** 320 mg TMP/1600 mg SMZ per day.	◉C ❋v **R** CI in pregnancy & nursing.

Septicemia, Bacterial

AMINOGLYCOSIDES

NAME	FORM/STRENGTH	DOSAGE	COMMENTS
Amikacin Sulfate	**Inj:** 50 mg/ml, 250 mg/ml	**IV: Adults, Children & Older Infants:** 7.5 mg/kg q12h or 5 mg/kg IM/IV q8h. **Max:** 1.5 gm/d. **Newborns: LD:** 10 mg/kg. **Maint:** 7.5 mg/kg q12h.	◉D ❋v **R W** [1]
Gentamicin Sulfate	**Inj:** 40 mg/ml	**IV: Adults:** 3 mg/kg/d given q8h. **Max:** 5 mg/kg/d in 3-4 doses. Reduce to 3 mg/kg/d as soon as clinically indicated. **Peds:** 2-2.5 mg/kg q8h. **Infants/Neonates:** 2.5 mg/kg q8h. **≤1 wk:** 2.5 mg/kg q12h.	◉N ❋>**R W** [1]
Tobramycin Sulfate	**Inj:** 10 mg/ml, 40 mg/ml, 1.2 gm	**IV: Adults:** 3 mg/kg/d given q8h. **Max:** 5 mg/kg/d in 3-4 doses. Reduce to 3 mg/kg/d as soon as clinically indicated. **Peds: >1 wk:** 2-2.5 mg/kg q8h or 1.5-1.89 mg/kg q6h. **<1 wk:** Up to 2 mg/kg q12h.	◉D ❋> **R W** [1]

Cefazolin	**Inj:** 500 mg, 1 gm, 10 gm, 20 gm	**IV: Adults:** 1-1.5 gm q6h. **Peds:** 100 mg/kg/d given as tid-qid.	◉B ❁> **R** Safety in prematures & neonates unknown.
Cefotaxime Sodium (Claforan)	**Inj:** 500 mg, 1 gm, 2 gm, 10 gm	**IV: Adults or >50 kg:** 2 gm q4h. **Max:** 12 gm/d. **1 mth-12 yo: <50 kg:** 50-180 mg/kg/d divided into 4-6 doses. **1-4 wks:** 50 mg/kg IV q8h. **0-1 wk:** 50 mg/kg IV q12h.	◉B ❁> **R**
Cefoxitin (Mefoxin)	**Inj:** (Generic) 1 gm, 1 gm/50 ml, 2 gm, 2 gm/ 50 ml, 10 gm, (Mefoxin) 1 gm/50 ml, 2 gm/ 50 ml	**IV: Adults:** 1 gm q4h or 2 gm q6-8h. **Peds: ≥3 mths:** 80-160 mg/kg/d given as q4-6h. **Max:** 12 gm/d.	◉B ❁> **R**
Ceftazidime (Fortaz)	**Inj:** 500 mg, 1 gm, 1 gm/ 50 ml, 2 gm, 2 gm/ 50 ml, 6 gm	**Adults:** 2 gm IV q8h. **Peds: 1 mth-12 yo:** 30-50 mg/kg IV q8h, up to 6 gm/d. **Neonates: 0-4 wks:** 30 mg/kg IV q12h.	◉B ❁> **R**
Ceftriaxone Sodium (Rocephin)	**Inj:** (Rocephin) 500 mg, 1 gm; (Generic) 250 mg, 500 mg, 1 gm, 2 gm, 10 gm, 1 gm/50 ml, 2 gm/50ml	**IV: Adults:** 1-2 gm qd (or in equally divided doses bid). **Max:** 4 gm/d. **Peds:** 50-75 mg/kg in divided doses q12h. **Max:** 2 gm/d.	◉B ❁>
Cefuroxime (Zinacef)	**Inj:** 750 mg, 1.5 gm, 7.5 gm	**IV: Adults:** 1.5 gm q6-8h. **Peds: >3 mths:** 100 mg/kg/d given q6-8h. **Max:** 4.5 gm/d.	◉B ❁> **R**

NAME	FORM/STRENGTH	DOSAGE	COMMENTS
MONOBACTAMS			
Aztreonam (Azactam)	**Inj:** 1 gm, 2 gm, 1 gm/50 ml, 2 gm/50 ml	**IV: Adults:** 2 gm q6-8h. **Peds:** 30 mg/kg q6-8h.	B v **R**
PENICILLINS			
Ticarcillin Disodium/ Clavulanate Potassium (Timentin)	**Inj:** 3 gm-100 mg, 3 gm-100 mg/100 ml, 30 gm-1 gm	**IV: Adults: ≥60 kg:** 300 mg/kg/d ticarcillin given q4h. **<60 kg:** 200-300 mg/kg/d ticarcillin given q4-6h. **Peds: ≥3 mths & <60 kg:** 50 mg/kg/d ticarcillin given q4h. **≥3 mths & ≥60 kg:** 3.1 gm q4h.	B > **R**
MISCELLANEOUS			
Clindamycin (Cleocin)	**Inj:** 150 mg/ml, 300 mg/50 ml, 600 mg/50 ml, 900 mg/50 ml	**IV: Adults:** 1200-2700 mg/d given bid-qid. Up to 4800 mg/d. **Peds: 1 mth-16 yo:** 20-40 mg/kg/d given tid-qid. **<1 mth:** 15-20 mg/kg/d given tid-qid.	B v **W** 84
Imipenem/Cilastatin (Primaxin I.V.)	**Inj:** 250-250 mg, 500-500 mg	**IV: Adults: ≥70 kg: Mild:** 250-500 mg q6h. **Moderate:** 500 mg q6-8h or 1 gm q8h. **Severe:** 500 mg q6h or 1 gm q6-8h. **Max:** 50 mg/kg/d or 4 gm/d, whichever is lower. **Peds: ≥3 mths:** 15-25 mg/kg q6h. **Max:** 4 gm/d. **4 wks-3 mths & ≥1500 gm:** 25 mg/kg q6h. **1-4 wks & ≥1500 gm:** 25 mg/kg q8h. **<1 wk & ≥1500 gm:** 25 mg/kg q12h.	C > **R**

Vancomycin HCl	**Inj:** 500 mg, 1 gm, 5 gm, 10 gm	**IV: Adults:** 500 mg q6h or 1 gm q12h. **Peds:** 10 mg/kg q6h. **Infants & Neonates:** 15 mg/kg x 1 dose, then 10 mg/kg q12h for 1st wk of life & q8h up to 1 mth of age.	◙C ❋v **R**

Skin/Skin Structure Infections

CARBAPENEM

Ertapenem Sodium (Invanz)	**Inj:** 1 gm	**Complicated SSSI: Adults/Peds: ≥13 yo:** 1 gm IM/IV qd. **3 mths-12 yo:** 15 mg/kg IM/IV bid (not to exceed 1 gm/d). **Duration:** 7-14d. May give IV up to 14d; IM up to 7d.	◙B ❋> **R**
Meropenem (Merrem)	**Inj:** 500 mg, 1 gm	**IV: Adults & Peds: ≥3 mths: >50 kg:** 500 mg q8h. **50 kg:** 10 mg/kg q8h. **Max:** 500 mg q8h.	◙B ❋> **R**

CEPHALOSPORINS

Cefaclor	**Cap:** 250 mg, 500 mg; **Susp:** 125 mg/5 ml, 187 mg/5 ml, 250 mg/5 ml, 375 mg/5 ml	**Adults: Cap/Susp: Usual:** 250 mg q8h. **Severe Infections:** 500 mg q8h. **Peds: ≥1 mth: Cap/Susp:** 20 mg/kg/d given q8h. **Serious Infections:** 40 mg/kg/d. **Max:** 1 gm/d.	◙B ❋>
Cefadroxil	**Cap:** 500 mg; **Susp:** 250 mg/5 ml, 500 mg/5 ml; **Tab:** 1 gm	**Adults:** 1 gm qd or 500 mg bid. **Peds:** 15 mg/kg q12h (or 30 mg/kg qd for impetigo).	◙B ❋> **R**
Cefdinir (Omnicef)	**Cap:** 300 mg; **Susp:** 125 mg/5 ml, 250 mg/5 ml	**Adults & Peds: ≥13 yo:** 300 mg cap q12h x 10d. **6 mths-12 yo:** 7 mg/kg susp q12h x 10d.	◙B ❋> **R**

NAME	FORM/STRENGTH	DOSAGE	COMMENTS
Cefepime HCl (Maxipime)	**Inj:** 500 mg, 1 gm, 2 gm	**Adults: Moderate-Severe:** 2 gm IV q12h x 10d. **Peds: 2 mths-16 yo: ≤40 kg:** 50 mg/kg IV q12h. **Max:** Do not exceed adult dose.	B > **R**
Cefpodoxime Proxetil (Vantin)	**Susp:** 50 mg/5 ml, 100 mg/5 ml; **Tab:** 100 mg, 200 mg	**Adults & Peds: ≥12 yo:** 400 mg q12h x 7-14d.	B v **R**
Cefprozil (Cefzil)	**Susp:** 125 mg/5 ml, 250 mg/5 ml; **Tab:** 250 mg, 500 mg	**Uncomplicated: Adults & Peds: ≥13 yo:** 250-500 mg q12h or 500 mg q24h x 10d. **2-12 yo:** 20 mg/kg q24h x 10d.	B > **R**
Ceftazidime (Fortaz)	**Inj:** 500 mg, 1 gm, 1 gm/50 ml, 2 gm, 2 gm/50 ml, 6 gm	**Adults:** 500-1000 mg IM/IV q8h. **Peds: 1 mth-12 yo:** 30-50 mg/kg IV q8h, up to 6 gm/d. **Neonates: 0-4 wks:** 30 mg/kg IV q12h.	B > **R**
Ceftriaxone Sodium (Rocephin)	**Inj:** (Rocephin) 500 mg, 1 gm; (Generic) 250 mg, 500 mg, 1 gm, 2 gm, 10 gm, 1 gm/50 ml, 2 gm/50ml	**IM/IV: Adults: Usual:** 1-2 gm qd (or in equally divided doses bid). **Max:** 4 gm/d. **Peds:** 50-75 mg/kg given qd (or in equally divided doses bid). **Max:** 2 gm/d.	B >
Cefuroxime Axetil (Ceftin)	**Susp:** 125 mg/5 ml, 250 mg/5 ml; **Tab:** 250 mg, 500 mg	**Adults & Peds: ≥13 yo: Tab:** 250-500 mg bid x 10d. **3 mths-12 yo: Susp:** 15 mg/kg/d bid x 10d for impetigo.	B v Tabs & susp not bioequivalent. **R**

Drug	Forms	Dosage	Ratings
Cephalexin (Keflex)	(Keflex) **Cap:** 250 mg, 500 mg, 750 mg; (Generic) **Cap:** 250 mg, 500 mg; **Susp:** 125 mg/5 ml, 250 mg/5 ml	**Adults:** 500 mg q12h. **Max:** 4 gm/d. **Peds:** 25-50 mg/kg/d given q12h.	◉B ✿>

MACROLIDES

Drug	Forms	Dosage	Ratings
Azithromycin (Zithromax)	**Susp:** 100 mg/5 ml, 200 mg/5 ml, 1 gm/pkt; **Tab:** 250 mg, 500 mg, 600 mg	**Adults:** **≥16 yo:** 500 mg qd x 1d, then 250 mg qd on Days 2-5.	◉B ✿>
Clarithromycin (Biaxin)	**Susp:** 125 mg/5 ml, 250 mg/5 ml; **Tab:** 250 mg, 500 mg	**Adults:** 250 mg q12h x 7-14d. **Peds:** **≥6 mths:** 7.5 mg/kg q12h x 10d.	◉C ✿> R
Erythromycin (Erythromycin Base)	**Tab:** 250 mg, 500 mg	**Adults: Usual:** 250 mg q6h or 500 mg q12h. **Peds: Usual:** 30-50 mg/kg/d in divided doses. **Max:** 4 gm/d.	◉B ✿>
Erythromycin Ethylsuccinate (E.E.S.)	**Susp:** 200 mg/5 ml, 400 mg/5 ml; **Tab:** 400 mg	**Adults: Usual:** 1600 mg/d in divided doses given q6h, q8h, or q12h. **Max:** 4 gm/d. **Peds: Usual:** 30-50 mg/kg/d in divided doses given q6h, q8h, or q12h. May double dose for more severe infections.	◉B ✿>
Erythromycin Ethylsuccinate (EryPed)	**Chewtab:** 200 mg; **Susp:** 100 mg/2.5 ml, 200 mg/5 ml, 400 mg/5 ml	**Adults: Usual:** 1600 mg/d in divided doses given q6h, q8h, or q12h. **Max:** 4 gm/d. **Peds: Usual:** 30-50 mg/kg/d in divided doses given q6h, q8h, or q12h. May double dose for more severe infections.	◉B ✿>

NAME	FORM/STRENGTH	DOSAGE	COMMENTS
Erythromycin Stearate (Erythrocin)	**Tab:** 250 mg, 500 mg	**Adults: Usual:** 250 mg q6h or 500 mg q12h. **Peds: Usual:** 30-50 mg/kg/d in divided doses. **Max:** 4 gm/d.	B >
Erythromycin (Ery-Tab)	**Tab,Delay:** 250 mg, 333 mg, 500 mg	**Adults: Usual:** 250 mg qid, 333 mg q8h, or 500 mg q12h. **Peds: Usual:** 30-50 mg/kg/d in divided doses. **Max:** 4 gm/d.	B >
Erythromycin (PCE)	**Tab,ER:** 333 mg, 500 mg	**Adults: Usual:** 333 mg q8h or 500 mg q12h. **Peds: Usual:** 30-50 mg/kg/d in divided doses. **Max:** 4 gm/d.	B >
OXAZOLIDINONE			
Linezolid (Zyvox)	**Inj:** 2 mg/ml; **Susp:** 100 mg/5 ml; **Tab:** 600 mg	**Complicated:** Treat x 10-14d. **Adults & Peds: ≥12 yo:** 600 mg IV/PO q12h. **Birth-11 yo:** 10 mg/kg IV/PO q8h. **Uncomplicated:** Treat x 10-14d. **Adults:** 400 mg PO q12h. **Peds: ≥12 yo:** 600 mg PO q12h. **5-11 yo:** 10 mg/kg PO q12h. **<5 yo:** 10 mg/kg PO q8h.	C >
PENICILLINS			
Amoxicillin/Clavulanate (Augmentin)	**Chewtab:** 200-28.5 mg, 250-62.5 mg, 400-57 mg; **Susp:** (per 5 ml) 125-31.25 mg, 200-28.5 mg, 250-62.5 mg, 400-57 mg; **Tab:** 250-125 mg,	Dose based on amoxicillin component. **Adults & Peds: ≥40 kg: Tab:** 500-875 mg q12h or 250-500 mg q8h, depending on severity. May use 125 mg/5 ml or 250 mg/5 ml susp in place of 500 mg tab & 200 mg/5 ml susp or 400 mg/5 ml susp in place of 875 mg tab. **≥12 wks: Chewtab/Susp:** 25-45 mg/kg/d given q12h or 20-40 mg/kg/d given q8h, depending on severity. **<12 wks: Susp:** 15 mg/kg q12h (use 125 mg/5 ml susp).	B > 2- 250 mg tabs are not equivalent to 1- 500 mg tab. Only use 250 mg tab if peds ≥40 kg. Chewtab & tab not

	500-125 mg, 875-125 mg		interchangeable. **H R**
Amoxicillin (Amoxil)	(Amoxil) **Cap:** 500 mg; **Sus:** 50 mg/ml, 250 mg/5 ml, 400 mg/5 ml. (Generic) **Cap:** 250 mg, 500 mg; **Sus:** 125 mg/5 ml, 200 mg/5 ml, 250 mg/5ml, 400 mg/5 ml; **Tab:** 500 mg, 875 mg; **Tab,Chew:** 125 mg, 200 mg, 250 mg, 400 mg	**Adults & Peds: >40 kg:** 500-875 mg q12h or 250-500 mg q8h, depending on severity. **>3 mths:** 25-45 mg/kg/d divided q12h or 20-40 mg/kg/d divided q8h, depending on severity. **≤3 mths: Max:** 15 mg/kg q12h.	B > **R**
Ampicillin Sodium/ Sulbactam Sodium (Unasyn)	**Inj:** 1-0.5 gm, 2-1 gm, 10-5 gm	**Adults & Peds: ≥1 yo:** 1.5-3 gm IV/IM q6h. **Max:** 4 gm sulbactam/d.	B > **R**
Penicillin V Potassium (Penicillin VK, Veetids)	**Susp:** 125 mg/5 ml, 250 mg/5 ml; **Tab:** 250 mg, 500 mg	**Adults & Peds: ≥12 yo:** 250-500 mg q6-8h.	B >
Piperacillin Sodium/ Tazobactam (Zosyn)	**Inj:** 40-5 mg/ml, 60-7.5 mg/ml, 2-0.25 gm, 3-0.375 gm, 4-0.5 gm, 4-0.5 gm/100 ml, 36-4.5 gm	**Adults:** 3.375 gm IV q6h x 7-10d.	B > **R**

NAME	FORM/STRENGTH	DOSAGE	COMMENTS
QUINOLONES			
Ciprofloxacin HCl (Cipro Oral)	**Susp:** 250 mg/5 ml, 500 mg/5 ml; **Tab:** 250 mg, 500 mg, 750 mg	**Adults: ≥18 yo: Mild-Moderate:** 500 mg PO q12h x 7-14d. **Severe/Complicated:** 750 mg PO q12h x 7-14d.	C v **R W** 98
Ciprofloxacin (Cipro IV)	**Inj:** 10 mg/ml, 200 mg/100 ml, 400 mg/200 ml	**Adults: ≥18 yo: Mild-Moderate:** 400 mg IV q12h x 7-14d. **Severe/Complicated:** 400 mg IV q8h x 7-14d.	C v **R W** 98
Levofloxacin (Levaquin)	**Inj:** 5 mg/ml, 25 mg/ml; **Sol:** 25 mg/ml; **Tab:** 250 mg, 500 mg, 750 mg	**Adults: ≥18 yo: Uncomplicated:** 500 mg IV/PO qd x 7-10d. **Complicated:** 750 mg IV/PO qd x 7-14d.	C v **R W** 98
Moxifloxacin HCl (Avelox)	**Inj:** 400 mg/250 ml; **Tab:** 400 mg	**Adults: ≥18 yo: Uncomplicated:** 400 mg IV/PO q24h x 7d. **Complicated:** 400 mg IV/PO q24h x 7-21d.	C v **W** 98
Ofloxacin (Floxin)	**Tab:** 200 mg, 300 mg, 400 mg	**Adults: ≥18 yo:** 400 mg q12h x 10d.	C v **H R W** 98
STREPTOGRAMIN AGENT			
Dalfopristin/Quinupristin (Synercid)	**Inj:** 350-150 mg; 420-180 mg	**Complicated: Adults & Peds: ≥16 yo:** 7.5 mg/kg IV q12h for at least 7d.	B > **H**

Doxycycline Hyclate (Doryx)	**Cap,Delay:** 75 mg, 100 mg	**Adults:** 100 mg q12h on Day 1, then 100 mg qd or 50 mg q12h. **Severe:** 100 mg q12h. **Peds: >8 yo & ≤100 lbs:** 1 mg/lb bid on Day 1, then 1 mg/lb qd or 0.5 mg/lb bid. **Severe:** 2 mg/lb. **>100 lbs:** Adult dose.	D v
Doxycycline Monohydrate (Monodox)	**Cap:** 50 mg, 100 mg	**Adults:** 100 mg q12h or 50 mg q6h on Day 1, then 100 mg qd or 50 mg q12h. **Severe:** 100 mg q12h. **Peds: >8 yo & ≤100 lbs:** 1 mg/lb bid on Day 1, then 1 mg/lb qd or 0.5 mg/lb bid. **Severe:** 2 mg/lb. **>100 lbs:** Adult dose.	D v
Doxycycline Monohydrate (Vibramycin)	**Cap:** (Vibramycin) 100 mg; **Tab:** (Vibra-Tabs) 100 mg	**Adults:** 100 mg q12h on Day 1, then 100 mg qd or 50 mg q12h. **Severe:** 100 mg q12h. **Peds: >8 yo & ≤100 lbs:** 1 mg/lb bid on Day 1, then 1 mg/lb qd or 0.5 mg/lb bid. **Severe:** 2 mg/lb. **>100 lbs:** Adult dose.	D v
Doxycycline Monohydrate (Vibramycin)	**Susp:** 25 mg/5 ml	**Adults:** 100 mg q12h or 50 mg q6h on Day 1, then 100 mg qd or 50 mg q12h. **Severe:** 100 mg q12h. **Peds: >8 yo & ≤100 lbs:** 1 mg/lb bid on Day 1, then 1 mg/lb qd or 0.5 mg/lb bid. **Severe:** 2 mg/lb. **>100 lbs:** Adult dose.	D v
Minocycline HCl (Dynacin)	**Tab:** 50 mg, 75 mg, 100 mg	**Adults:** 200 mg PO, then 100 mg q12h or 50 mg qid. **Peds: >8 yo:** 4 mg/kg PO, then 2 mg/kg q12h.	D v **R**
Minocycline HCl (Minocin)	**Cap:** 50 mg, 100 mg; **Inj:** 100 mg	**Adults:** 200 mg PO/IV, then 100 mg q12h or 50 mg qid. **Peds: >8 yo:** 4 mg/kg PO/IV, then 2 mg/kg q12h.	D v **R**

NAME	FORM/STRENGTH	DOSAGE	COMMENTS
MISCELLANEOUS			
Clindamycin (Cleocin)	**Cap:** 75 mg, 150 mg, 300 mg; **Inj:** 150 mg/ml, 300 mg/50 ml, 600 mg/50 ml, 900 mg/50 ml; **Susp:** 75 mg/5 ml	**IM/IV: Adults:** 600-2700 mg/d in 2-4 doses. **Max:** 600 mg IM single dose. **Peds: 1 mth-16 yo:** 20-40 mg/kg/d in 3-4 doses. **<1 mth:** 15-20 mg/kg/d in 3-4 doses. **PO: Adults:** 150-450 mg q6h. **Peds:** 8-20 mg/kg/d given 3-4 doses.	B v(IV) > (PO) **W** 84
Daptomycin (Cubicin)	**Inj:** 250 mg, 500 mg	**Adults: ≥18 yo:** 4 mg/kg IV infusion over 30 min once q24h x 7-14d.	B > **R**
Tigecycline (Tygacil)	**Inj:** 50 mg/5 ml	**Adults:** 100 mg IV, followed by 50 mg IV q12h x 5-14d.	D > **H**

Tuberculosis

NAME	FORM/STRENGTH	DOSAGE	COMMENTS
Aminosalicylic Acid (Paser)	**Granule:** 4 gm/pkt	**Adults:** 4 gm tid. May sprinkle on applesauce, yogurt, or swirl in tomato or orange juice.	C >
Ethambutol HCl (Myambutol)	**Tab:** 100 mg, 400 mg	**Adults & Peds: ≥13 yo: Initial:** 15 mg/kg q24h. **Retreatment:** 25 mg/kg q24h x 60d, then decrease to 15 mg/kg q24h.	N > **R**
Isoniazid/ Pyrazinamide/ Rifampin (Rifater)	**Tab:** 50-300-120 mg	**Adults & Peds: ≥15 yo: Usual: ≤44 kg:** 4 tabs qd, **45-54 kg:** 5 tabs qd. **≥55 kg:** 6 tabs qd. Take 1h before or 2h after a meal. Give pyridoxine to the malnourished, adolescents, or if predisposed to neuropathy.	C v **W** 14

Isoniazid/Rifampin (Rifamate)	**Cap:** 150-300 mg	**Adults: Usual:** 2 caps qd, 1h before or 2h after a meal. Give pyridoxine to the malnourished, if predisposed to neuropathy & adolescents.	N > **W**[14]
Isoniazid (Nydrazid)	**Inj:** 100 mg/ml; **Syr:** 50 mg/5 ml; **Tab:** 100 mg, 300 mg	**Active TB: Adults:** 5 mg/kg, up to 300 mg qd. **Peds:** 10-20 mg/kg, up to 300-500 mg qd. **Prevention: Adults:** 300 mg qd. **Peds:** 10 mg/kg qd, up to 300 mg qd.	N > **W**[14]
Pyrazinamide	**Tab:** 500 mg	**Adults & Peds: Usual:** 15-30 mg/kg qd. **Max:** 3 gm/d. CDC recommends max 2 gm/d w/ daily regimen. **Alternate Regimen:** 50-70 mg/kg BIW. Continue x 2 mths.	C >
Rifampin (Rifadin)	**Cap:** 150 mg, 300 mg; **Inj:** 600 mg	**PO/IV: Adults:** 10 mg/kg qd. **Max:** 600 mg/d. **Peds:** 10-20 mg/kg qd. **Max:** 600 mg/d. Take PO 1h before or 2h after a meal w/ full glass of water. Continue x 2 mths.	C v

Upper Respiratory Tract Infection

CEPHALOSPORINS

Cefaclor	**Cap:** 250 mg, 500 mg; **Susp:** 125 mg/5 ml, 187 mg/5 ml, 250 mg/5 ml, 375 mg/5 ml	**Pharyngitis/Tonsillitis: Adults: Cap/Susp:** 250 mg q8h. **Severe Infections:** 500 mg q8h. **Peds: ≥1 mth: Cap/Susp:** 20 mg/kg/d given q8h. **Serious Infections:** 40 mg/kg/d. **Max:**1 gm/d.	B >
Cefadroxil	**Cap:** 500 mg; **Susp:** 250 mg/5 ml, 500 mg/5 ml; **Tab:** 1 gm	**Adults:** 1 gm qd or 500 mg bid x 10d. **Peds:** 15 mg/kg q12h or 30 mg/kg qd.	B > **R**

NAME	FORM/STRENGTH	DOSAGE	COMMENTS
Cefdinir (Omnicef)	**Cap:** 300 mg; **Susp:** 125 mg/5 ml; 250 mg/5 ml	**Pharyngitis/Tonsillitis: Adults & Peds: ≥13 yo: Cap:** 300 mg q12h x 5-10d or 600 mg q24h x 10d. **6 mths-12 yo: Susp:** 7 mg/kg q12h x 5-10d or 14 mg/kg q24h x 10d. **Sinusitis: Adults & Peds: ≥13 yo: Cap:** 300 mg q12h or 600 mg q24h x 10d. **6 mths-12 yo: Susp:** 7 mg/kg q12h or 14 mg/kg q24h x 10d.	B > **R**
Cefixime (Suprax)	**Susp:** 100 mg/5 ml	**Pharyngitis/Tonsillitis: Adults & Peds: >12 yo or >50 kg: Tab/Susp:** 400 mg qd or 200 mg bid. **≤50 kg or >6 mths: Susp:** 8 mg/kg qd or 4 mg/kg bid.	B v **R**
Cefpodoxime Proxetil (Vantin)	**Susp:** 50 mg/5 ml, 100 mg/5 ml; **Tab:** 100 mg, 200 mg	**Pharyngitis/Tonsillitis: Adults & Peds: ≥12 yo:** 100 mg q12h x 5-10d. **2 mths-11 yo:** 5 mg/kg q12h x 5-10d. **Sinusitis: Adults & Peds: ≥12 yo:** 200 mg q12h x 10d. **2 mths-11 yo:** 5 mg/kg q12h x 10d.	B v **R**
Cefprozil (Cefzil)	**Susp:** 125 mg/5 ml, 250 mg/5 ml; **Tab:** 250 mg, 500 mg	**Pharyngitis/Tonsillitis: Adults & Peds: ≥13 yo:** 500 mg q24h x 10d. **2-12 yo:** 7.5 mg/kg q12h x 10d. **Max:** Adult dose. **Sinusitis: Adults & Peds: ≥13 yo:** 250-500 mg q12h x 10d. **6 mths-12 yo:** 7.5-15 mg/kg q12h x 10d. **Max:** Adult dose.	B > **R**
Cefuroxime Axetil (Ceftin)	**Susp:** 125 mg/5 ml, 250 mg/5 ml; **Tab:** 250 mg, 500 mg	**Pharyngitis/Tonsillitis/Sinusitis: Adults & Peds: ≥13 yo: Tab:** 250 mg bid x 10d. **3 mths-12 yo: Pharyngitis/Tonsillitis: Tab:** 125 mg bid x 10d. **Susp:** 10 mg/kg bid x 10d. **Max:** 500 mg/d. **Sinusitis: Tab:** 250 mg bid x 10d. **Susp:** 15 mg/kg bid x 10d. **Max:** 1 gm/d.	B v Tabs & susp not bioequivalent. **R**

Cephalexin (Keflex)	(Keflex) **Cap:** 250 mg, 500 mg, 750 mg; (Generic) **Cap:** 250 mg, 500 mg; **Susp:** 125 mg/5 ml, 250 mg/5 ml	**Adults: Usual:** 250 mg q6h. **Streptococcal Pharyngitis:** 500 mg q12h. **Max:** 4 gm/d. **Peds: >1 yo: Usual:** 25-50 mg/kg/d given q12h.	B >
MACROLIDES			
Azithromycin (Zithromax)	**Susp:** 100 mg/5 ml, 200 mg/5 ml, 1 gm/pkt; **Tab:** 250 mg, 500 mg, 600 mg	**Pharyngitis/Tonsillitis: Adults:** 500 mg on Day 1, then 250 mg qd on Days 2-5. **Peds: ≥2 yo:** 12 mg/kg qd x 5d. **Acute Bacterial Sinusitis: Adults:** 500 mg qd x 3d. **Peds: ≥6 mths:** 10 mg/kg qd x 3d.	B >
Azithromycin (Zmax)	**Susp,ER:** 2 gm (27 mg/ml)	**Acute Bacterial Sinusitis: Adults:** 2 gm single dose. Take on empty stomach.	B >
Clarithromycin (Biaxin XL)	**Tab,ER:** 500 mg	**Adults: Sinusitis:** 1 gm qd x 14d.	C > **R**
Clarithromycin (Biaxin)	**Susp:** 125 mg/5 ml, 250 mg/5 ml; **Tab:** 250 mg, 500 mg	**Adults: Pharyngitis/Tonsillitis:** 250 mg q12h x 10d. **Sinusitis:** 500 mg q12h x 14d. **Peds: ≥6 mths: Usual:** 7.5 mg/kg q12h x 10d.	C > **R**
Erythromycin (Erythromycin Base)	**Tab:** 250 mg, 500 mg	**Adults: Usual:** 250 mg q6h or 500 mg q12h. **Peds: Usual:** 30-50 mg/kg/d in divided doses. **Max:** 4 gm/d.	B >

NAME	FORM/STRENGTH	DOSAGE	COMMENTS
Erythromycin Ethylsuccinate (E.E.S.)	**Susp:** 200 mg/5 ml, 400 mg/5 ml; **Tab:** 400 mg	**Adults: Usual:** 1600 mg/d in divided doses given q6h, q8h, or q12h. **Max:** 4 gm/d. **Peds: Usual:** 30-50 mg/kg/d in divided doses given q6h, q8h, or q12h. May double dose for more severe infections.	B >
Erythromycin Ethylsuccinate (EryPed)	**Chewtab:** 200 mg; **Susp:** 100 mg/2.5 ml, 200 mg/5 ml, 400 mg/5 ml	**Adults: Usual:** 1600 mg/d in divided doses given q6h, q8h, or q12h. **Max:** 4 gm/d. **Peds: Usual:** 30-50 mg/kg/d in divided doses given q6h, q8h, or q12h. May double dose for more severe infections.	B >
Erythromycin Stearate (Erythrocin)	**Tab:** 250 mg, 500 mg	**Adults: Usual:** 250 mg q6h or 500 mg q12h. **Peds: Usual:** 30-50 mg/kg/d in divided doses. **Max:** 4 gm/d.	B >
Erythromycin (Ery-Tab)	**Tab,Delay:** 250 mg, 333 mg, 500 mg	**Adults: Usual:** 250 mg qid, 333 mg q8h, or 500 mg q12h. **Peds: Usual:** 30-50 mg/kg/d in divided doses. **Max:** 4 gm/d.	B >
Erythromycin (PCE)	**Tab,ER:** 333 mg, 500 mg	**Adults: Usual:** 333 mg q8h or 500 mg q12h. **Peds: Usual:** 30-50 mg/kg/d in divided doses. **Max:** 4 gm/d.	B >

PENICILLINS

NAME	FORM/STRENGTH	DOSAGE	COMMENTS
Amoxicillin/Clavulanate (Augmentin XR)	**Tab,ER:** 1000-62.5 mg	**Sinusitis: Adults & Peds: ≥16 yo:** 2 tabs q12h x 10d.	B >
Amoxicillin/Clavulanate (Augmentin)	**Chewtab:** 200-28.5 mg, 250-62.5 mg, 400-57 mg; **Susp:** (per 5 ml) 125-31.25 mg,	Dose based on amoxicillin component. **Adults & Peds: ≥40 kg: Tab:** 500-875 mg q12h or 250-500 mg q8h, depending on severity. May use 125 mg/5 ml or 250 mg/5 ml susp in place of 500 mg tab & 200 mg/5 ml	B > 2- 250 mg tabs are not equivalent

	200-28.5 mg, 250-62.5 mg, 400-57 mg; **Tab:** 250-125 mg, 500-125 mg, 875-125 mg	susp or 400 mg/5 ml susp in place of 875 mg tab. **≥12 wks: Chewtab/Susp:** 25-45 mg/kg/d given q12h or 20-40 mg/kg/d given q8h, depending on severity. **<12 wks: Susp:** 15 mg/kg q12h (use 125 mg/5 ml susp).	to 1- 500 mg tab. Only use 250 mg tab if peds ≥40 kg. Chewtab & tab not interchangeable. **H R**
Amoxicillin (Amoxil)	(Amoxil) **Cap:** 500 mg; **Sus:** 50 mg/ml, 250 mg/5 ml, 400 mg/5 ml. (Generic) **Cap:** 250 mg, 500 mg; **Sus:** 125 mg/5 ml, 200 mg/5 ml, 250 mg/5ml, 400 mg/5 ml; **Tab:** 500 mg, 875 mg; **Tab,Chew:** 125 mg, 200 mg, 250 mg, 400 mg	**Adults & Peds: >40 kg:** 500-875 mg q12h or 250-500 mg q8h, depending on severity. **>3 mths:** 25-45 mg/kg/d divided q12h or 20-40 mg/kg/d divided q8h, depending on severity. **≤3 mths: Max:** 15 mg/kg q12h.	B > **R**
Ampicillin Sodium	**Inj:** 250 mg, 500 mg, 1 gm, 2 gm,	**IM/IV: Adults & Peds: ≥40 kg:** 250-500 mg q6h. **<40 kg:** 25-50 mg/kg/d given q6-8h.	B >
Ampicillin	**Cap:** 250 mg, 500 mg; **Susp:** 125 mg/5 ml, 250 mg/5 ml	**Adults & Peds: >20 kg:** 250 mg qid. **≤20 kg:** 50 mg/kg/d given tid-qid.	B >

NAME	FORM/STRENGTH	DOSAGE	COMMENTS
Penicillin V Potassium (Penicillin VK, Veetids)	**Susp:** 125 mg/5 ml, 250 mg/5 ml; **Tab:** 250 mg, 500 mg	**Adults & Peds: ≥12 yo: Streptococcal:** 125-250 mg q6-8h x 10d. **Fusospirochetosis:** (Oropharnyx) 250-500 mg q6-8h. **Pneumococcal:** 250-500 mg q6h until afebrile x 2d.	B >
QUINOLONES			
Ciprofloxacin HCl (Cipro Oral)	**Susp:** 250 mg/5 ml, 500 mg/5 ml; **Tab:** 250 mg, 500 mg, 750 mg	**Mild/Moderate Acute Sinusitis: Adults: ≥18 yo:** 500 mg PO q12h x 10d.	C v **R W** 98
Ciprofloxacin (Cipro IV)	**Inj:** 10 mg/ml, 200 mg/100 ml, 400 mg/200 ml	**Mild/Moderate Acute Sinusitis: Adults: ≥18 yo:** 400 mg IV q12h x 10d.	C v **R W** 98
Levofloxacin (Levaquin)	**Inj:** 5 mg/ml, 25 mg/ml; **Sol:** 25 mg/ml; **Tab:** 250 mg, 500 mg, 750 mg	**Sinusitis: Adults: ≥18 yo:** 500 mg IV/PO qd x 10-14d or 750 mg IV/PO qd x 5d.	C v **R W** 98
Moxifloxacin HCl (Avelox)	**Inj:** 400 mg/250 ml; **Tab:** 400 mg	**Sinusitis: Adults: ≥18 yo:** 400 mg PO/IV qd x 10d.	C v **W** 98
TETRACYCLINES			
Demeclocycline (Declomycin)	**Tab:** 150 mg, 500 mg	**Adults:** 150 mg qid or 300 mg bid. **Peds: ≥8 yo:** 3-6 mg/lb/d given bid-qid.	N v

Doxycycline Hyclate (Doryx)	**Cap,Delay:** 75 mg, 100 mg	**Adults:** 100 mg q12h on Day 1, then 100 mg qd or 50 mg q12h. **Severe:** 100 mg q12h. **Peds: >8 yo & ≤100 lbs:** 1 mg/lb bid on Day 1, then 1 mg/lb qd or 0.5 mg/lb bid. **Severe:** 2 mg/lb. **>100 lbs:** Adult dose.	D v
Doxycycline Monohydrate (Monodox)	**Cap:** 50 mg, 100 mg	**Adults:** 100 mg q12h or 50 mg q6h on Day 1, then 100 mg qd or 50 mg q12h. **Peds: >8 yo & ≤100 lbs:** 1 mg/lb bid on Day 1, then 1 mg/lb qd or 0.5 mg/lb bid. **>100 lbs:** Adult dose.	D v
Doxycycline Monohydrate (Vibramycin)	**Cap:** (Vibramycin) 100 mg; **Tab:** (Vibra-Tabs) 100 mg	**Adults:** 100 mg q12h on Day 1, then 100 mg qd or 50 mg q12h. **Severe:** 100 mg q12h. **Peds: >8 yo & ≤100 lbs:** 1 mg/lb bid on Day 1, then 1 mg/lb qd or 0.5 mg/lb bid. **Severe:** 2 mg/lb. **>100 lbs:** Adult dose.	D v
Doxycycline Monohydrate (Vibramycin)	**Susp:** 25 mg/5 ml	**Adults:** 100 mg q12h or 50 mg q6h on Day 1, then 100 mg qd or 50 mg q12h. **Peds: >8 yo & ≤100 lbs:** 1 mg/lb bid on Day 1, then 1 mg/lb qd or 0.5 mg/lb bid. **>100 lbs:** Adult dose.	D v
Minocycline HCl (Dynacin)	**Tab:** 50 mg, 75 mg, 100 mg	**Adults:** 200 mg PO, then 100 mg q12h or 50 mg qid. **Peds: >8 yo:** 4 mg/kg PO, then 2 mg/kg q12h.	D v **R**
Minocycline HCl (Minocin)	**Cap:** 50 mg, 100 mg; **Inj:** 100 mg	**Adults:** 200 mg PO/IV, then 100 mg q12h or 50 mg qid. **Peds: >8 yo:** 4 mg/kg PO/IV, then 2 mg/kg q12h.	D v **R**
Tetracycline HCl (Sumycin)	**Cap:** 250 mg, 500 mg; **Susp:** 125 mg/5 ml	**Adults:** 250 mg qid or 500 mg bid. **Peds: >8 yo:** 25-50 mg/kg divided bid-qid.	D v **R**

NAME	FORM/STRENGTH	DOSAGE	COMMENTS

Urinary Tract Infection

CARBAPENEM

NAME	FORM/STRENGTH	DOSAGE	COMMENTS
Doripenem (Doribax)	**Inj:** 500 mg	**Complicated UTI/Pyelonephritis: Adults: ≥18 yo:** 500 mg IV q8h x 10d. Infuse over 1h. **Renal Impairment: CrCl: >50 mL/min:** No dose adjustment. **CrCl 30-50 mL/min:** 250 mg IV q8h. **CrCl >10 to < 30 mL/min:** 250mg IV q12h.	◉B ❋> R
Ertapenem Sodium (Invanz)	**Inj:** 1 gm	**Complicated UTI/Acute Pelvic Infections: Adults/Peds: ≥13 yo:** 1 gm IM/IV qd. **3 mths-12 yo:** 15 mg/kg IM/IV bid (not to exceed 1 gm/d). **Duration: Complicated UTI:** 10-14d. **Acute Pelvic Infections:** 3-10d. May give IV up to 14d; IM up to 7d.	◉B ❋> R

CEPHALOSPORINS

NAME	FORM/STRENGTH	DOSAGE	COMMENTS
Cefaclor	**Cap:** 250 mg, 500 mg; **Susp:** 125 mg/5 ml, 187 mg/5 ml, 250 mg/5 ml, 375 mg/5 ml	**Adults:** 250 mg q8h. **Severe Infections:** 500 mg q8h. **Peds: ≥1 mth:** 20 mg/kg/d q8h. **Serious Infections:** 40 mg/kg/d. **Max:**1 gm/d.	◉B ❋>
Cefadroxil	**Cap:** 500 mg; **Susp:** 250 mg/5 ml, 500 mg/5 ml; **Tab:** 1 gm	**Adults: Uncomplicated Lower UTI:** 1-2 gm/d given qd-bid. **Other UTIs:** 1 gm bid. **Peds:** 15 mg/kg q12h.	◉B ❋> R
Cefepime HCl (Maxipime)	**Inj:** 500 mg, 1 gm, 2 gm	**Adults: Mild-Moderate:** 0.5-1 gm IM/IV q12h x 7-10d. **Severe:** 2 gm IV q12h x 10d. **Peds: 2 mths-16 yo: ≤40 kg:** 50 mg/kg IV q12h. **Max:** Do not exceed adult dose.	◉B ❋> R

Cefixime (Suprax)	**Susp:** 100 mg/5 ml	**Adults & Peds: >12 yo or >50 kg: Tab/Susp:** 400 mg qd or 200 mg bid. **≤50 kg or >6 mths: Susp:** 8 mg/kg qd or 4 mg/kg bid.	⊙B ❁v **R**
Cefpodoxime Proxetil (Vantin)	**Susp:** 50 mg/5 ml, 100 mg/5 ml; **Tab:** 100 mg, 200 mg	**Adults & Peds: ≥12 yo: Uncomplicated UTI:** 100 mg q12h x 7d.	⊙B ❁v **R**
Ceftazidime (Fortaz)	**Inj:** 500 mg, 1 gm, 1 gm/50 ml, 2 gm, 2 gm/50 ml, 6 gm	**Adults: Uncomplicated UTI:** 250 mg IM/IV q12h. **Complicated UTI:** 500 mg IM/IV q8-12h. **Peds: 1 mth-12 yo:** 30-50 mg/kg IV q8h, up to 6 gm/d. **Neonates: 0-4 wks:** 30 mg/kg IV q12h.	⊙B ❁> **R**
Ceftriaxone Sodium (Rocephin)	**Inj:** (Rocephin) 500 mg, 1 gm; (Generic) 250 mg, 500 mg, 1 gm, 2 gm, 10 gm, 1 gm/50 ml, 2 gm/50ml	**Adults: IM/IV:** 1-2 gm qd (or in equally divided doses bid). **Max:** 4 gm/d.	⊙B ❁>
Cefuroxime (Zinacef)	**Inj:** 750 mg, 1.5 gm, 7.5 gm	**IM/IV: Adults: Uncomplicated UTI:** 750 mg q8h x 5-10d. **Severe/Complicated UTI:** 1.5 gm q8h x 5-10d. **Peds: >3 mths:** 50-100 mg/kg/d given q6-8h. **Max:** 4.5 gm/d.	⊙B ❁> **R**
Cefuroxime Axetil (Ceftin)	**Tab:** 250 mg, 500 mg	**Adults & Peds: ≥13 yo:** 125-250 mg bid x 7-10d.	⊙B ❁v **R**

NAME	FORM/STRENGTH	DOSAGE	COMMENTS
Cephalexin (Keflex)	(Keflex) **Cap:** 250 mg, 500 mg, 750 mg; (Generic) **Cap:** 250 mg, 500 mg; **Susp:** 125 mg/5 ml, 250 mg/5 ml	**Adults: Usual:** 250 mg q6h. **Uncomplicated Cystitis:** 500 mg q12h x 7-14d. **Max:** 4 gm/d. **Peds: Usual:** 25-50 mg/kg/d in divided doses.	B >
PENICILLINS			
Amoxicillin/Clavulanate (Augmentin)	**Chewtab:** 200-28.5 mg, 250-62.5 mg, 400-57 mg; **Susp:** (per 5 ml) 125-31.25 mg, 200-28.5 mg, 250-62.5 mg, 400-57 mg; **Tab:** 250-125 mg, 500-125 mg, 875-125 mg	Dose based on amoxicillin component. **Adults & Peds: ≥40 kg: Tab:** 500 mg q12h or 250 mg q8h. May use 125 mg/5 ml or 250 mg/5 ml susp in place of 500 mg tab & 200 mg/5 ml or 400 mg/5 ml susp in place of 875 mg tab. **≥12 wks: Chewtab/Susp:** 25 mg/kg/d given q12h or 20 mg/kg/d given q8h. **<12 wks: Susp:** 15 mg/kg q12h (use 125 mg/5 ml susp).	B > 2- 250 mg tabs are not equivalent to 1- 500 mg tab. Only use 250 mg tab if peds ≥40 kg. Chewtab & tab not interchangeable. **H R**

Amoxicillin (Amoxil)	(Amoxil) **Cap:** 500 mg; **Sus:** 50 mg/ml, 250 mg/5 ml, 400 mg/5 ml. (Generic) **Cap:** 250 mg, 500 mg; **Sus:** 125 mg/5 ml, 200 mg/5 ml, 250 mg/5ml, 400 mg/5 ml; **Tab:** 500 mg, 875 mg; **Tab,Chew:** 125 mg, 200 mg, 250 mg, 400 mg	**Adults & Peds: >40 kg:** 500-875 mg q12h or 250-500 mg q8h, depending on severity. **>3 mths:** 25-45 mg/kg/d divided q12h or 20-40 mg/kg/d divided q8h, depending on severity. ≤**3 mths: Max:** 15 mg/kg q12h.	◙B ❃> **R**
Ampicillin	**Cap:** 250 mg, 500 mg; **Susp:** 125 mg/5 ml, 250 mg/5 ml	**GU Tract: Adults & Peds: >20 kg:** 500 mg qid. ≤**20 kg:** 25 mg/kg qid.	◙B ❃>

QUINOLONES

Ciprofloxacin HCl (Cipro Oral)	**Inj:** 10 mg/ml, 200 mg/100 ml, 400 mg/200 ml; **Susp:** 250 mg/5 ml, 500 mg/5 ml; **Tab:** 250 mg, 500 mg, 750 mg	**Adults: Acute Uncomplicated UTI:** 250 mg PO q12h x 3d. **Mild/Moderate UTI:** 250 mg PO q12h or 200 mg IV q12h x 7-14d. **Severe/Complicated UTI:** 500 mg PO q12h or 400 mg IV q12h x 7-14d. **Chronic Bacterial Prostatitis:** 500 mg PO q12h or 400 mg IV q12h x 28d. **Urethral & Cervical Gonococcal Infections:** 250 mg PO as single dose. **Peds: 1-17 yo: Complicated UTI/Pyelonephritis:** 10-20 mg/kg PO q12h or 6-10 mg/kg IV q8h x 10-21d. **Max:** 750 mg PO or 400 mg IV per dose.	◙C ❃v **R W** 98

NAME	FORM/STRENGTH	DOSAGE	COMMENTS
Ciprofloxacin HCl (Proquin XR)	**Tab,ER:** 500 mg	**Adults:** 500 mg qd x 3 days.	◙C ❁v **W**[98]
Ciprofloxacin (Cipro IV)	**Inj:** 10 mg/ml, 200 mg/ 100 ml, 400 mg/200 ml	**Adults: Mild/Moderate UTI:** 200 mg IV q12h x 7-14d. **Severe/Complicated UTI:** 400 mg IV q12h x 7-14d. **Chronic Bacterial Prostatitis:** 400 mg IV q12h x 28d. **Peds: 1-17 yo: Complicated UTI/Pyelonephritis:** 6-10 mg/kg IV q8h x 10-21d. **Max:** 400 mg IV per dose.	◙C ❁v **R W**[98]
Ciprofloxacin (Cipro XR)	**Tab,ER:** 500 mg, 1000 mg	**Adults: ≥18 yo: Uncomplicated UTI:** 500 mg qd x 3d. **Complicated UTI:** 1000 mg qd x 7-14d. **Acute Uncomplicated Pyelonephritis:** 1000 mg qd x 7-14d.	◙C ❁v **R W**[98]
Levofloxacin (Levaquin)	**Inj:** 5 mg/ml, 25 mg/ml; **Sol:** 25 mg/ml; **Tab:** 250 mg, 500 mg, 750 mg	**Adults: ≥18 yo: Complicated UTI/Acute Pyelonephritis:** 250 mg IV/PO qd x 10d. **Uncomplicated UTI:** 250 mg IV/ PO qd x 3d. **Chronic Bacterial Prostatitis:** 500 mg IV/ PO qd x 28d.	◙C ❁v **R W**[98]
Lomefloxacin (Maxaquin)	**Tab:** 400 mg	**Adults: ≥18 yo: Complicated UTI:** 400 mg qd x 14d. **Uncomplicated Cystitis:** 400mg qd x 3d (*E.coli*) or 10d (*K.pneumoniae, P.mirabilis,* or *S.saprophyticus*).	◙C ❁v **R W**[98]
Norfloxacin (Noroxin)	**Tab:** 400 mg	**Adults: ≥18 yo: Uncomplicated UTI:** 400 mg q12h x 3d (*K.pneumoniae, E.coli,* or *P.mirabilis*), or x 7-10d (other organisms). **Complicated UTI:** 400 mg q12h x 10-21d. **Acute/Chronic Prostatitis:** 400 mg q12h x 28d.	◙C ❁v **R W**[98]

Ofloxacin (Floxin)	**Tab:** 200 mg, 300 mg, 400 mg	**Adults: ≥18 yo: Nongonococcal Cervicitis/Urethritis (*C.trachomatis*) or Mixed Infection of Urethra & Cervix (*C.trachomatis* & *N.gonorrhoeae*):** 300 mg q12h x 7d. **Acute PID:** 400 mg q12h x 10-14d. **Uncomplicated Cystitis:** 200 mg q12h x 3d (*E.coli* or *K.pneumoniae*) or 7d (other pathogens). **Complicated UTI:** 200 mg q12h x 10d. **Prostatitis (*E.coli*):** 300 mg q12h x 6 wks. **Acute Uncomplicated Urethral & Cervical Gonorrhea:** 400 mg as single dose.	C v **H R W** [98]

SULFONAMIDE

Sulfisoxazole (Gantrisin Pediatric)	**Susp:** 500 mg/5 ml	**Peds: >2 mths: Initial:** 1/2 of 24h dose. **Maint:** 150 mg/kg/d or 4 gm/m^2/d in divided doses. **Max:** 6 gm/d.	C v CI in pregnancy & nursing.

SULFONAMIDES AND COMBINATIONS

Sulfamethoxazole/ Trimethoprim (Septra, Septra DS, Sulfatrim Pediatric)	**Susp:** 200-40 mg/5 ml; **Tab:** (SS) 400-80 mg, (DS) 800-160 mg	**PO: Adults:** 800 mg SMX & 160 mg TMP (1 DS tab, 2 SS tabs, or 20 ml) q12h x 10-14d. **Peds: ≥2 mths:** 4 mg/kg TMP & 20 mg/kg SMX q12h x 10d. **Severe: Adults & Peds: IV:** 8-10 mg/kg/d (based on TMP) given q6-12h up to 14d.	C v **R** CI in pregnancy & nursing.

NAME	FORM/STRENGTH	DOSAGE	COMMENTS
TETRACYCLINES			
Doxycycline Hyclate (Doryx)	**Cap,Delay:** 75 mg, 100 mg	**Adults:** 100 mg q12h on Day 1, then 100 mg qd or 50 mg q12h. **Peds: >8 yo & ≤100 lbs:** 1 mg/lb bid on Day 1, then 1 mg/lb qd or 0.5 mg/lb bid. **>100 lbs:** Adult dose.	D v
Doxycycline Monohydrate (Monodox)	**Cap:** 50 mg, 100 mg	**Adults:** 100 mg q12h or 50 mg q6h on Day 1, then 100 mg qd or 50 mg q12h. **Peds: >8 yo & ≤100 lbs:** 1 mg/lb bid on Day 1, then 1 mg/lb qd or 0.5 mg/lb bid. **>100 lbs:** Adult dose.	D v
Doxycycline Monohydrate (Vibramycin)	**Cap:** (Vibramycin) 100 mg; **Tab:** (Vibra-Tabs) 100 mg	**Adults:** 100 mg q12h on Day 1, then 100 mg qd or 50 mg q12h. **Peds: >8 yo & ≤100 lbs:** 1 mg/lb bid on Day 1, then 1 mg/lb qd or 0.5 mg/lb bid. **>100 lbs:** Adult dose.	D v
Doxycycline Monohydrate (Vibramycin)	**Susp:** 25 mg/5 ml	**Adults:** 100 mg q12h or 50 mg q6h on Day 1, then 100 mg qd or 50 mg q12h. **Peds: >8 yo & ≤100 lbs:** 1 mg/lb bid on Day 1, then 1 mg/lb qd or 0.5 mg/lb bid. **>100 lbs:** Adult dose.	D v
Minocycline HCl (Dynacin)	**Tab:** 50 mg, 75 mg, 100 mg;	**Adults:** 200 mg PO, then 100 mg q12h or 50 mg qid. **Peds: >8 yo:** 4 mg/kg PO, then 2 mg/kg q12h.	D v **R**
Minocycline HCl (Minocin)	**Cap:** 50 mg, 100 mg; **Inj:** 100 mg	**Adults:** 200 mg PO/IV, then 100 mg q12h or 50 mg qid. **Peds: >8 yo:** 4 mg/kg PO/IV, then 2 mg/kg q12h.	D v **R**
Tetracycline HCl (Sumycin)	**Cap:** 250 mg, 500 mg; **Susp:** 125 mg/5 ml	**Adults:** 250 mg qid or 500 mg bid. **Peds: >8 yo:** 25-50 mg/kg divided bid-qid.	D v **R**

MISCELLANEOUS

Nitrofurantoin, Macrocrystals (Macrobid)	**Cap:** 100 mg	**Adults & Peds: >12 yo:** 100 mg q12h x 7d.	B v **R**
Nitrofurantoin, Macrocrystals (Macrodantin)	**Cap:** 25 mg, 50 mg, 100 mg	**Adults:** 50-100 mg qid x 7d. **Peds: ≥1 mth:** 5-7 mg/kg/d given as qid x 7d.	B v **R**
Nitrofurantoin (Furadantin)	**Susp:** 25 mg/5 ml	**Adults:** 50-100 mg qid x 7d. **Peds: >1 mth:** 5-7 mg/kg/d given as qid x 7d.	B v **R**

Miscellaneous Anti-Infectives

Tinidazole (Tindamax)	**Tab:** 250 mg, 500 mg	**Giardiasis: Adults:** 2 gm single dose. **>3 yo:** 50 mg/kg single dose. **Max:** 2 gm/d. **Amebiasis: Intestinal: Adults:** 2 gm qd x 3d. **>3 yo:** 50 mg/kg qd x 3d. **Max:** 2 gm/d. **Amebic Liver Abscess: Adults:** 2 gm qd x 3-5d. **>3 yo:** 50 mg/kg qd x 3-5d. **Max:** 2 gm/d. May crush tabs in cherry syrup. Take w/ food.	X (1st trimester) C (2nd/3rd trimester) v **R** Avoid unnecessary use.

ANTINEOPLASTICS

Antineoplastics

Anastrozole (Arimidex)	**Tab:** 1 mg	**Adjuvant/Advanced/Metastatic Breast Cancer: Adults:** 1 mg qd.	X >

NAME	FORM/STRENGTH	DOSAGE	COMMENTS
Bendamustine HCl (Treanda)	**Inj:** 25 mg, 100 mg	**CLL: Adults:** 100 mg/m^2 IV over 30 min on Days 1 & 2, of 28d cycle. **Max:** 6 cycles. Delay treatment for Grade 4 hematologic toxicity or clinically significant ≥Grade 2 non-hematologic toxicity. **For ≥Grade 3 Hematologic Toxicity:** Reduce dose to 50 mg/m^2 on Days 1 & 2 of each cycle; if ≥Grade 3 toxicity recurs, reduce dose to 25mg/m^2 on Days 1 & 2. **For ≥Grade 3 Nonhematologic Toxicity:** Reduce dose to 50 mg/m^2 on Days 1 & 2 of each cycle. Consider dose re-escalation in subsequent cycles.	◉D ❋v
Bicalutamide (Casodex)	**Tab:** 50 mg	**Stage D2 Metastatic Carcinoma of Prostate: Adults:** 50 mg qd. Intiate w/ LHRH analogue therapy. **Peds: Initial:** 12.5 mg. **Titrate:** May adjust dose until trough levels reach 5-15 mcg/ml.	◉X ❋> **W** 3
Busulfan (Myleran)	**Tab:** 2 mg	**CML (Palliation): Adults & Peds:** 60 mcg/kg/d or 1.8 mg/m^2/d.	◉D ❋v Bone marrow hypoplasia. **W** 3
Capecitabine (Xeloda)	**Tab:** 150 mg, 500 mg	**Metastatic Breast Cancer/Colorectal Cancer: Adults ≥18 yo:** 1250 mg/m^2 bid x 2 wks, then 1 wk rest period. Give as 3 wk cycles. **Dukes' C Colon Cancer: Adjuvant Treatment:** 3 wk cycles for 8 cycles (24 wks). Interrupt and/or reduce dose if toxicity occurs. Re-adjust according to adverse effects.	◉D ❋v **R** Bleeding & death reported w/ coumarin.

Cetuximab (Erbitux)	**Inj:** 2 mg/ml	**Adults:** Pre-medication w/ H_1 antagonist (eg, diphenhydramine 50 mg IV) recommended. **Metastatic Colorectal Carcinoma: Initial:** 400 mg/m^2 IV infusion over 120 min. **Maint:** 250 mg/m^2 IV infusion over 60 min once wkly. **Squamous Cell Carcinoma of Head & Neck: Combination Therapy: Initial:** 400 mg/m^2 IV over 120 min 1 wk prior to initiation of a course of radiation treatment. **Maint:** 250 mg/m^2 over 60 min wkly for duration of radiation therapy. **Recurrent/Metastatic Squamous Cell Carcinoma of Head & Neck: Monotherapy: Initial:** 400 mg/m^2. **Maint:** 250 mg/m^2 until disease progression or unacceptable toxicity. Adjust dose based on infusion reactions or dermatologic toxicity. **Max Infusion Rate:** 5 ml/min.	C v Infusion reactions.
Chlorambucil (Leukeran)	**Tab:** 2 mg	**Adults: CLL/Malignant Lymphoma/Hodgkin's Disease: Usual:** 0.1-0.2 mg/kg/d x 3-6 wks. **Lymphocytic Infiltration of Bone Marrow/Hypoplastic Bone Marrow: Max:** 0.1 mg/kg/d.	D v Bone marrow suppression. Infertility. Carcinogenic.
Conjugated Estrogens (Premarin Tablets)	**Tab:** 0.3 mg, 0.45 mg, 0.625 mg, 0.9 mg, 1.25 mg	**Adults: Advanced Prostate Cancer (Palliation):** 1.25-2.5 mg tid. **Metastatic Breast Cancer (Palliation):** 10 mg tid x minimum of 3 mths.	X > **W** [4, 28]

NAME	FORM/STRENGTH	DOSAGE	COMMENTS
Cyclophosphamide (Cytoxan)	**Inj:** 500 mg, 1 gm, 2 gm; **Tab:** 25 mg, 50 mg	**Adults & Peds: Malignant Lymphomas/Leukemias/ Multiple Myeloma/ Mycosis Fungoides/Neuroblastoma/ Ovary Adenocarcinoma/Retinoblastoma/Breast Carcinoma: IV:** 40-50 mg/kg in divided doses over 2-5d, or 10-15 mg/kg q7-10d, or 3-5 mg/kg BIW. **PO:** 1-5 mg/kg/d. **Nonmalignant Disease - Biopsy Proven (Minimal Changes) Nephrotic Syndrome: Peds:** 2.5-3 mg/kg qd x 60-90d.	D v
Dasatinib (Sprycel)	**Tab:** 20 mg, 50 mg, 70 mg	**Adults: Chronic Phase CML:** 100 mg qd. **Accelerated Phase CML/Myeloid or Lymphoid Blast Phase CML/ Ph+ ALL:** 70 mg bid. Swallow whole. **Concomitant Strong CYP3A4 Inducers:** Consider dose increase. **Concomitant Strong CYP3A4 Inhibitors:** Consider dose decrease to 20 mg daily.	D v Severe thromocytopenia, neutropenia, anemia.
Doxorubicin HCl Liposome (Doxil)	**Inj:** 2 mg/ml	**Adults:** Administer as IV infusion at initial rate of 1 mg/ min to minimize risk of infusion-related reactions; if no reactions, may increase rate to complete infusion over 1h. **Ovarian Cancer:** 50 mg/m^2 IV q4wks x min of 4 courses. **AIDS-related Kaposi's Sarcoma:** 20 mg/m^2 IV once q3wks. **Multiple Myeloma:** Give bortezomib 1.3 mg/m^2 IV bolus on Days 1, 4, 8 and 11, q3wks. Give doxorubicin 30 mg/m^2 IV on Day 4 following bortezomib. **Max:** 8 cycles.	D vH **W** [93]

Erlotinib (Tarceva)	**Tab:** 25 mg, 100 mg, 150 mg	**Adults: Non-Small Cell Lung Cancer:** 150 mg ≥1 h before or 2 h after ingestion of food. **Pancreatic Cancer:** 100 mg at least 1 h before or 2 h after ingestion of food, in combination w/ gemcitabine. Continue until disease progression or unacceptable toxicity.	◉D ❁v
Exemestane (Aromasin)	**Tab:** 25 mg	**Advanced Breast Cancer in Postmenopausal Women/ Adjuvant Treatment in Early Breast Cancer: Adults:** 25 mg qd after a meal. Continue in absence of recurrence until completion of 5 yrs of adjuvant endocrine therapy in early breast cancer treated w/ 2-3 yrs of tamoxifen. Continue until tumor progression evident in advanced breast cancer. **Concomitant Potent CYP3A4 Inducers:** 50 mg qd after a meal.	◉D ❁>
Flutamide	**Cap:** 125 mg	**Stage B2-C Prostatic Carcinoma/Stage D2 Metastatic Carcinoma: Adults:** 250 mg tid at 8h intervals.	◉D ❁> Hepatic injury.
Fulvestrant (Faslodex)	**Inj:** 50 mg/ml	**Hormone Receptor Positive Metastatic Breast Cancer in Postmenopausal Women: Adults:** 250 mg IM into buttock monthly. Give as either single 5 ml inj or 2 concurrent 2.5 ml inj.	◉D ❁v
Hydroxyurea (Hydrea)	**Cap:** 500 mg	**Adults: Solid Tumors: Intermittent Therapy/Concomitant Therapy w/ Irradiation (Head/Neck Carcinoma):** 80 mg/kg PO as single dose q 3rd day. **Continuous Therapy/Resistant CML:** 20-30 mg/kg PO as single dose.	◉D ❁v **R**

NAME	FORM/STRENGTH	DOSAGE	COMMENTS
Imatinib Mesylate (Gleevec)	**Tab:** 100 mg, 400 mg	**Adults: CML: Chronic Phase:** 400 mg/d, may increase to 600 mg qd. **Accelerated Phase/Blast Crisis:** 600 mg/d, may increase to 400 mg bid. **Relapsed/Refractory Ph+ ALL:** 600 mg/d. **Myelodysplastic or Myeloproliferative Diseases/Aggressive Systemic Mastocytosis (ASM)/ Hypereosinophilic Syndrome (HES) and/or Chronic Eosinophilic Leukemia (CEL):** 400 mg/d. **ASM w/ Eosinophilia/HEM or CEL w/ FIP1L1-PDGFRα: Initial:** 100 mg/d. **Titrate:** May increase up to 400 mg/d. **Dermatofibrosarcoma Protuberans:** 800 mg/d. **GIST:** 400 mg/d. **Titrate:** May increase up to 800 mg/d (as 400 mg bid). **Peds: Ph+ CML: Newly Diagnosed:** 340 mg/m^2/d. **Chronic Phase: Recurrent after Stem Cell Transplant or Resistant to Interferon-Alpha Therapy:** 260 mg/m^2/d given qd or split into 2 doses (am & pm). **Co-administration w/ Strong CYP3A4 Inducers:** Increase dose by at least 50% & monitor carefully. **Hepatotoxicity/ Neutropenia/Thrombocytopenia/Non-Hematologic Adverse Reaction:** See PI. Take w/ food & plenty of water.	◙D ❃v **H**
Interferon alfa-2b (Intron A)	**Inj:** 10 MIU, 18 MIU, 50 MIU, 10 MIU/ml, 3 MIU/0.2 ml, 5 MIU/0.2 ml, 10 MIU/0.2 ml	**Adults: ≥18 yo: Hairy Cell Leukemia:** 2 MIU/m^2 SC/IM TIW up to 6 mths. **Malignant Melanoma: Induction:** 20 MIU/m^2 IV x 5d/wk x 4 wks. **Maint:** 10 MIU/m^2 SC TIW x 48 wks. **Follicular Lymphoma:** 5 MIU SC TIW up to 18 mths. **Condylomata Acuminata:** 1 MIU into lesions TIW	◙C ❃v **W** 13

		x 3 wks. **Kaposi's Sarcoma:** 30 MIU/m^2 SC/IM TIW x 16 wks.	
Lapatinib (Tykerb)	**Tab:** 250 mg	**Advanced/Metastatic Breast Cancer: Adults: Usual:** 1250 mg qd on Days 1-21 continuously w/ capecitabine 2000 mg/m^2/d on Days 1-14 in repeating 21-day cycle.	D v
Lenalidomide (Revlimid)	**Cap:** 5 mg, 10 mg, 15 mg, 25 mg	**Multiple Myeloma: Adults: ≥18 yo:** 25 mg daily w/ water. Administer as single dose on Days 1-21 of repeated 28-day cycles. Do not break, chew, or open caps. Adjust dose based on platelet and/or neutrophil counts.	X v **W** [56]
Megestrol Acetate	(Generic) **Susp:** 40 mg/ml; **Tab:** 20 mg, 40 mg; (Megace) **Susp:** 40 mg/ml	**Adults: Advanced Breast Carcinoma (Palliation):** 40 mg qid. **Advanced Endometrial Carcinoma (Palliation):** 40-320 mg qd in divided doses. Treat for min of 2 mths. **Anorexia/Cachexia/Significant Weight Loss in AIDS: Susp: Initial:** 800 mg/d.	X v
Melphalan (Alkeran)	**Inj:** 50 mg; **Tab:** 2 mg	**Adults: Multiple Myeloma (Palliation): IV** 16 mg/m^2 q2wks x 4 doses, then q4wks after recovery from toxicity. **PO:** 6 mg qd x 2-3 wks, then 2 mg qd after WBC & platelets are rising. **Epithelial Ovary Carcinoma (Palliation):** 0.2 mg/kg/d x 5d. May repeat q4-5wks.	D v **R** (Inj) **W** [3, 23]
Mercaptopurine (Purinethol)	**Tab:** 50 mg	**Adults & Peds: ALL: Induction: Initial:** 2.5 mg/kg/d. Calculate to nearest multiple of 25 mg. **Titrate:** May increase to 5 mg/kg/d after 4 wks if needed. **Maint:** 1.5-2.5 mg/kg/d. Dose peds in pm.	D v **H R W** [3]

NAME	FORM/STRENGTH	DOSAGE	COMMENTS
Methotrexate Sodium	**Inj:** 20 mg, 25 mg/ml, 1 gm; **Tab:** 2.5 mg	**Adults: Burkitt's Lymphoma: Stages I-II: PO:**10-25 mg/d x 4-8d for several courses; separate by 7-10d rest period. **Lymphosarcomas: Stage III: PO:** 0.625-2.5 mg/kg/d. **Leukemia: Induction:** 3.3 mg/m^2 w/ prednisone qd. **Remission Maint:** 15 mg/m^2 PO/IM twice wkly or 2.5 mg/kg IV q14d. **Mycosis Fungoides:** 5-50 mg qwk. If poor response, give 15-37.5 mg twice wkly. **Osteosarcoma: Initial:** 12 g/m^2 IV, increase to 15 g/m^2 if peak levels of 1000 micromolar not reached at end of infusion. **Choriocarcinoma/Trophoblastic Diseases: PO/IM:** 15-30 mg qd x 5d, rest ≥1 wk & repeat 3-5x. **Peds: Meningeal Leukemia: Intrathecal:** Dilute preservative free MTX to 1 mg/ml. Dose q2-5d. ≥**3 yo:** 12 mg. **2 yo:** 10 mg. **1 yo:** 8 mg. **<1 yo:** 6 mg.	X v **W** [3, 19]
Nilotinib (Tasigna)	**Cap:** 200 mg	**Adults: CML:** 400 mg PO bid, 12h apart. Swallow whole w/ water. Avoid food for at least 2h before & 1h after dosing. Adjust dose based on toxicities & drug interactions (see PI).	D v **H**
Paclitaxel Protein-bound Particles (Abraxane)	**Inj:** 100 mg	**Breast Cancer: Adults: IV:** 260 mg/m^2 q3wks. Severe neutropenia or severe sensory neuropathy reduce to 220 mg/m^2; recurrence reduce to 180 mg/m^2.	D v

Paclitaxel (Taxol)	**Inj:** 6 mg/ml	**Adults: IV: Ovary Carcinoma: Previously Untreated:** 175 mg/m^2 over 3h or 135 mg/m^2 over 24h q3wks followed by Cisplatin 75 mg/m^2. **Treated:** 135 or 175 mg/m^2 over 3h q3wks. **Breast Cancer:** 175 mg/m^2 over 3h q3wks. **Non-Small Cell Lung Cancer:** 135 mg/m^2 over 24h q3wks. **Kaposi's Sarcoma:** 135 mg/m^2 over 3h q3wks or 100 mg/m^2 over 3h q2wks.	D v Anaphylaxis & severe hypersensitivity reactions. **W** [3]
Pemetrexed Disodium (Alimta)	**Inj:** 100 mg, 500 mg	**Adults: Combination Use: Non-Small Cell Lung Cancer/ Malignant Pleural Mesothelioma:** 500 mg/m^2 IV over 10 min on Day 1 of each 21d cycle w/ cisplatin 75 mg/m^2 infused over 2h beginning 30 min after pemetrexed. **Single-Agent Use: Non-Small Cell Lung Cancer:** 500 mg IV over 10 min on Day 1 of each 21d cycle.	D v **R**
Raloxifene HCl (Evista)	**Tab:** 60 mg	**Reduction of Breast Cancer in Postmenopausal Women w/ Osteoporosis & Postmenopausal Women at High Risk for Invasive Breast Cancer: Adults: Female:** 60 mg qd.	X v
Sorafenib (Nexavar)	**Tab:** 200 mg	**Advanced Renal Cell Carcinoma/Unresectable Hepatocellular Carcinoma: Adults:** 400 mg bid w/o food (1h before or 2h after eating). Continue until no clinical benefit or unacceptable toxicity. Temporary interruption or reduction to 400 mg qd or qod if serious adverse events suspected.	D v

NAME	FORM/STRENGTH	DOSAGE	COMMENTS
Sunitinib Maleate (Sutent)	**Cap:** 12.5 mg, 25 mg, 50 mg	**Adults:** 50 mg qd; 4 wks on, 2 wks off. Dose increase/ reduction in 12.5 mg increments is recommended. **Concomitant Strong CYP3A4 Inhibitors:** Consider dose reduction to minimum of 37.5 mg qd. **Concomitant CYP3A4 Inducer:** Consider dose increase to max of 87.5 mg qd.	D v
Tamoxifen Citrate	**Tab:** 10 mg, 20 mg	**Adults: Breast Cancer Treatment:** 20 mg qd or qam & qpm. **Ductal Carcinoma in Situ or Reduction of Breast Cancer (High Risk):** 20 mg qd x 5 yrs.	D v Uterine malignancies, stroke & PE reported.
Tamoxifen Citrate (Soltamox)	**Sol:** 10 mg/5 ml	**Adults: Breast Cancer Treatment:** 20 mg qd or qam & qpm. **Ductal Carcinoma in Situ or Reduction of Breast Cancer (High Risk):** 20 mg qd x 5 yrs.	D v Uterine malignancies, stroke & PE reported.
Temozolomide (Temodar)	**Cap:** 5 mg, 20 mg, 100 mg, 140 mg, 180 mg, 250 mg; **Inj:** 100 mg	**Adults:** Adjust according to nadir neutrophil & platelet counts of previous cycle & at time of initiating next cycle. **Glioblastoma Multiforme:** 75 mg/m^2 qd x 42d w/ focal radiotherapy. **Maint: Cycle 1 (28d):** 150 mg/m^2 qd x 5d. **Cycles 2-6 (28d):** If Cycle 1 toxicity Grade ≤2, ANC ≥1.5 x 10^9/L & platelets ≥100 x 10^9/L, increase to 200 mg/m^2/d x 5 consecutive days per 28d cycle. Do not increase dose in subsequent cycles if dose not escalated at Cycle 2.	D v

		Anaplastic Astrocytoma: Initial: 150 mg/m^2 qd x 5 consecutive days per 28d cycle. If ANC ≥1.5 x 10^9/L & platelets ≥100 x 10^9/L for both nadir & Day 29 (Day 1 of next cycle), may increase to 200 mg/m^2/d x 5 consecutive days per 28d cycle. Start next cycle when ANC >1.5 x 10^9/L & platelets >100 x 10^9/L . If ANC <1 x 10^9/L or platelets <50 x 10^9/L during any cycle, reduce next cycle by 50 mg/m^2, but not <100 mg/m^2. Swallow whole w/ water.	
Topotecan (Hycamtin Injection)	**Cap:** 0.25 mg, 1 mg; **Inj:** (as HCl) 4 mg	**Adults:** Adjust dose based on neutrophil/platelet counts (See PI). **Inj: Ovarian Carcinoma/Small-Cell Lung Cancer:** 1.5 mg/m^2 IV over 30 min x 5d. Start Day 1 of 21d course x min of 4 courses. **Cervical Cancer:** 0.75 mg/m^2 IV qd over 30 min on Days 1, 2, & 3; followed by cisplatin 50 mg/m^2 IV on Day 1 of every 21-day course. **PO: Relapsed Small Cell Lung Cancer:** 2.3 mg/m^2/d PO qd x 5 consecutive days. Repeat q21d.	D v Monitor blood cell counts. **R W** [3]
Vorinostat (Zolinza)	**Cap:** 100 mg	**Cutaneous T-Cell Lymphoma: Adults:** 400 mg PO qd w/ food. **Intolerant to Therapy:** May reduce dose to 300 mg PO qd w/ food. If necessary, may further reduce dose to 300 mg PO qd w/ food x 5 consecutive days each wk.	D v

CARDIOVASCULAR AGENTS

Angina

BETA BLOCKERS

NAME	FORM/STRENGTH	DOSAGE	COMMENTS
Atenolol (Tenormin)	**Tab:** 25 mg, 50 mg, 100 mg	**Angina Pectoris: Adults: Initial:** 50 mg qd. **Titrate:** May increase to 100 mg qd after 1 wk. **Max:** 200 mg/d.	D > **R W** [17]
Metoprolol Succinate (Toprol-XL)	**Tab,ER:** 25 mg, 50 mg, 100 mg, 200 mg	**Angina Pectoris: Adults: Initial:** 100 mg qd. **Titrate:** May increase qwk. **Max:** 400 mg/d.	C >
Metoprolol Tartrate (Lopressor)	**Tab:** 50 mg, 100 mg	**Angina Pectoris: Adults: Initial:** 50 mg bid. **Titrate:** May increase qwk. **Maint:** 100-400 mg/d. **Max:** 400 mg/d.	C >
Nadolol (Corgard)	**Tab:** 20 mg, 40 mg, 80 mg, 120 mg, 160 mg	**Angina Pectoris: Adults: Initial:** 40 mg qd. **Titrate:** Increase by 40-80 mg q3-7d. **Usual:** 40-80 mg qd. **Max:** 240 mg/d.	C v **R W** [17]
Propranolol HCl (Inderal)	**Tab:** 10 mg, 20 mg, 40 mg, 60 mg, 80 mg	**Angina Pectoris: Adults:** 80-320 mg/d given bid-qid.	C >

CALCIUM CHANNEL BLOCKERS (DIHYDROPYRIDINES)

NAME	FORM/STRENGTH	DOSAGE	COMMENTS
Amlodipine Besylate (Norvasc)	**Tab:** 2.5 mg, 5 mg, 10 mg	**Chronic Stable/Vasospastic Angina: Adults:** 5-10 mg qd.	C v **H**
Nicardipine	**Cap:** 20 mg, 30 mg	**Chronic Stable Angina: Adults: Initial:** 20 mg tid. **Maint:** 20-40 mg tid.	C v **H**

Nifedipine (Procardia XL)	**Tab,ER:** 30 mg, 60 mg, 90 mg	**Vasospastic/Chronic Stable: Adults: Initial:** 30-60 mg qd. **Titrate:** May increase over 7-14d. **Max:** 120 mg/d. Caution if dose >90 mg.	C >
Nifedipine (Procardia)	**Cap:** (Generic) 10 mg, 20 mg, (Procardia) 10 mg	**Vasospastic/Chronic Stable: Adults: Initial:** 10 mg tid. **Titrate:** May increase over 7-14d. **Usual:** 10-20 mg tid. **Max:** 180 mg/d.	C >

CALCIUM CHANNEL BLOCKER (NON-DIHYDROPYRIDINES)

Diltiazem HCl (Cardizem CD, Cardizem LA, Cartia XT)	**Cap,ER:** (Cardizem CD/Cartia XT) 120 mg, 180 mg, 240 mg, 300 mg, (Cardizem CD) 360 mg; **Tab,ER:** (Cardizem LA) 120 mg, 180 mg, 240 mg, 300 mg, 360 mg, 420 mg	**Chronic Stable Angina/Angina Due To Coronary Artery Spasm: Adults: Cardizem CD/Cartia XT: Initial:** 120-180 mg qd. **Titrate:** Adjust at 1-2 wk intervals. **Max:** 480 mg/d. **Cardizem LA: Initial:** 180 mg qd. **Titrate:** Adjust at 1-2 wk intervals.	C v
Diltiazem HCl (Cardizem)	**Tab:** 30 mg, 60 mg, 90 mg, 120 mg	**Chronic Stable Angina/Angina Due To Coronary Artery Spasm: Adults: Initial:** 30 mg qid (before meals & qhs). **Titrate:** Adjust at 1-2d intervals. **Usual:** 180-360 mg/d.	C v
Diltiazem HCl (Dilacor XR, Diltia XT)	**Cap,ER:** 120 mg, 180 mg, 240 mg	**Chronic Stable Angina: Adults: Initial** 120 mg qd. **Titrate:** Adjust at 1-2 wk intervals. **Max:** 480 mg/d.	C v

NAME	FORM/STRENGTH	DOSAGE	COMMENTS
Diltiazem HCl (Taztia XT, Tiazac)	**Cap,ER:** (Taztia XT/ Tiazac) 120 mg, 180 mg, 240 mg, 300 mg, 360 mg, (Tiazac) 420 mg	**Chronic Stable Angina: Adults: Initial:** 120-180 mg qd. **Titrate:** Adjust over 7-14 days. **Max:** 540 mg/d.	C v
Verapamil (Calan)	**Tab:** 40 mg, 80 mg, 120 mg	**Vasospastic/Unstable/Chronic Stable: Adults: Calan: Usual:** 80-120 mg tid. **Titrate:** Increase by qd or qwk intervals.	C v **H**
Verapamil (Covera-HS)	**Tab,ER:** 180 mg, 240 mg	**Vasospastic/Unstable/Chronic Stable: Adults: Initial:** 180 mg qhs. **Titrate:** Increase to 240 qhs, then 360 mg qhs, then 480 mg qhs.	C v

CALCIUM CHANNEL BLOCKER/HMG-COA REDUCTASE INHIBITOR

NAME	FORM/STRENGTH	DOSAGE	COMMENTS
Amlodipine Besylate/ Atorvastatin Calcium (Caduet)	**Tab:** 2.5-10 mg, 2.5-20 mg, 2.5-40 mg, 5-10 mg, 5-20 mg, 5-40 mg, 5-80 mg, 10-10 mg, 10-20 mg, 10-40 mg, 10-80 mg	Dosing is based on appropriate combination of recommendations for monotherapies. **Adults: Amlodipine:** 5-10 mg qd. **Elderly/Hepatic Dysfunction:** 5 mg qd. **Atorvastatin:** See under Antilipidemic Agents for dosing.	X v **H**

VASODILATORS

NAME	FORM/STRENGTH	DOSAGE	COMMENTS
Isosorbide Dinitrate (Dilatrate-SR)	**Cap,ER:** 40 mg	**Adults: Prevention: Dilatrate-DR: Usual:** 40 mg bid. Separate doses by 6h. **Max:** 160 mg/d. Take at least 18h nitrate-free interval.	C >

Isosorbide Dinitrate (Isordil, Isordil Titradose)	**Tab,SL:** (Generic) 2.5 mg, 5 mg; **Tab:** (Generic) 5 mg, 10 mg, 20 mg, 30 mg, 40 mg, (Isordil Titradose) 5 mg, 10 mg, 40 mg	**Adults: Prevention: Isordil (Titradose): Initial:** 5-20 mg bid-tid. **Maint:** 10-40 mg bid-tid. Take at least 14h nitrate-free interval. **Acute Episode/Prevention: Isordil:** 2.5-5 mg SL 15 min before expected episode or to abort acute episode after failure of SL NTG.	C >
Isosorbide Mononitrate (Imdur)	**Tab,ER:** 30 mg, 60 mg, 120 mg	**Prevention: Adults: Initial:** 30-60 mg qam. **Titrate:** May increase after several days to 120 mg/d. **Elderly:** Start at low end of dosing range.	B >
Nitroglycerin (Minitran, Nitrek, Nitro-Dur)	**Patch:** (mg/h) (Minitran) 0.1, 0.2, 0.4, 0.6; (Nitrek) 0.2, 0.4, 0.6; (Nitro-Dur) 0.1, 0.2, 0.4, 0.6, 0.8	**Prevention: Initial:** 0.2-0.4 mg/h for 12-14h. Remove for 10-12h.	C >
Nitroglycerin (Nitro-Bid)	**Oint:** 2% (15 mg/inch)	**Prevention: Initial:** 0.5 inch qam & 6h later. **Titrate:** May increase to 1 inch bid, then to 2 inches bid. Should have 10-12h nitrate-free period.	C >
Nitroglycerin (Nitroquick, Nitrostat)	**Tab,SL:** 0.3 mg, 0.4 mg, 0.6 mg	**Treatment:** 1 tab SL q5min, up to 3 tabs/15 min. **Prophylaxis:** Take tab or spr 5-10 min before precipitating activity.	C >

MISCELLANEOUS

Ranolazine (Ranexa)	**Tab,ER:** 500 mg, 1000 mg	**Chronic Angina: Adults: Initial:** 500 mg bid. **Max:** 1000 mg bid. Swallow whole.	C v **H**

NAME	FORM/STRENGTH	DOSAGE	COMMENTS

Antiarrhythmics

GROUP IA

NAME	FORM/STRENGTH	DOSAGE	COMMENTS
Disopyramide Phosphate (Norpace, Norpace CR)	**Cap:** 100 mg, 150 mg; **Cap,ER:** 100 mg, 150 mg	**Adults: <50 kg: Cap:** 100 mg q6h. **Cap,ER:** 200 mg q12h. **≥50 kg: Cap:** 150 mg q6h. **Cap,ER:** 300 mg q12h. **Peds: 12-18 yo:** 6-15 mg/kg/d. **4-12 yo:** 10-15 mg/kg/d. **1-4 yo:** 10-20 mg/kg/d. **<1 yo:** 10-30 mg/kg/d.	C v **H R W**[5]
Quinidine Sulfate	**Tab, ER:** 300 mg	**Adults: A-Fib/Flutter Conversion: Initial:** 300 mg q8-12h. **Titrate:** Increase cautiously if no result & levels within therapeutic range. **A-Fib/Flutter Relapse Reduction:** 300 mg q8-12h. **Titrate:** Increase cautiously if needed. **Ventricular Arrhythmia:** Dosing regimens not adequately studied. Monitor ECG for QTc prolongation.	C v

GROUP IB

NAME	FORM/STRENGTH	DOSAGE	COMMENTS
Lidocaine HCl (Xylocaine, Xylocaine-MPF)	**Inj:** 0.5%, 1%, 2%	**Adults: Initial:** 50-100 mg IV given 25-50 mg/min, may repeat after 5 min. **Max:** 200-300 mg/h. Following bolus, initiate w/ 1-4 mg min continuous infusion. **Maint:** Adjust according to cardiac rhythm & toxicity. **Peds:** 1 mg/kg bolus, then 30 mcg/kg/min.	B >
Mexiletine HCl	**Cap:** 150 mg, 200 mg, 250 mg	**Adults: Initial:** 200 mg q8h. **Titrate:** Increase by 50-100 mg q2-3d. **Max:** 1200 mg/d.	C v **H W**[5]

GROUP IC

Flecainide Acetate (Tambocor)	**Tab:** 50 mg, 100 mg, 150 mg	**Adults: PSVT/PAF: Initial:** 50 mg q12h. **Titrate:** Increase by 50 mg bid q4d. **Max:** 300 mg/d. **Sustained VT: Initial:** 100 mg q12h. **Titrate:** Increase by 50 mg bid q4d. **Max:** 400 mg/d. **Peds: <6 mths: Initial:** 50 mg/m^2/d given bid-tid. **>6 mths:** 100 mg/m^2/d given bid-tid. **Max:** 200 mg/m^2/d.	◉C ❋> **R**
Propafenone HCl (Rythmol SR)	**Cap,ER:** 225 mg, 325 mg, 425 mg	**Adults: Initial:** 225 mg q12h. **Titrate:** May increase at minimum 5d intervals to 325 mg q12h, then to 425 mg q12h if needed.	◉C ❋> **H W** [5]

GROUP II

Acebutolol HCl (Sectral)	**Cap:** 200 mg, 400 mg	**Ventricular Arrhythmia: Adults: Initial:** 200 mg bid. **Maint:** Increase gradually to 600-1200 mg/d.	◉B ❋v **R**
Propranolol HCl (Inderal)	**Inj:** 1 mg/ml; **Tab:** 10 mg, 20 mg, 40 mg, 60 mg, 80 mg	**Adults: PO:** 10-30 mg tid-qid, given ac & qhs. **IV:** 1-3 mg IV at 1 mg/min.	◉C ❋>

GROUP III

Amiodarone HCl (Cordarone)	**Tab:** 200 mg	**Adults:** Give LD in hospital. **LD:** 800-1600 mg/d in divided doses x 1-3 wks. After control achieved, give 600-800 mg/d x 1 mth. **Maint:** 400 mg/d (up to 600 mg/d if needed). Use lowest effective dose. Take w/ meals. **Elderly:** Start at low end of dosing range.	◉D ❋v

NAME	FORM/STRENGTH	DOSAGE	COMMENTS
Sotalol HCl (Betapace AF)	**Cap:** 80 mg, 120 mg, 160 mg	**Adults: NSR Maint in A-Fib/Flutter:** Dose according to CrCl (see PI). **Peds: Betapace AF: ≥2 yo: Initial:** 30 mg/m^2 tid. **Titrate:** Wait ≥36h between dose increases. Guide dose by response, HR & QT_c. **Max:** 60 mg/m^2. **<2 yo:** See dosing chart in PI. Reduce dose or d/c if QT_c >550 msec.	B v Should be inpatient at least 3d when initiated. Monitor ECG & CrCl. **R W** 5
Sotalol HCl (Betapace)	**Tab:** 80 mg, 120 mg, 160 mg, 240 mg	**Adults: Life-Threatening Ventricular Arrhythmia: Initial:** 80 mg bid. **Titrate:** Increase q3d prn to 120-160 mg bid. **Usual:** 160-320 mg/d given bid-tid. **Peds: Betapace: ≥2 yo: Initial:** 30 mg/m^2 tid. **Titrate:** Wait ≥36h between dose increases. Guide dose by response, HR & QT_c. **Max:** 60 mg/m^2. **<2 yo:** See dosing chart in PI. Reduce dose or d/c if QT_c >550 msec.	B v Should be inpatient at least 3d when initiated. Monitor ECG & CrCl. **R W** 5
GROUP IV			
Verapamil HCl (Calan)	**Tab:** 40 mg, 80 mg, 120 mg	**Adults: A-Fib (Digitalized): Usual:** 240-320 mg/d given tid-qid. **PSVT Prophylaxis (Non-Digitalized):** 240-480 mg/d given tid-qid. **Max:** 480 mg/d.	C v

MISCELLANEOUS

Digoxin (Digitek, Lanoxicaps, Lanoxin, Lanoxin Pediatric)	**Cap:** (Lanoxicaps) 0.05 mg, 0.1 mg, 0.2 mg; **Inj:** (Lanoxin Pediatric) 0.1 mg/ml, (Lanoxin) 0.25 mg/ml; **Sol:** (Lanoxin Pediatric) 0.05 mg/ml; **Tab:** (Digitek, Lanoxin) 0.125 mg, 0.25 mg	**A-Fib: Adults:** Titrate to minimum effective dose for desired response.	◙C ❁> **R**

Antilipidemic Agents

BILE ACID SEQUESTRANTS

Cholestyramine (Questran, Questran Light, Prevalite)	**Pow:** 4 gm/pkt or scoopful	**Adults: Initial:** 1 pkt or scoopful qd or bid. **Maint:** 2-4 pkts or scoopfuls/d divided into 2 doses. **Max:** 6 pkts or scoopfuls/d. **Peds: Usual:** 240 mg/kg/d of anhydrous cholestyramine resin in 2-3 divided doses. **Max:** 8 g/d.	◙C ❁> May decrease vitamin content in breast milk.
Colesevelam HCl (WelChol)	**Tab:** 625 mg	**Adults: Initial:** 3 tabs bid or 6 tabs qd. Take w/ a meal & liquid.	◙B ❁>
Colestipol Hydrochloride (Colestid)	**Granules:** 5 gm/pkt or scoopful; **Tab:** 1 gm	**Adults: Initial:** 2 gm (tabs) or 5 gm (1 pkt or scoopful) qd-bid. **Titrate:** Increase by 2 gm qd or bid at 1-2 mth intervals. **Usual:** 2-16 gm/d (tab) or 1-6 pkts or scoopfuls qd or in divided doses.	◙N ❁>

NAME	FORM/STRENGTH	DOSAGE	COMMENTS
CALCIUM CHANNEL BLOCKER/HMG-COA REDUCTASE INHIBITOR			
Amlodipine Besylate/ Atorvastatin Calcium (Caduet)	**Tab:** 2.5-10 mg, 2.5-20 mg, 2.5-40 mg, 5-10 mg, 5-20 mg, 5-40 mg, 5-80 mg, 10-10 mg, 10-20 mg, 10-40 mg, 10-80 mg	Dosing based on appropriate combination of recommendations for monotherapies. **Amlodipine:** See under Angina & Hypertension for dosing. **Atorvastatin: Adults: Hypercholesterolemia/Mixed Dyslipidemia: Initial:** 10-20 mg qd (or 40 mg qd for LDL-C reduction >45%). **Titrate:** Adjust dose at 2-4 wk intervals. **Usual:** 10-80 mg qd. **Homozygous Familial Hypercholesterolemia:** 10-80 mg qd. **Peds: 10-17 yo (postmenarchal): Heterozygous Familial Hypercholesterolemia: Initial:** 10 mg/d. **Titrate:** Adjust dose at ≥4 wks intervals. **Max:** 20 mg/d.	X v **H**
CHLOESTEROL ABSORPTION INHIBITOR/HMG-COA REDUCTASE INHIBITOR			
Ezetimibe/Simvastatin (Vytorin)	**Tab:** 10/10 mg, 10/20 mg, 10/40 mg, 10/80 mg	**Adults:** Take once daily in evening. **Initial:** 10/20 mg qd. **Less Aggressive LDL-C Reductions: Initial:** 10/10 mg qd. **LDL-C Reduction >55%: Initial:** 10/40 mg qd. **Titrate:** Adjust at ≥2 wks. **Homozygous Familial Hypercholesterolemia:** 10/40 mg or 10/80 mg qd. **Concomitant Bile Acid Sequestrant:** Take either ≥2 hrs before or ≥4 hrs after bile acid sequestrant. **Concomitant Cyclosporine:** Avoid unless tolerant of ≥5 mg of simvastatin. **Max:** 10/10 mg/d. **Concomitant Amiodarone/ Verapamil: Max:** 10/20 mg/d.	X v **R**

CHOLESTEROL ABSORPTION INHIBITOR

Ezetimibe (Zetia)	**Tab:** 10 mg	**Adults:** 10 mg qd. May give w/ HMG-CoA reductase inhibitor (primary hypercholesterolemia) or fenofibrate (mixed hyperlipidemia) for incremental effect. Give either ≥2h before or ≥4h after bile acid sequestrant.	◉C ❁v

FIBRIC ACIDS

Fenofibrate (Tricor)	**Tab:** 48 mg, 145 mg	**Adults: Hypercholesterolemia/Mixed Dyslipidemia: Initial:** 145 mg/d. **Hypertriglyceridemia: Initial:** 48-145 mg/d. **Titrate:** May adjust dose at 4-8 wk intervals. **Max:** 145 mg/d. **Elderly/Renal Dysfunction: Initial:** 48 mg/d.	◉C ❁v **H R**
Gemfibrozil (Lopid)	**Tab:** 600 mg	**Adults:** 600 mg bid 30 min ac.	◉C ❁v **H R**

HMG-COA REDUCTASE INHIBITOR/NICOTINIC ACID

Lovastatin/Niacin (Advicor)	**Tab:** 20-500 mg, 20-750 mg, 20-1000mg, 40-1000 mg	**Adults: ≥18 yo: Initial:** 20-500 mg qhs. **Titrate:** Increase by ≤500 mg of niacin q4wks. **Max:** 40-2000 mg. Adjust w/ cyclosporine or fibrates. May pretreat w/ ASA/NSAID to reduce flushing.	◉X ❁v **H**

NAME	FORM/STRENGTH	DOSAGE	COMMENTS
Niacin/Simvastatin (Simcor)	**Tab,ER:** 500-20 mg, 750-20 mg, 1000-20 mg	**Adults: Patients Not Currently on ER Niacin or Switching from IR Niacin: Initial:** 500-20 mg qd hs, w/ low fat snack. **Titrate:** Adjust dose at ≥4 wks. After Wk 8, titrate to response & tolerance. **Maint:** 1000-20 mg to 2000-40 mg qd. **Max:** 2000-40 mg qd. Do not break, crush or chew before swallowing.	X v **H**

HMG-COA REDUCTASE INHIBITORS

NAME	FORM/STRENGTH	DOSAGE	COMMENTS
Atorvastatin Calcium (Lipitor)	**Tab:** 10 mg, 20 mg, 40 mg, 80 mg	**Adults: Hypercholesterolemia/Mixed Dyslipidemia: Initial:** 10-20 mg qd (or 40 mg qd for LDL-C reduction >45%). **Titrate:** Adjust at 2-4 wk intervals. **Usual:** 10-80 mg qd. **Homozygous Familial Hypercholesterolemia:** 10-80 mg qd. **Peds: 10-17 yo (postmenarchal): Heterozygous Familial Hypercholesterolemia: Initial:** 10 mg/d. **Titrate:** Adjust at ≥4 wk intervals. **Max:** 20 mg/d.	X v
Fluvastatin Sodium (Lescol, Lescol XL)	**Cap:** (Lescol) 20 mg, 40 mg; **Tab,ER:** (Lescol XL) 80 mg	**Adults: ≥18 yo: Initial:** (LDL-C reduction ≥25%) 40 mg cap qpm or 80 mg XL tab at anytime of day or 40 mg cap bid. (LDL-C reduction <25%) l20 mg cap qpm. **Range:** 20-80 mg/d. Take 2h after bile-acid resins qhs. **Peds: 10-16 yo (≥1 yr post-menarche): Heterozygous Familial Hypercholesterolemia:** Individualize dose: **Initial:** 20 mg cap. **Titrate:** Adjust dose at 6 wk intervals. **Max:** 40 mg cap bid or 80 mg XL tab qd.	X v **H**

Lovastatin (Mevacor)	**Tab:** 20 mg, 40 mg	**Adults: Initial:** 20 mg qd w/ pm meal (10 mg/d if need LDL-C reduction <20%). **Usual:** 10-80 mg/d as qd-bid. **Peds: 10-17 yo: Heterozygous Familial Hypercholesterolemia: Initial:** 20 mg qd (10 mg qd if need LDL-C reduction <20%). **Titrate:** May adjust q4wks. **Max:** 40 mg/d. Adjust w/ cyclosporine, fibrates, niacin, verapamil, or amiodarone.	X v **H R**
Pravastatin Sodium (Pravachol)	**Tab:** 10 mg, 20 mg, 40 mg, 80 mg	**Adults: ≥18 yo: Initial:** 40 mg qd. **Titrate:** Increase to 80 mg qd. **Heterozygous Familial Hypercholesterolemia: Peds: 14-18 yo:** 40 mg qd. **8-13 yo:** 20 mg qd. **Concomitant Immunosuppressives (eg, cyclosporine): Initial:**10 mg qhs. **Max:** 20 mg/d. Take at least 1h before or 4h after resins.	X v **H R**
Rosuvastatin (Crestor)	**Tab:** 5 mg, 10 mg, 20 mg, 40 mg	**Adults: Hypercholesterolemia/Mixed Dyslipidemia: Initial:** 10 mg qd (or 5 mg qd for less aggressive LDL-C reductions; 20 mg qd w/ LDL-C >190 mg/dL). **Titrate:** Adjust dose if needed at 2-4 wk intervals. **Range:** 5-40 mg qd. **Homozygous Familial Hypercholesterolemia:** 20 mg qd. **Max:** 40 mg qd. Adjust w/ cyclosporine, gemfibrozil.	X v **H R**

NAME	FORM/STRENGTH	DOSAGE	COMMENTS
Simvastatin (Zocor)	**Tab:** 5 mg, 10 mg, 20 mg, 40 mg, 80 mg	**Adults: Initial:** 20-40 mg qpm. **Usual:** 5-80 mg/d. **Titrate:** Adjust at ≥4 wk intervals. **High Risk for CHD Events: Initial:** 40 mg/d. **Homozygous Familial Hypercholesterolemia:** 40 mg qpm or 80 mg/d given as 20 mg bid plus 40 mg qpm. **Peds: 10-17 yo (≥1-yr postmenarchal): Heterozygous Familial Hypercholesterolemia: Initial:** 10 mg qpm. **Usual:** 10-40 mg/d. **Titrate:** Adjust at ≥4 wk intervals. **Max:** 40 mg/d. Adjust w/ cyclosporine, fibrates, amiodarone, verapamil, or niacin.	X v **H R**
NICOTINIC ACID			
Niacin (Niaspan)	**Tab,ER:** 500 mg, 750 mg, 1000 mg	**Adults: Initial:** 500 mg qhs. **Titrate:** Increase by 500 mg q4wks. **Maint:** 1-2 gm qhs. May pretreat w/ ASA/NSAID to reduce flushing.	C v **H**
MISCELLANEOUS			
Omega-3-Acid Ethyl Esters (Lovaza)	**Cap:** 1 gm	**Adults:** 4 gm qd. Given as a single 4-gm dose or as two 2-gm doses.	C >

LOW MOLECULAR WEIGHT HEPARINS

Dalteparin Sodium (Fragmin)	**Inj:** (Syringe) 2500 IU/0.2 ml, 5000 IU/0.2 ml, 7500 IU/0.3 ml, 10,000 IU/0.4ml, 10,000 IU/ml, 12,500 IU/0.5ml, 15,000 IU/0.6 ml, 18,000 IU/0.72 ml; (MDV) 95,000 IU/3.8ml, 95,000 IU/9.5ml	**Adults: SC: Unstable Angina/Non-Q-Wave MI:** 120 U/kg, up to 10,000 IU q12h w/ 75-165 mg/d ASA x 5-8d. **Hip Replacement Surgery: Pre-Op Start: Initial (if start 2h pre-op):** 2500 IU within 2h pre-op, then 2500 IU 4-8h post-op. **Initial (if start 10-14h pre-op):** 5000 IU 10-14h pre-op, then 5000 IU 4-8h post-op. **Maint (for either dose):** 5000 IU qd x 5-10d post-op (up to 14d). **Post-Op Start:** 2500 IU 4-8h post-op. **Maint:** 5000 IU qd. **Abdominal Surgery: Initial:** 2500 IU 1-2h pre-op. **Maint:** 2500 IU qd x 5-10d post-op. **Abdominal Surgery w/ High Risk: Initial:** 5000 IU evening before surgery. **Maint:** 5000 IU qd x 5-10d post-op. **Abdominal Surgery w/ Malignancy: Initial:** 2500 IU 1-2h pre-op, then 2500 IU 12h later. **Maint:** 5000 IU qd x 5-10d post-op. **Severely Restricted Mobility During Acute Illness:** 5000 IU qd x 12-14d. **Symptomatic VTE in Cancer Patients:** 200 IU/kg qd x 1st 30 days, then 150 IU/kg qd for mths 2-6. **Max:** 18,000 IU/d. Adjust dose based on platelet count & anti-Xa levels.	◉B ❄> **R** **W** [6]

NAME	FORM/STRENGTH	DOSAGE	COMMENTS
Enoxaparin (Lovenox)	**Inj:** 30 mg/0.3 ml, 40 mg/0.4 ml, 60 mg/0.6 ml, 80 mg/0.8 ml, 100 mg/ml, 120 mg/0.8 ml, 150 mg/ml, 300 mg/3 ml	**Adults: SC: Hip/Knee Replacement Surgery:** 30 mg q12h 12-24h post-op x 7-10d (up to 14d). **Hip (alternative dosing):** 40 mg qd 12h pre-op, then 40 mg qd x 3 wks. **Abdominal Surgery:** 40 mg qd, 2h pre-op x 7-10d (up to 14d). **DVT Outpatient Treatment:** 1 mg/kg q12h w/ warfarin (goal INR 2-3) x 7d (up to 17d). **DVT/PE Inpatient Treatment:** 1 mg/kg q12h or 1.5 mg/kg qd w/ warfarin (goal INR 2-3) x 7d (up to 17d). **Unstable Angina/Non-Q-Wave MI:** 1 mg/kg q12h w/ 100-325 mg/d ASA x 2-8d (up to 12.5d). **Acute Illness:** 40 mg qd x 6-11d (up to 14d). **Acute STEMI: <75 yo:** 30 mg single IV bolus plus a 1 mg/kg SC dose followed by 1 mg/kg SC qd. **Acute STEMI: ≥75 yo:** 1 mg/kg SC qd (no initial bolus).	B > **R W** [6]

PHOSPHODIESTERASE/PLATELET AGGREGATION-ADHESION INHIBITORS

NAME	FORM/STRENGTH	DOSAGE	COMMENTS
Anagrelide HCl (Agrylin)	**Cap:** 0.5 mg, 1 mg	**Thrombocythemia: Initial: Adults:** 0.5 mg qid or 1 mg bid x 1 wk. **Peds:** 0.5 mg qd. **Titrate:** May increase by 0.5 mg/d qwk. Adjust based on platelet count. **Max:** 10 mg/d or 2.5 mg/dose.	C v **H R**
Aspirin (Bayer Aspirin)	**Chewtab:** 81 mg; **Tab:** 81 mg, 325 mg; **Tab,Delay:** 81 mg, 325 mg, 500 mg	**Adults: Stroke/TIA:** 50-325 mg qd. **Suspected AMI: Initial:** 160-162.5 mg qd as soon as suspect MI. **Maint:** 160-162.5 mg x 30d post-infarct. **Prevention or Recurrent MI:** 75-325 mg qd.	N v Avoid use during 3rd trimester. **H R**

Aspirin (Ecotrin)	**Chewtab:** 81 mg; **Tab:** 81 mg, 325 mg; **Tab,Delay:** 81 mg, 325 mg, 500 mg	**Adults: Stroke/TIA:** 50-325 mg qd. **Suspected AMI: Initial:** 160-162.5 mg qd as soon as suspect MI. **Maint:** 160-162.5 mg x 30d post-infarct. **Prevention or Recurrent MI:** 75-325 mg qd.	◉N ❈> Avoid use during 3rd trimester. **H R**
Cilostazol (Pletal)	**Tab:** 50 mg, 100 mg	**Intermittent Claudication: Adults:** 100 mg bid, 1/2h before or 2h after breakfast & dinner. Dose 50 mg bid w/ certain drugs.	◉C ❈v CI in CHF.
Clopidogrel Bisulfate (Plavix)	**Tab:** 75 mg, 300 mg	**Adults: MI/Stroke/Peripheral Arterial Disease:** 75 mg qd. **Acute Coronary Syndrome: Non-ST-Segment Elevation (Unstable Angina/Non-Q-Wave MI): LD:** 300 mg. **Maint:** 75 mg qd. Take w/ 75-325 mg ASA qd. **ST-Segment Elevation MI:** 75 mg qd. Take w/ 75-325 mg ASA & w/ or w/o LD.	◉B ❈v
Dipyridamole/ASA (Aggrenox)	**Cap,ER:** 200-25 mg	**Risk Reduction of Stroke: Adults:** 1 cap qam & qpm.	◉D ❈> **R** Avoid if CrCl <10ml/min.
Dipyridamole (Persantine)	**Tab:** 25 mg, 50 mg, 75 mg	**Prophylaxis to Thromboembolism after Cardiac Valve Replacement: Adults:** 75-100 mg qid as an adjunct to warfarin.	◉B ❈>
Ticlopidine HCl (Ticlid)	**Tab:** 250 mg	**Adults: Stroke:** 250 mg bid. **Coronary Artery Stenting:** 250 mg bid w/ ASA up to 30d after stent implant. Take w/ food.	◉B ❈v **H R W** [15]

NAME	FORM/STRENGTH	DOSAGE	COMMENTS
SPECIFIC FACTOR XA INHIBITOR			
Fondaparinux Sodium (Arixtra)	**Inj:** 2.5 mg/0.5 ml, 5 mg/ 0.4 ml, 7.5 mg/0.6 ml, 10 mg/0.8 ml	**Adults: SC: DVT Prophylaxis for Hip Fracture or Replacement Surgery/Knee Replacement Surgery/ Abdominal Surgery:** 2.5 mg qd, starting 6-8h post-op x 5-9d (Hip/Knees: up to 11d; Abdominal: up to 10d). **Hip Fracture Surgery:** Extended prophylaxis up to 24 additional days. **DVT/PE Treatment: <50 kg:** 5 mg qd. **50-100 kg:** 7.5 mg qd. **>100 kg:** 10 mg qd. Add concomitant warfarin ASAP (usually within 72h) & continue x 5-9d (up to 26d) until INR=2-3.	B > R W [6]
THROMBOLYTICS			
Reteplase (Retavase)	**Inj:** 10.4 U	**Acute MI: Adults:** 10 U IV over 2 min, repeat in 30 min.	C >
Streptokinase (Streptase)	**Inj:** 250,000 IU, 750,000 IU, 1.5 MIU	**Adults: Acute MI:** 1.5 MIU IV within 60 min. **PE/DVT:** 250,000 IU over 30 min, then 100,000 IU/h x 24h (72h if DVT). **Thrombosis/Embolism:** 250,000 IU over 30 min, then 100,000 IU/h x 24-72h.	C >
Urokinase (Abbokinase)	**Inj:** 250,000 IU	**PE: Adults: LD:** 4400 IU/kg IV at 90 ml/h over 10 min. **Maint:** 4400 IU/kg/h IV at 15 ml/h for 12h. Flush line after each cycle.	B >

Warfarin Sodium (Coumadin, Jantoven)	**Inj:** (Coumadin) 5 mg; **Tab:** (Coumadin, Jantoven) 1 mg, 2 mg, 2.5 mg, 3 mg, 4 mg, 5 mg, 6 mg, 7.5 mg, 10 mg	**Adults: ≥18 yo:** Adjust dose based on PT/INR. Give IV as alternate to PO. **Initial:** 2-5 mg qd. **Maint:** 2-10 mg qd. **Venous Thromboembolism (including PE):** INR of 2-3. **A-Fib:** INR of 2-3. **Post-MI:** Initiate 2-4 wks post-infarct & maintain INR of 2.5-3.5. **Mechanical Heart Valve:** INR of 2.5-3.5. **Bioprosthetic Heart Valve:** INR of 2-3 x 12 wks after valve insertion.	X > **H** May cause major/fatal bleeding.

Heart Failure

ACE INHIBITORS

Captopril (Capoten)	**Tab:** 12.5 mg, 25 mg, 50 mg, 100 mg	**Adults: CHF: Initial:** 25 mg tid. **Usual:** 50-100 mg tid. **Max:** 450 mg/d. **Left Ventricular Dysfunction Following MI: Initial:** 6.25 mg single dose, then 12.5 mg tid. **Titrate:** Increase to 25 mg tid over next several days, then to 50 mg tid over next several wks. **Usual:** 50 mg tid.	C (1st trimester) D (2nd/3rd trimester) v **R W** [7]
Enalapril Maleate (Vasotec)	**Tab:** 1.25 mg, 2.5 mg, 5 mg, 10 mg, 20 mg	**Adults: Initial:** 2.5 mg qd. **Titrate:** Increase over few days or wks. **Usual:** 2.5-20 mg given bid. **Max:** 40 mg/d.	C (1st trimester) D (2nd/3rd trimester) v **R W** [7]

NAME	FORM/STRENGTH	DOSAGE	COMMENTS
Fosinopril Sodium (Monopril)	**Tab:** 10 mg, 20 mg, 40 mg	**Adults: Initial:** 10 mg qd. **Titrate:** Increase over several wks. **Usual:** 20-40 mg qd. **Max:** 40mg/d.	C (1st trimester) D (2nd/3rd trimester) v **R W** [7]
Lisinopril (Prinivil)	**Tab:** 5 mg, 10 mg, 20 mg	**Adults: Initial:** 5 mg qd. **Usual:** 5-20 mg qd. **Hyponatremia or CrCl ≤30 ml/min: Initial:** 2.5 mg qd.	C (1st trimester) D (2nd/3rd trimester) v **R W** [7]
Lisinopril (Zestril)	**Tab:** 2.5 mg, 5 mg, 10 mg, 20 mg, 30 mg, 40 mg	**Adults: Initial:** 5 mg qd. **Usual:** 5-40 mg qd. May increase by 10 mg q2wks. **Max:** 40 mg/d. **Hyponatremia or CrCl ≤30 ml/min or SrCr >3 mg/dL: Initial:** 2.5 mg qd.	C (1st trimester) D (2nd/3rd trimester) v **R W** [7]
Quinapril HCl (Accupril)	**Tab:** 5 mg, 10 mg, 20 mg, 40 mg	**Adults: Initial:** 5 mg bid. **Titrate:** Increase at wkly intervals. **Usual:** 10-20 mg bid. **Max:** 40 mg/d.	C (1st trimester) D (2nd/3rd trimester) v **R W** [7]

Ramipril (Altace)	**Cap:** 1.25 mg, 2.5 mg, 5 mg, 10 mg	**Adults: Post-MI CHF: Initial:** 2.5 mg bid, 1.25 mg bid if hypotensive. **Titrate:** Increase to 5 mg bid. **CrCl <40 ml/min: Initial:** 1.25 mg qd. **Titrate:** May increase to 1.25 mg bid. **Max:** 2.5 mg bid. Reduce or d/c diuretic if possible. **Volume Depletion/Renal Artery Stenosis: Initial:** 1.25 mg qd.	C (1st trimester) D (2nd/3rd trimester) v **H R W** [7]
Trandolapril (Mavik)	**Tab:** 1 mg, 2 mg, 4 mg	**Post-MI CHF: Adults: Initial:** 1 mg qd. **Usual:** 4 mg qd. **Max:** 4 mg/d.	C (1st trimester) D (2nd/3rd trimester) v **R W** [7]

ALDOSTERONE BLOCKER

Eplerenone (Inspra)	**Tab:** 25 mg, 50 mg	**CHF Post-MI: Adults: Initial:** 25 mg qd. **Titrate:** To 50 mg qd within 4 wks. **Maint:** 50 mg qd. **Adjust dose based on K^+ level:** See PI.	B v **R**

ALPHA/BETA BLOCKERS

Carvedilol (Coreg, Coreg CR)	**Cap,ER:** 10 mg, 20 mg, 40 mg, 80 mg; **Tab:** 3.125 mg, 6.25 mg, 12.5 mg, 25 mg	**Adults:** Individualize dose. Take w/ food. Monitor dose increases. Take extended-release caps in am & swallow whole. **CHF: Tab: Initial:** 3.125 mg bid x 2 wks. **Titrate:** May double dose q2wks as tolerated. **Max:** 50 mg bid if >85 kg. Reduce dose if HR <55 beats/min. **Cap,ER: Initial:**	C v

Continued on Next Page

NAME	FORM/STRENGTH	DOSAGE	COMMENTS
Carvedilol (Coreg, Coreg CR) *Continued*		10 mg qd x 2 wks. **Titrate:** May double dose q2wks as tolerated. **Max:** 80 mg/d. Reduce dose if HR <55 beats/min. **LVD Post-MI: Tab: Initial:** 6.25 mg bid x 3-10d. **Titrate:** May double dose q3-10d to target of 25 mg bid. May begin w/ 3.125 mg bid & slow up-titration rate if clinically indicated. **Cap,ER: Initial:** 20 mg qd x 3-10d. **Titrate:** May double dose q3-10d to target of 80 mg qd.	
ANGIOTENSIN II RECEPTOR ANTAGONISTS			
Candesartan Cilexetil (Atacand)	**Tab:** 4 mg, 8 mg, 16 mg, 32 mg	**Adults: Initial:** 4 mg qd. **Titrate:** Double dose at 2 wk intervals. **Target:** 32 mg qd.	◙C (1st trimester) ◙D (2nd/3rd trimester) ❋v **R W** [9]
Valsartan (Diovan)	**Tab:** 40 mg, 80 mg, 160 mg, 320 mg	**Adults: CHF: Initial:** 40 mg bid. **Titrate:** May increase to 80 mg or 160 mg bid (use highest dose tolerated). **Max:** 320 mg/d in divided doses. **Hepatic/Severe Renal Impairment:** Use w/ caution.	◙D ❋v **W** [9]
BETA BLOCKERS			
Metoprolol Succinate (Toprol-XL)	**Tab,ER:** 25 mg, 50 mg, 100 mg, 200 mg	**Adults: Initial: Class II HF:** 25 mg qd x 2 wks. **Severe HF:** 12.5 mg qd x 2 wks. **Titrate:** Double dose q2wks as tolerated. **Max:** 200 mg/d.	◙C ❋>

Bumetanide (Bumex)	(Bumex) **Tab:** 0.5 mg, 1 mg, 2 mg; (Generic) **Inj:** 0.25 mg/ml; **Tab:** 0.5 mg, 1 mg, 2 mg	**Adults:** **≥18 yo:** **PO:** **Usual:** 0.5-2 mg qd. **Maint:** Give qod or q3-4d. **Max:** 10 mg/d. **IV/IM:** **Initial:** 0.5-1 mg, may repeat q2-3h x 2-3 doses. **Max:** 10 mg/d.	C v **W** [8]
Furosemide (Lasix)	(Generic) **Inj:** 10 mg/ml; **Sol:** 10 mg/ml, 40 mg/5 ml; **Tab:** 20 mg, 40 mg, 80 mg; (Lasix) **Tab:** 20 mg, 40 mg, 80 mg	**Adults:** **PO:** **Usual:** 20-80 mg as single dose, may repeat or increase by 20-40 mg after 6-8h. **Max:** 600 mg/d. **IV/IM:** 20-40 mg. May repeat or increase by 20 mg after 2h. **Peds:** **PO:** **Usual:** 2 mg/kg as single dose, may increase by 1-2 mg/kg after 6-8h. **Max:** 6 mg/kg. **IV/IM:** 1 mg/kg single dose. May increase by 1 mg/kg after 2h. **Max:** 6 mg/kg.	C > **W** [8]
Torsemide (Demadex)	**Tab:** 5 mg, 10 mg, 20 mg, 100 mg	**Adults:** **Initial:** 10-20 mg qd. **Titrate:** Double dose until desired diuretic response. **Max:** 200 mg/d.	B >

DIURETICS (POTASSIUM SPARING)

Spironolactone (Aldactone)	**Tab:** 25 mg, 50 mg, 100 mg	**Adults:** **Initial:** 100 mg/d in single or divided doses. **Usual:** 25-200 mg/d.	C v **W** [16]
Triamterene (Dyrenium)	**Cap:** 50 mg, 100 mg	**Adults:** **Initial:** 100 mg bid. **Max:** 300 mg/d.	C v **W** [88]

NAME	FORM/STRENGTH	DOSAGE	COMMENTS
DIURETICS (POTASSIUM SPARING/THIAZIDE)			
Spironolactone/ Hydrochlorothiazide (Aldactazide)	**Tab:** 25-25 mg, 50-50 mg	**Adults: Usual:** 100 mg/d per component qd or in divided doses. **Maint:** 25-200 mg/d per component.	C v Not for initial therapy. **W** [16]
Triamterene/ Hydrochlorothiazide (Maxzide, Maxzide-25)	**Tab:** 37.5-25 mg, 75-50 mg	**Adults: Usual:** (37.5-25 mg) 1-2 tabs qd. (75-50 mg) 1 tab qd.	C v
DIURETICS (QUINAZOLINE)			
Metolazone (Zaroxolyn)	**Tab:** 2.5 mg, 5 mg, 10 mg	**Adults: Initial:** 5-20 mg qd. **Elderly:** Start at low end of dosing range.	B v Rapid & slow formulations not equivalent.
DIURETICS (THIAZIDE)			
Chlorothiazide (Diuril, Diuril IV)	(Diuril) **Inj:** (Na salt) 0.5 gm; **Susp:** 250 mg/5 ml; (Generic) **Tab:** 250 mg, 500 mg	**Adults: PO/IV:** 0.5-1 gm qd-bid. May give qod or 3-5d/wk. **Peds: PO: Usual:** 10-20 mg/kg/d given qd-bid. **Max: 2-12 yo:** 1 gm/d. **≤2 yo:** 375 mg/d. **<6 mths:** 15 mg/kg bid.	C v
Hydrochlorothiazide	**Cap:** 12.5 mg; **Tab:** 25 mg, 50 mg, 100 mg	**Adults: Usual:** 25-100 mg qd. May give qod or 3-5d per wk. **Peds:** 1-2 mg/kg/d given qd-bid. **Max: 2-12 yo:** 100 mg/d. **≤2 yo:** 37.5 mg/d. **<6 mths:** 1.5 mg/kg bid.	B v

Digoxin (Digitek, Lanoxicaps, Lanoxin, Lanoxin Pediatric)	**Cap:** (Lanoxicaps) 0.05 mg, 0.1 mg, 0.2 mg; **Inj:** (Lanoxin Pediatric) 0.1 mg/mL, (Lanoxin) 0.25 mg/mL; **Sol:** (Lanoxin Pediatric) 0.05 mg/mL; **Tab:** (Digitek, Lanoxin) 0.125 mg, 0.25 mg	**HF: Adults: Rapid Digitalization: LD:** (Cap/Inj) 0.4-0.6 mg PO/IV or (Tab) 0.5-0.75 mg PO. May give additional (Cap/Inj) 0.1-0.3 mg or (Tab) 0.125-0.375 mg at 6-8h intervals until clinical effect. **Maint:** (Tab) 0.125-0.5 mg qd. **Peds: Sol/Ped Inj: Digitalizing Dose: Premature Infants:** 20-30 mcg/kg PO or 15-25 mcg/kg IV. **Full-Term Infants:** 25-35 mcg/kg PO or 20-30 mcg/kg IV. **1-24 mths:** 35-60 mcg/kg PO or 30-50 mcg/kg IV. **2-5 yo:** 30-40 mcg/kg PO or 25-35 mcg/kg IV. **5-10 yo:** 20-35 mcg/kg PO or 15-30 mcg/kg IV. **>10 yo:** 10-15 mcg/kg PO or 8-12 mcg/kg IV. **Maint: Premature Infants:** 20-30% of digitalizing dose. **Full-Term Infants to >10 yo:** 25-35% of digitalizing dose. **Cap: Digitalizing Dose: 2-5 yo:** 25-35 mcg/kg. **5-10 yo:** 15-30 mcg/kg. **>10 yo:** 8-12 mcg/kg. **Maint: ≥2 yo:** 25-35% of digitalizing dose. **Tab: Maint: 2-5 yo:** 10-15 mcg/kg. **5-10 yo:** 7-10 mcg/kg. **>10 yo:** 3-5 mcg/kg.	◙C ❊> **R**

MISCELLANEOUS

Isosorbide Dinitrate/ Hydralazine HCl (BiDil)	**Tab:** 20-37.5 mg	**Adults: Initial:** 1 tab bid. **Max:** 2 tabs tid.	◙C ❊>

Hypertension

ACE INHIBITORS

NAME	FORM/STRENGTH	DOSAGE	COMMENTS
Benazepril HCl (Lotensin)	**Tab:** 5 mg, 10 mg, 20 mg, 40 mg	**Adults: Initial:** 10 mg qd or 5 mg qd if on diuretic. **Maint:** 20-40 mg/d as qd-bid. **Max:** 80 mg/d. **Peds: ≥6 yo: Initial:** 0.2 mg/kg qd. **Max:** 0.6 mg/kg.	D v **R W** [7]
Captopril (Capoten)	**Tab:** 12.5 mg, 25 mg, 50 mg, 100 mg	**Adults: Initial:** 25 mg bid-tid. **Titrate:** Increase to 50 mg bid-tid after 1-2 wks. **Usual:** 25-150 mg bid-tid. **Max:** 450 mg/d.	C (1st trimester) D (2nd/3rd trimester) v **R W** [7]
Enalapril Maleate (Vasotec)	**Tab:** 1.25 mg, 2.5 mg, 5 mg, 10 mg, 20 mg	**Adults: Initial:** 5 mg qd, 2.5 mg if on diuretic. **Usual:** 10-40 mg/d as qd-bid. **Peds: 1 mth-16 yo: Initial:** 0.08 mg/kg (up to 5 mg) qd. **Max:** 0.58 mg/kg/dose (or 40 mg/dose).	C (1st trimester) D (2nd/3rd trimester) v **R W** [7]
Enalaprilat (Vasotec I.V.)	**Inj:** 1.25 mg/ml	**Adults: Usual:** 1.25 mg over 5 min q6h. **Max:** 20 mg/d. **Concomitant Diuretic: Initial:** 0.625 mg over 5 min, may repeat after 1h. **Maint:** 1.25 mg q6h. **PO/IV Conversion:** 5 mg/d PO or 1.25 mg IV q6h & 2.5 mg/d PO or 0.625 mg q6h IV.	C (1st trimester) D (2nd/3rd trimester) v **R W** [7]

Fosinopril Sodium (Monopril)	**Tab:** 10 mg, 20 mg, 40 mg	**Adults: Initial:** 10 mg qd. **Usual:** 20-40 mg qd. **Max:** 80 mg/d. **Peds: >50 kg:** 5-10 mg qd.	◙C (1st trimester) ◙D (2nd/3rd trimester) ❃v **W** [7]
Lisinopril (Prinivil)	**Tab:** 5 mg, 10 mg, 20 mg	**Adults:** If possible, d/c diuretic 2-3d prior to therapy. **Initial:** 10 mg qd; 5 mg qd w/ diuretic. **Usual:** 20-40 mg qd. Resume diuretic if BP not controlled. **Max:** 80 mg/d. **Peds: ≥6 yo: Initial:** 0.07 mg/kg qd (up to 5 mg total). Adjust dose based on BP response. **Max:** 0.61 mg/kg qd (40 mg/d).	◙C (1st trimester) ◙D (2nd/3rd trimester) ❃v **R W** [7]
Lisinopril (Zestril)	**Tab:** 2.5 mg, 5 mg, 10 mg, 20 mg, 30 mg, 40 mg	**Adults:** If possible, d/c diuretic 2-3d prior to therapy. **Initial:** 10 mg qd; 5 mg qd w/ diuretic. **Usual:** 20-40 mg qd. Resume diuretic if BP not controlled. **Max:** 80 mg/d. **Peds: ≥6 yo: Initial:** 0.07 mg/kg qd (up to 5 mg total). Adjust dose based on BP response. **Max:** 0.61 mg/kg qd (40 mg/d).	◙C (1st trimester) ◙D (2nd/3rd trimester) ❃v **R W** [7]
Quinapril HCl (Accupril)	**Tab:** 5 mg, 10 mg, 20 mg, 40 mg	**Adults: Initial:** 10-20 mg qd; 5 mg qd if on diuretic. **Usual:** 20-80 mg/d given qd-bid.	◙C (1st trimester) ◙D (2nd/3rd trimester) ❃v **R W** [7]

NAME	FORM/STRENGTH	DOSAGE	COMMENTS
Ramipril (Altace)	**Tab:** 1.25 mg, 2.5 mg, 5 mg, 10 mg	**Adults: Initial:** 2.5 mg bid, 1.25 mg bid if on diuretic. **Usual:** 2.5-20 mg/d given qd-bid.	◙C (1st trimester) ◙D (2nd/3rd trimester) ❋v **R W** [7]
ACE INHIBITORS/CALCIUM CHANNEL BLOCKERS			
Amlodipine/Benazepril (Lotrel)	**Cap:** 2.5-10 mg, 5-10 mg, 5-20 mg, 5-40 mg, 10-20 mg, 10-40 mg	**Adults: Usual:** If not controlled on monotherapy, or unacceptable edema w/ amlodipine, then 2.5-10 mg amlodipine & 10-80 mg benazepril per day.	◙C (1st trimester) ◙D (2nd/3rd trimester) ❋v **H R W** [7, 24]
ACE INHIBITORS/THIAZIDES			
Enalapril/Hydrochlorothiazide (Vaseretic)	**Tab:** 5-12.5 mg, 10-25 mg	**Adults: Initial (if not controlled on enalapril/HCTZ monotherapy):** 5-12.5 mg tab or 10-25 mg tab qd. **Titrate:** May increase after 2-3 wks. **Max:** 20 mg enalapril/50 mg HCTZ per day. **Replacement Therapy:** Substitute combination for titrated components.	◙C (1st trimester) ◙D (2nd/3rd trimester) ❋v **R W** [7, 24]
Lisinopril/ Hydrochlorothiazide (Prinzide)	**Tab:** 10-12.5 mg, 20-12.5 mg, 20-25 mg	**Adults: Initial (if not controlled w/ lisinopril/HCTZ monotherapy):** 10-12.5 mg tab or 20-12.5 mg tab daily. **Titrate:** May increase after 2-3 wks. **Initial (if controlled on 25 mg HCTZ/d w/ hypokalemia):** 10-12.5 mg tab.	◙C (1st trimester) ◙D (2nd/3rd trimester) ❋v **R W** [7, 24]

		Replacement Therapy: Substitute combination for titrated components.	
Lisinopril/ Hydrochlorothiazide (Zestoretic)	**Tab:** 10-12.5 mg, 20-12.5 mg, 20-25 mg	**Adults: Initial (if not controlled w/ lisinopril/HCTZ monotherapy):** 10-12.5 mg tab or 20-12.5 mg tab daily. **Titrate:** May increase after 2-3 wks. **Initial (if controlled on 25 mg HCTZ/d w/ hypokalemia):** 10-12.5 mg tab. **Replacement Therapy:** Substitute combination for titrated components.	◉C (1st trimester) ◉D (2nd/3rd trimester) ❊v **R W** [7, 24]
Quinapril/Hydrochlorothiazide (Accuretic)	**Tab:** 10-12.5 mg, 20-12.5 mg, 20-25 mg	**Adults: Initial (if not controlled on quinapril monotherapy):** 10-12.5 mg or 20-12.5 mg tab qd. **Titrate:** May increase after 2-3 wks. **Initial (if controlled on 25 mg HCTZ/d w/ hypokalemia):** 10-12.5 mg or 20-12.5 mg tab qd.	◉C (1st trimester) ◉D (2nd/3rd trimester) ❊v **W** [7, 24]

ALDOSTERONE BLOCKER

Eplerenone (Inspra)	**Tab:** 25 mg, 50 mg	**Adults: Initial:** 50 mg qd. May increase to 50 mg bid if inadequate effect. **With Weak CYP3A4 Inhibitors: Initial:** 25 mg qd.	◉B ❊v **R**

ALPHA ADRENERGIC BLOCKERS

Methyldopa	**Tab:** 125 mg, 250 mg, 500 mg	**Adults: Initial:** 250 mg bid-tid x 48h. **Titrate:** Adjust to desired response q2d. **Maint:** 500 mg-2 gm/d given bid-qid. **Max:** 3 gm/d. **Peds: Initial:** 10 mg/kg/d given bid-qid. **Max:** 65 mg/kg/d or 3 gm/d.	◉B ❊>**R**

NAME	FORM/STRENGTH	DOSAGE	COMMENTS
ALPHA/BETA BLOCKERS			
Carvedilol (Coreg, Coreg CR)	**Cap,ER:** 10 mg, 20 mg, 40 mg, 80 mg; **Tab:** 3.125 mg, 6.25 mg, 12.5 mg, 25 mg	**Adults:** Individualize dose. **Tab: Initial:** 6.25 mg bid x 7-14d. **Titrate:** May double dose at 7-14 day intervals. **Max:** 50 mg/d. **Cap,ER: Initial:** 20 mg qd x 7-14d. **Titrate:** May double dose q7-14d as tolerated. **Max:** 80 mg/d. Take w/ food. Monitor dose increases. Take extended-release caps in am & swallow whole.	◙C ❁v
Labetalol HCl	**Inj:** 5 mg/ml; **Tab:** 100 mg, 200 mg, 300 mg	**Adults: PO: Initial:** 100 mg bid. **Titrate:** Increase by 100 mg bid q2-3d. **Maint:** 200-400 mg bid. **Max:** 2400 mg/d. **IV: Initial:** 20 mg over 2 min, then may give 40-80 mg q10min until desired response. **Max:** 300 mg.	◙C ❁>
ANGIOTENSIN II RECEPTOR ANTAGONISTS			
Candesartan Cilexetil (Atacand)	**Tab:** 4 mg, 8 mg, 16 mg, 32 mg	**Adults: Initial:** 16 mg qd. **Usual:** 8-32 mg/d, given qd-bid.	◙C (1st trimester) ◙D (2nd/3rd trimester) ❁v **R W** [9]
Irbesartan (Avapro)	**Tab:** 75 mg, 150 mg, 300 mg	**Adults & Peds: ≥17 yo: Initial:** 150 mg qd. **Titrate:** May increase to 300 mg qd. **Intravascular Volume/Salt Depletion: Initial:** 75 mg qd.	◙C (1st trimester) ◙D (2nd/3rd trimester) ❁v **W** [9]

Losartan Potassium (Cozaar)	**Tab:** 25 mg, 50 mg, 100 mg	**Adults: HTN: Initial:** 50 mg qd. **Usual:** 25-100 mg given qd-bid. **HTN w/ LVH: Initial:** 50 mg qd. Add HCTZ 12.5 mg qd and/or increase losartan to 100 mg qd, followed by an increase in HCTZ to 25 mg qd based on BP response.	C (1st trimester) D (2nd/3rd trimester) v **H W** [9]
Olmesartan Medoxomil (Benicar)	**Tab:** 5 mg, 20 mg, 40 mg	**Adults: Monotherapy Without Volume Depletion: Initial:** 20 mg qd. **Titrate:** May increase to 40 mg qd after 2 wks if needed. May add diuretic if BP not controlled. **Intravascular Volume Depletion (eg, w/ diuretics, impaired renal function):** Lower initial dose; monitor closely.	C (1st trimester) D (2nd/3rd trimester) v **W** [9]
Telmisartan (Micardis)	**Tab:** 20 mg, 40 mg, 80 mg	**Adults: Initial:** 40 mg qd. **Usual:** 20-80 mg qd.	C (1st trimester) D (2nd/3rd trimester) v **W** [9]
Valsartan (Diovan)	**Tab:** 40 mg, 80 mg, 160 mg, 320 mg	**Adults: Initial:** 80 or 160 mg qd. **Titrate:** May increase to 320 mg qd or add diuretic (greater effect than increasing dose >80 mg). **Peds: 6-16 yo: Initial:** 1.3 mg/kg qd (up to 40 mg total). Adjust dose according to BP response. **Max:** 2.7 mg/kg (up to 160 mg) qd. **Hepatic/Severe Renal Impairment:** Use w/ caution. Avoid use in peds w/ GFR <30 ml/min/1.73m^2.	D v **W** [9]

NAME	FORM/STRENGTH	DOSAGE	COMMENTS
ANGIOTENSIN II RECEPTOR ANTAGONISTS/THIAZIDES			
Irbesartan/ Hydrochlorothiazide (Avalide)	**Tab:** 150-12.5 mg, 300-12.5 mg, 300-25 mg	**Adults: Initial:** 150 mg irbesartan qd. **Max:** 300 mg irbesartan qd. **Elderly:** Start at low end of dosing range. **Intravascular Volume/Salt Depletion: Initial:** 75 mg irbesartan qd. Avoid w/ CrCl ≤30 ml/min.	C (1st trimester) D (2nd/3rd trimester) v **R W** [9]
Losartan/Hydrochlorothiazide (Hyzaar)	**Tab:** 50-12.5 mg, 100-12.5, 100-25 mg	**Adults: HTN:** If BP uncontrolled on losartan monotherapy, HCTZ alone or controlled w/ HCTZ 25 mg/d but hypokalemic: 50-12.5 mg tab qd. **Titrate/Max:** If uncontrolled after 3 wks, increase to 2 tabs of 50-12.5 mg qd or 1 tab of 100-25 mg qd. If uncontrolled on losartan 100 mg monotherapy, may switch to 100-12.5 mg qd. **Severe HTN: Initial:** 50-12.5 mg qd. **Titrate/Max:** If inadequate response after 2-4 wks, increase to 1 tab of 100-25 mg qd. **HTN w/ Left Ventricular Hypertrophy: Initial:** Losartan 50 mg qd. If BP reduction inadequate, add HCTZ 12.5 mg or substitute losartan/HCTZ 50-12.5 mg. If additional BP reduction is needed, losartan 100 mg & HCTZ 12.5 mg or losartan/HCTZ 100-12.5 mg may be substituted, followed by losartan 100 mg & HCTZ 25 mg or losartan/HCTZ 100-25 mg.	C (1st trimester) D (2nd/3rd trimester) v **H R W** [9, 24]

Telmisartan/ Hydrochlorothiazide (Micardis HCT)	**Tab:** 40-12.5 mg, 80-12.5 mg, 80-25 mg	**Initial:** If not controlled on 80 mg telmisartan, or 25 mg HCTZ/d, or controlled on 25 mg HCTZ/d but serum K^+ decreased, 80-12.5 mg tab qd. **Max:** 160 mg telmisartan-25 mg HCTZ/d.	C (1st trimester) D(2nd/3rd trimester) > **H R W** [9, 24]
Valsartan/ Hydrochlorothiazide (Diovan HCT)	**Tab:** 80-12.5 mg, 160-12.5 mg, 160-25 mg, 320-12.5 mg, 320-25 mg	**Adults: Add-On/Initial Therapy:** 160-12.5 mg qd. **Titrate:** May increase after 1-2 wks of therapy. **Max:** 320-25 mg. **Replacement Therapy:** May be substituted for titrated components. **CrCl ≤30 ml/min:** Use not recommended.	D v **R W** [9, 24]
BETA BLOCKERS			
Atenolol (Tenormin)	**Tab:** 25 mg, 50 mg, 100 mg	**Adults: Initial:** 50 mg qd. **Titrate:** May increase after 1-2 wks. **Max:** 100 mg qd.	D > **R W** [17]
Bisoprolol Fumarate (Zebeta)	**Tab:** 5 mg, 10 mg	**Adults: Initial:** 2.5-5 mg qd. **Max:** 40 mg/d.	C > **H R**
Metoprolol Succinate (Toprol-XL)	**Tab,ER:** 25 mg, 50 mg, 100 mg, 200 mg	**Adults: Usual:** 25-100 mg qd. **Titrate:** Increase wkly. **Max:** 400 mg qd.	C >
Metoprolol Tartrate (Lopressor)	**Tab:** 50 mg, 100 mg	**Adults: Initial:** 100 mg qd or 50 mg bid. **Titrate:** May increase at wkly (or longer) intervals. **Usual:** 100-450 mg/d. **Max:** 450 mg/d.	C > **W** [17]
Nadolol (Corgard)	**Tab:** 20 mg, 40 mg, 80 mg, 120 mg, 160 mg	**Adults: Initial:** 40 mg qd. **Titrate:** Increase by 40-80 mg. **Max:** 320 mg/d.	C v **R W** [17]

NAME	FORM/STRENGTH	DOSAGE	COMMENTS
Nebivolol (Bystolic)	**Tab:** 2.5 mg, 5 mg, 10 mg, 20 mg	**Adults: Monotherapy/Combination Therapy: Initial:** 5 mg qd. **Titrate:** May increase dose at 2 wk intervals if needed. **Max:** 40 mg qd. **Hepatic Impairment/CrCl <30 ml/min:** 2.5 mg qd; upward titration may be performed cautiously.	C v **H R**
Propranolol HCl (Inderal)	**Tab:** 10 mg, 20 mg, 40 mg, 60 mg, 80 mg	**Adults: Initial:** 40 mg bid. **Maint:** 120-240 mg qd. **Peds: Initial:** 1mg/kg/d. **Usual:** 1-2mg/kg bid. **Max:** 16 mg/kg/d.	C >

BETA BLOCKERS/THIAZIDES

NAME	FORM/STRENGTH	DOSAGE	COMMENTS
Atenolol/Chlorthalidone (Tenoretic)	**Tab:** 50-25 mg, 100-25 mg	**Initial:** 50-25 mg tab qd. **Titrate:** May increase to 100-25 mg tab qd.	D > **R**

CALCIUM CHANNEL BLOCKER/ANGIOTENSIN II RECEPTOR ANTAGONIST

NAME	FORM/STRENGTH	DOSAGE	COMMENTS
Amlodipine Besylate/ Olmesartan Medoxomil (Azor)	**Tab:** 5-20mg, 10-20mg, 5-40mg, 10-40mg	**Adults: Replacement Therapy:** May substitute for individually titrated components for patients on amlodipine & olmesartan. When substituting for individual components, the dose of 1 or both components may be increased if needed. **Add-On Therapy:** May use as add-on therapy when not adequately controlled on amlodipine or olmesartan. May increase dose after 2 wks to max of 10-40mg qd.	C (1st trimester) D (2nd/3rd trimester) v **W** [9]

Amlodipine Besylate/ Valsartan (Exforge)	**Tab:** 5-160 mg, 5-320 mg, 10-160 mg, 10-320 mg	**Adults: Initial Therapy:** 5-160 mg qd. **Add-On/ Replacement Therapy:** May be substituted for titrated components. **Titrate:** If inadequate control, may increase after 1-2 wks of therapy. **Max:** 10-320 mg qd. **Elderly: Initial:** 2.5 mg amlodipine.	D v **W** [9]

CALCIUM CHANNEL BLOCKER/HMG-COA REDUCTASE INHIBITOR

Amlodipine Besylate/ Atorvastatin Calcium (Caduet)	**Tab:** 2.5-10 mg, 2.5-20 mg, 2.5-40 mg, 5-10 mg, 5-20 mg, 5-40 mg, 5-80 mg, 10-10 mg, 10-20 mg, 10-40 mg, 10-80 mg	Dosing based on appropriate combination of recommendations for monotherapies. **Amlodipine: Adults: Initial:** 5 mg qd. Titrate over 7-14d. **Max:** 10 mg qd. **Small, Fragile, or Elderly/Hepatic Dysfunction/ Concomitant Antihypertensive: Initial:** 2.5 mg qd. **Peds: ≥10 yo (postmenarchal):** 2.5-5 mg qd. **Atorvastatin:** See under Antilipidemic Agents for dosing.	X v **H**

CALCIUM CHANNEL BLOCKERS (DIHYDROPYRIDINES)

Amlodipine Besylate (Norvasc)	**Tab:** 2.5 mg, 5 mg, 10 mg	**Adults: Initial:** 5 mg qd. **Max:** 10 mg qd. **Peds: 6-17 yo:** 2.5-5 mg qd.	C v**H**
Isradipine (DynaCirc, DynaCirc CR)	**Cap:** 2.5 mg, 5 mg; **Tab,ER:** (CR) 5 mg, 10 mg	**Adults: Initial: Cap:** 2.5 mg bid. **Tab,ER:** 5 mg qd. **Titrate:** Increase by 5 mg/d q2-4wks. **Max:** 20 mg/d.	C v
Nicardipine (Cardene SR)	**Cap:** 20 mg, 30 mg; **Cap,ER:** (SR) 30 mg, 45 mg, 60 mg	**Adults: Initial:** 20 mg tid. **Usual:** 20-40 mg tid. **Cap,ER: Initial:** 30 mg bid. **Usual:** 30-60 mg bid.	C v **H**

NAME	FORM/STRENGTH	DOSAGE	COMMENTS
Nifedipine (Procardia XL)	**Tab,ER:** 30 mg, 60 mg, 90 mg	**Adults: Initial:** 30-60 mg qd. **Titrate:** May increase over 7-14d. **Max:** 120 mg/d	C >
CALCIUM CHANNEL BLOCKERS (NON-DIHYDROPYRIDINES)			
Diltiazem HCl (Cardizem CD, Cardizem LA, Cartia XT)	**Cap,ER:** (Cardizem CD/Cartia XT) 120 mg, 180 mg, 240 mg, 300 mg, (Cardizem CD) 360 mg; **Tab,ER:** (Cardizem LA) 120 mg, 180 mg, 240 mg, 300 mg, 360 mg, 420 mg	**Adults: Cardizem CD/Cartia XT: Initial:** 180-240 mg qd. **Titrate:** Adjust at 2-wk intervals. **Usual:** 240-360 mg/d. **Max:** 480 mg/d. **Cardizem LA: Initial:** 180-240 mg qd. **Titrate:** Adjust at 2-wk intervals. **Max:** 540 mg qd.	C v
Diltiazem HCl (Dilacor XR, Diltia XT)	**Cap,ER:** 120 mg, 180 mg, 240 mg	**Adults: Initial:** 180-240 mg qd. **Usual:** 180-480 mg qd. **Max:** 540 mg/d. **≥60 yo: Initial:** 120 mg qd.	C v
Diltiazem HCl (Taztia XT, Tiazac)	**Cap,ER:** (Taztia XT/Tiazac) 120 mg, 180 mg, 240 mg, 300 mg, 360 mg, (Tiazac) 420 mg	**Adults: Initial:** 120-240 mg qd. Titrate: Adjust at 2-wk intervals. **Usual:** 120-540 mg qd. **Max:** 540 mg/d.	C v
Verapamil (Calan SR)	**Tab,ER:** 120 mg, 180 mg, 240 mg	**Adults: Initial:** 180 mg qam. **Titrate:** Increase to 240 mg qam, then 180 mg bid; or 240 mg + 120 mg qpm, then 240 mg q12h.	C v
Verapamil (Calan)	**Tab:** 40 mg, 80 mg, 120 mg	**Adults: Initial:** 80 mg tid. **Usual:** 360-480 mg/d.	C v H

Drug	Forms	Dosage	Ratings
Verapamil (Covera-HS)	**Tab,ER:** 180 mg, 240 mg	**Adults: Initial:** 180 mg qhs. **Titrate:** Increase to 240 mg qhs, then 360 mg qhs, then 480 mg qhs.	C v
Verapamil (Verelan PM)	**Cap,ER:** 100 mg, 200 mg, 300 mg	**Adults: Initial:** 200 mg qhs. **Titrate:** Increase to 300 mg qhs, then 400 mg qhs.	C v **H**
Verapamil (Verelan)	**Cap,ER:** 120 mg, 180 mg, 240 mg, 360 mg,	**Adults: Usual:** 240 mg qam. **Titrate:** Increase by 120 mg qam. **Max:** 480 mg qam.	C v **H**
DIURETIC (LOOP)			
Furosemide (Lasix)	(Generic) **Inj:** 10 mg/ml; **Sol:** 10 mg/ml, 40 mg/ 5 ml; **Tab:** 20 mg, 40 mg, 80 mg; (Lasix) **Tab:** 20 mg, 40 mg, 80 mg	**Adults: Initial:** 40 mg bid. **Maint:** Adjust according to response.	C > **W** 8
Torsemide (Demadex)	**Tab:** 5 mg, 10 mg, 20 mg, 100 mg	**Adults: Initial:** 5 mg qd. **Maint:** May increase to 10 mg qd after 4-6 wks.	B >
DIURETICS (POTASSIUM SPARING)			
Spironolactone (Aldactone)	**Tab:** 25 mg, 50 mg, 100 mg	**Adults: Initial:** 50-100 mg/d as single or divided doses. **Maint:** After 2 wks, adjust by response.	C v **W** 16
Triamterene (Dyrenium)	**Cap:** 50 mg, 100 mg	**Adults: Initial:** 100 mg bid. **Max:** 300 mg/d.	C v **W** 88

NAME	FORM/STRENGTH	DOSAGE	COMMENTS
DIURETICS (POTASSIUM SPARING/THIAZIDE)			
Spironolactone/ Hydrochlorothiazide (Aldactazide)	**Tab:** 25-25 mg, 50-50 mg	**Adults:** 50-100 mg/d per component qd or in divided doses.	C v Not for initial therapy. **W** [16]
Triamterene/ Hydrochlorothiazide (Maxzide, Maxzide-25)	**Tab:** 37.5-25 mg, 75-50 mg	**Adults: Usual:** (37.5-25 mg) 1-2 tabs qd. (75-50 mg) 1 tab qd.	C v
DIURETICS (QUINAZOLINE)			
Metolazone (Zaroxolyn)	**Tab:** 2.5 mg, 5 mg, 10 mg	**Adults: Initial:** 2.5-5 mg qd. **Elderly:** Start at low end of dosing range.	B v Rapid & slow formulations not equivalent.
DIURETICS (THIAZIDE)			
Chlorothiazide (Diuril)	**Susp:** (Diuril) 250 mg/ 5 ml; **Tab:** (Generic) 250 mg, 500 mg	**Adults: Initial:** 0.5-1 gm qd or in divided doses. **Max:** 2 gm/d. **Peds: Usual:** 10-20 mg/kg/d given qd-bid. **Max: 2-12 yo:** 1 gm/d. **≤2 yo:** 375 mg/d. **<6 mths:** 15 mg/kg bid.	C v
Hydrochlorothiazide	**Cap:** 12.5 mg; **Tab:** 25 mg, 50 mg, 100 mg	**Adults: Initial:** 25 mg qd. **Max:** 50 mg/d. **Peds:** 1-2 mg/kg/d given qd-bid. **Max: Infants up to 2 yo:** 37.5 mg/d. **2-12 yrs:** 100 mg/d. **<6 mths:** Up to 1.5 mg/kg bid may be required.	B v

RENIN INHIBITORS

Aliskiren (Tekturna)	**Tab:** 150 mg, 300 mg	**Adults: Usual:** 150 mg qd. **Titrate:** May increase to 300 mg/d if needed. High-fat meals decrease absorption.	◉C (1st trimester) ◉D (2nd/3rd trimester) ❊v **W**[9]

RENIN INHIBITORS/THIAZIDES

Aliskiren/Hydrochlorothiazide (Tekturna HCT)	**Tab:** 150-12.5 mg, 150-25 mg, 300-12.5 mg, 300-25 mg	**Adults: Usual:** 150 mg qd. **Titrate:** May increase to 300 mg/d if needed. High-fat meals decrease absorption.	◉D ❊v **W**[9]

VASODILATORS (PERIPHERAL)

Hydralazine	**Inj:** 20 mg/ml; **Tab:** 10 mg, 25 mg, 50 mg, 100 mg	**Adults: PO: Initial:** 10 mg qid x 2-4d. **Titrate:** Increase to 25 mg qid x 3-5d, then 50 mg qid. **Max:** 300 mg/d. **IM/IV:** 20-40 mg, repeat as necessary. **Peds: Initial:** 0.75 mg/kg/d given qid. **Titrate:** Increase gradually over 3-4 wks. **Max:** 7.5 mg/kg/d or 200 mg/d.	◉C ❊>
Minoxidil	**Tab:** 2.5 mg, 10 mg	**Adults & Peds: >12 yo: Initial:** 5 mg qd. **Maint:** 10-40 mg qd. **Max:** 100 mg/d. **<12 yo: Initial:** 0.2 mg/kg qd. **Maint:** 0.25-1 mg/kg/d. **Max:** 50 mg/d.	◉C ❊v Pericardial effusion. Exacerbates angina.

NAME	FORM/STRENGTH	DOSAGE	COMMENTS
Clonidine HCl (Catapres, Catapres-TTS)	**Tab:** 0.1 mg, 0.2 mg, 0.3 mg; **Patch:** (TTS) 0.1 mg/24 h, 0.2 mg/24 h, 0.3 mg/24 h	**Adults: Patch: Initial:** 0.1 mg/24h patch wkly. **Titrate:** May increase after 1-2 wks. **Max:** 0.6 mg/24h. **Tab: Initial:** 0.1 mg bid. **Titrate:** May increase by 0.1 mg wkly. **Usual:** 0.2-0.6 mg/d. **Max:** 2.4 mg/d.	C > R
Doxazosin Mesylate (Cardura)	**Tab:** 1 mg, 2 mg, 4 mg, 8 mg	**Adults: Initial:** 1 mg qd. **Titrate:** May double dose q1-2wks. **Max:** 8 mg/d.	C >
Terazosin HCl (Hytrin)	**Cap:** 1 mg, 2 mg, 5 mg, 10 mg	**Adults: Initial:** 1 mg qhs. **Titrate:** Increase stepwise as needed. **Usual:** 10 mg qd. May increase to 20 mg/d after 4-6 wks. **Max:** 20 mg/d. If d/c for several days, restart at initial dose.	C > Syncope w/ 1st dose.

DERMATOLOGY

Acne Preparations

ANTIBACTERIAL/KERATOLYTIC

NAME	FORM/STRENGTH	DOSAGE	COMMENTS
Adapalene/Benzoyl Peroxide (Epiduo)	**Gel:** 0.1%-2.5%	**Adults & Peds: ≥12 yo:** Apply pea-sized amount to affected area(s) of face and/or trunk qd after washing.	C >
Benzoyl Peroxide (Benzac AC)	**Gel:** 5%, 10%	**Adults:** Apply to clean affected area(s) qd-bid.	C >
Benzoyl Peroxide (Benzac AC)	**Sol:** 5%, 10%	**Adults:** Wash area qd-bid; rinse & dry.	C >

Benzoyl Peroxide (Brevoxyl)	**Gel:** 4%, 8%; **Lot (Cleanser/Wash):** 4%, 8%	**Adults & Peds: ≥12 yo: Gel:** Apply to clean affected area(s) qd-bid. **Lot:** Shake well. Wet affected area(s) & wash qd x 1st wk, then bid as tolerated.	C >
Benzoyl Peroxide (Triaz)	**Cleanser, Pads:** 3%, 6%, 9%; **Foaming Cloths:** 6%	**Adults:** (Cleanser) Wash affected area(s) for 10-20 sec qd-bid. Pat dry. (Foaming Cloths/Pads) Apply qd-bid to affected area(s) after washing w/ mild cleanser.	C >

ANTI-INFECTIVES AND COMBINATIONS

Benzoyl Peroxide/ Clindamycin (BenzaClin)	**Gel:** 5%-1%	**Adults & Peds: ≥12 yo:** Apply to affected area bid.	C v
Benzoyl Peroxide/ Clindamycin (Duac)	**Gel:** 5%-1%	**Adults & Peds: ≥12 yo:** Apply qpm.	C v
Clindamycin Phosphate/ Benzoyl Peroxide (Acanya)	**Gel:** 1.2%-2.5%	**Adults & Peds: ≥12 yo:** Apply pea-sized amount to face qd. Minimize sun exposure. Not for oral, ophthalmic, or intravaginal use.	C v
Clindamycin Phosphate/ Tretinoin (Ziana)	**Gel:** 1.2%-0.025%	**Adults & Peds: ≥12 yo:** Apply pea-sized amt to entire face qd at bedtime. Avoid eyes, mouth, angles of nose, or mucous membranes. Not for oral, ophthalmic, or intravaginal use.	C v
Clindamycin Phosphate (Evoclin)	**Foam:** 1%	**Adults & Peds ≥12 yo:** Apply to affected area once daily.	B >

NAME	FORM/STRENGTH	DOSAGE	COMMENTS
Clindamycin (Cleocin T)	**Gel, Lot, Sol, Swab:** 1%	**Adults & Peds: ≥12 yo:** Apply to affected area bid.	B v
Dapsone (Aczone)	**Gel:** 5%	**Adults & Peds: ≥12 yo:** Apply to affected area bid.	C v
Erythromycin	**Swabs:** 2%	**Adults:** Apply to affected area bid (qam & qpm).	B >
Minocycline HCl (Solodyn)	**Tab,ER:** 45 mg, 90 mg, 135 mg	**Acne Vulgaris: Adults & Peds: ≥12 yo:** 1 mg/kg qd x 12 wks.	D v **R**
Sodium Sulfacetamide/Sulfur (Rosac)	**Cre:** 10%-5%	**Adults & Peds: ≥12 yo:** Apply thin film qd-tid.	C >
Sodium Sulfacetamide/Sulfur (Plexion, Plexion SCT, Plexion TS)	**Cleanser:** 10%-5%; **Cre:** (SCT) 10%-5%; **Sus,Top:** (TS) 10%-5%; **Pads:** 10%-5%	**Adults & Peds: ≥12 yo: Cleanser/Pads:** Wash qd-bid. Massage into skin x 10-20 sec, then rinse & dry. **TS:** Apply qd-tid. **SCT:** Apply to wet skin. Rinse off w/ water after 10 min or if dry.	C > CI in kidney disease.
Sodium Sulfacetamide/Sulfur (Rosula)	**Cleanser, Gel:** 10%-5%	**Adults & Peds: ≥12 yo: Gel:** Apply thin film qd-tid. **Cleanser:** Wash for 10-20 sec qd-bid.	C >
Sodium Sulfacetamide/Urea (Rosula NS)	**Swab:** 10%-10%	**Adults & Peds: ≥12 yo:** Apply to affected area qd-bid.	C >
Tetracycline HCl (Sumycin)	**Cap:** 250 mg, 500 mg; **Susp:** 125 mg/5 ml	**Severe Acne: Adults & Peds: >8 yo:** 1 gm/d in divided doses. **Maint:** After improvement, 125-500 mg/d.	D v **R**

DICARBOXYLIC ACID

Azelaic Acid (Azelex)	**Cre:** 20%	**Adults & Peds: ≥12 yo:** Apply to affected area bid (qam & qpm).	B >
Azelaic Acid (Finacea)	**Gel:** 15%	**Adults:** Wash & dry skin. Apply to affected area bid (qam & qpm) x up to 12 wks.	B >

ESTROGEN/PROGESTIN COMBINATION

Ethinyl Estradiol/ Drospirenone (YAZ)	**Tab:** 0.02-3 mg	**Moderate Acne Vulgaris: Adults & Peds: ≥14 yo:** 1 tab qd x 28d, then repeat. Start 1st Sunday after menses begin or 1st day of menses.	X v
Ethinyl Estradiol/ Norethindrone (Estrostep FE)	**Tab:** (Phase 1) 35 mcg-1 mg; (Phase 2) 30 mcg-1 mg; (Phase 3) 20 mcg-1 mg and 75 mg ferrous fumarate	**Women: ≥15 yo:** 1 tab qd. See PI for initiation instructions.	X v
Ethinyl Estradiol/ Norgestimate (Ortho Tri-Cyclen)	**Tab:** (Phase 1) 35 mcg-0.18 mg; (Phase 2) 35 mcg-0.215 mg; (Phase 3) 35 mcg-0.25 mg	**Women: ≥15 yo:** 1 tab qd x 28d, then repeat. Start 1st Sunday after menses begin or 1st day of menses.	X v

NAME	FORM/STRENGTH	DOSAGE	COMMENTS
RETINOID-LIKE AGENTS			
Adapalene (Differin)	**Cre, Gel, Sol:** 0.1%	**Adults & Peds: ≥12 yo:** Apply to affected area qhs. Avoid eyes, lips & mucous membranes.	C >
RETINOIDS			
Isotretinoin (Accutane, Amnesteem, Claravis, Sotret)	**Cap:** (Accutane) 10 mg, 20 mg, 40 mg; (Sotret) 10 mg, 20 mg, 30 mg, 40 mg	**Adults & Peds: ≥12 yo: Initial:** 0.5-1 mg/kg/d given bid x 15-20 wks w/ food. Repeat if needed after 2 mths off of drug.	X v **W** [52]
Tazarotene (Tazorac)	**Cre:** 0.1%; **Gel:** 0.1%	**Adults & Peds: ≥12 yo:** Apply to affected area qpm.	X >
Tretinoin (Retin-A, Retin-A Micro)	**Cre:** 0.025%, 0.05%, 0.1%; **Gel:** 0.01%, 0.025%, (Micro) 0.04%, 0.1%; **Sol:** 0.05%	**Retin-A: Adults:** Apply to affected area qhs. **Retin-A Micro: Adults & Peds: ≥12 yo:** Apply to affected area qhs.	C >

Anti-Infective Agents

ANTIBACTERIALS

NAME	FORM/STRENGTH	DOSAGE	COMMENTS
Gentamicin	**Cre, Oint:** 0.1%	**Adults & Peds: >1 yo:** Apply to lesions tid-qid.	N >

Metronidazole (MetroCream, MetroGel, MetroLotion)	**Cre, Lot:** 0.75%; **Gel:** 0.75%, 1%	**Rosacea: Adults:** (Cre, Gel 0.75%, Lot) Wash affected area(s) then apply bid (am & pm). (Gel 1%) Wash affected area(s) then apply qd.	B v
Mupirocin Calcium (Bactroban Nasal)	**Oint:** 2%	**Nasal Colonization w/ MRSA: Adults & Peds: ≥12 yo:** Apply 1/2 tube per nostril bid x 5d.	B v
Mupirocin (Bactroban)	**Cre, Oint:** 2%	**S.aureus/S.pyogenes: Adults & Peds ≥2 mths: Oint:** Apply tid. **≥3 mths: Cre:** Apply tid x 10d.	B v
Polymyxin B Sulfate/ Bacitracin Zinc/Neomycin (Neosporin Ointment)	**Oint:** 5,000 U-400 U-3.5 mg/gm	**Prevent Infection in Minor Cuts, Scrapes, & Burns: Adults & Peds:** Apply to affected area qd-tid.	N >
Retapamulin (Altabax)	**Oint:** 1%	**Impetigo: Adults & Peds: ≥9 mths:** Apply thin layer (up to 100 cm^2 in total area for adults or 2% total BSA for peds) bid x 5d. May cover w/ sterile bandage or gauze.	B >
Sodium Sulfacetamide/Sulfur (Plexion, Plexion SCT, Plexion TS)	**Cleanser:** 10%-5%; **Cre:** (SCT) 10%-5%; **Sus,Top:** (TS) 10%-5%; **Pads:** 10%-5%	**Adults & Peds: ≥12 yo: Seborrheic Dermatitis: Cleanser/ Pads:** Wash qd-bid. Massage into skin x 10-20 sec, then rinse & dry. **TS:** Apply qd-tid. **SCT:** Apply to wet skin. Rinse off w/ water after 10 min or if dry.	C > CI in kidney disease.
Sodium Sulfacetamide/Sulfur (Rosula)	**Cleanser, Gel:** 10%-5%	**Seborrheic Dermatitis: Adults & Peds: ≥12 yo: Gel;** Apply thin film qd-tid. **Cleanser:** Wash for 10-20 sec qd-bid.	C >

NAME	FORM/STRENGTH	DOSAGE	COMMENTS
ANTIFUNGALS			
Butenafine (Mentax)	**Cre:** 1%	**Adults & Peds: ≥12 yo: Interdigital Tinea Pedis:** Apply bid x 7d or qd x 4 wks. **Tinea Corporis/Tinea Cruris/Tinea Versicolor:** Apply qd x 2 wks.	B >
Ciclopirox (Loprox, Loprox TS)	**Cre, Gel:** 0.77%; **Shampoo:** 1%; **Susp:** (TS) 0.77%	**Seborrheic Dermatitis: Adults:** (Shampoo) Apply about 5 ml (up to 10 ml for long hair) to wet scalp. Lather & rinse off after 3 min. Repeat twice weekly x 4 wks, at least 3 days apart. **Tinea Pedis/Tinea Cruris/Tinea Corporis/Cutaneous Candidiasis/Tinea Versicolor: Adults:** (Cre/Gel/Susp) Massage affected & surrounding areas bid (am & pm) up to 4 wks. **Peds: ≥10 yo:** (Cre/Susp) Massage affected & surrounding areas bid (am & pm) up to 4 wks. Gel or Shampoo not recommended in peds <16 yo.	B >
Clotrimazole	**Cre, Sol:** 1%	**Candidiasis/Tinea Versicolor: Adults & Peds:** Apply qam & qpm.	B >
Ketoconazole	**Cre:** 2%	**Adults: Tinea Cruris/Tinea Corporis/Tinea Versicolor/Cutaneous Candidiasis:** Apply qd x 2 wks. **Tinea Pedis:** Apply qd x 6 wks. **Seborrheic Dermatitis:** Apply bid x 4 wks.	C v
Ketoconazole (Extina)	**Foam:** 2%	**Seborrheic Dermatitis: Adults/Peds: ≥12 yo:** Apply to affected area(s) bid x 4 wks.	C >
Ketoconazole (Nizoral A-D)	**Shampoo:** 1%	**Dandruff: Adults & Peds: >12 yo:** Apply to wet hair q3-4d x up to 8 wks if needed.	C >

Ketoconazole (Nizoral Shampoo)	**Shampoo:** 2%	**Tinea Versicolor: Adults:** Apply to damp skin of affected area, lather & rinse off after 5 min.	◉C ❋>
Ketoconazole (Xolegel)	**Gel:** 2%	**Adults & Peds: ≥12 yo:** Apply qd to affected area x 2 wks.	◉C ❋>
Miconazole (Monistat-Derm)	**Cre:** 2%	**Adults: Tinea Cruris/Tinea Corporis/Cutaneous Candidiasis:** Apply qam & qpm x 2 wks. **Tinea Pedis:** Apply qam & qpm x 4 wks. **Tinea Versicolor:** Apply qd x 2 wks.	◉N ❋>
Naftifine (Naftin)	**Cre, Gel:** 1%	**Tinea Pedis/Tinea Cruris/Tinea Corporis: Adults: Cre:** Apply qd. **Gel:** Apply qam & qpm.	◉B ❋>
Nystatin (Nystop)	**Pow:** 100,000 U/gm	***Candida* Species: Adults & Peds:** Apply to lesions bid-tid.	◉N ❋>
Oxiconazole (Oxistat)	**Cre, Lot:** 1%	**Adults: Tinea Cruris/Tinea Corporis: Cre/Lot:** Apply qd-bid x 2 wks. **Tinea Pedis: Cre/Lot:** Apply qd-bid x 4 wks. **Tinea Versicolor: Cre:** Apply qd x 2 wks. **Peds: ≥12 yo: Cre:** Same as adult dose.	◉B ❋>
Sertaconazole Nitrate (Ertaczo)	**Cre:** 2%	**Interdigital Tinea Pedis: Adults & Peds: ≥12 yo:** Apply bid x 4 wks. Re-evaluate if no improvement after 2 wks.	◉C ❋>
Terbinafine (Lamisil AT)	**Cre:** 1%	**Adults & Peds: ≥12 yo: Tinea Pedis:** Apply to area bid x 1 wk (interdigital) or x 2 wks (bottom/sides of foot). **Tinea Cruris/Tinea Corporis:** Apply to area qd x 1 wk. Wash & dry area before applying.	◉N ❋>

NAME	FORM/STRENGTH	DOSAGE	COMMENTS
ANTIVIRALS			
Acyclovir (Zovirax Ointment)	**Oint:** 5%	**Herpes Genitalis/Herpes Labialis: Adults:** Apply q3h, 6x/d x 7d. Initiate w/ 1st sign/symptom.	B >
Acyclovir Cre (Zovirax Cream)	**Cre:** 5%	**Herpes Labialis: Adults & Peds: ≥12 yo:** Apply 5x/d x 4d.	B >
Imiquimod (Aldara)	**Cre:** 5%	**Actinic Keratosis: Adults:** Apply 2x/wk qhs to area on face/scalp (but not both concurrently). Wash off after 8h. **Max:** 16 wks of therapy. **Genital/Perianal Warts (Condyloma Acuminata): Adults & Peds: ≥12 yo:** Apply 3x/wk qhs. Wash off after 6-10h. Use until warts clear. **Max:** 16 wks of therapy. Do not occlude treatment area.	C >
Penciclovir (Denavir)	**Cre:** 1%	**Recurrent Herpes Labialis (Cold Sores): Adults:** Apply q2h w/a x 4d. Start w/ earliest sign or symptom.	B v
Podofilox (Condylox)	**Gel, Sol:** 0.5%	**External Genital Warts (Condyloma Acuminata) (Gel/Sol), Perianal Warts (Gel): Adults:** Apply q12h x 3d, then withhold x 4d. May repeat up to 4 treatment cycles. **Max:** 0.5 gm/d or 0.5 ml/d & <10 cm^2 of wart tissue.	C v

Anti-Infective Combinations

NAME	FORM/STRENGTH	DOSAGE	COMMENTS
ANTIBIOTIC/ANTI-INFLAMMATORY AGENTS			
Clotrimazole/Betamethasone (Lotrisone)	**Cre, Lot:** 1%-0.05%	**Adults: ≥17 yo: Tinea Cruris/Tinea Corporis:** Apply bid x 2 wks. **Tinea Pedis:** Apply bid x 4 wks.	C >

Hydrocortisone/Iodoquinol (Alcortin)	**Gel:** 2%-1%	**Adults & Peds:** **≥12 yo:** Apply to affected area(s) tid-qid.	C v
Neomycin/Polymyxin B/ Bacitracin/Hydrocortisone (Cortisporin)	**Oint:** 3.5 mg-5,000 U-400 U-1%	**Adults:** Apply to affected area bid-qid up to 7d.	C >
Neomycin/Polymyxin B/ Hydrocortisone (Cortisporin)	**Cre:** 3.5 mg-10,000 U- 0.5%	**Adults:** Apply to affected area bid-qid up to 7d.	C >
Nystatin/Triamcinolone	**Cre, Oint:** 100,000 U-1 mg/gm	**Adults & Peds:** Apply to affected area bid.	C >

Antipruritics/Anti-Inflammatory Agents

HISTAMINE RECEPTOR BLOCKER & COMBINATIONS

Doxepin HCl (Zonalon)	**Cre:** 5%	**Adults:** Apply thin film qid up to 8d. Wait at least 3-4h between applications. Avoid occlusive dressings.	B v

TOPICAL CORTICOSTEROIDS/LOCAL ANESTHETIC AGENTS

Hydrocortisone Acetate/ Pramoxine HCl (Analpram-HC)	**Aer:** 1%-1%; **Cre:** 1%-1%, 1%-2.5%; **Lot:** 1%-2.5%	**Anal Dermatoses: Adults & Peds:** Apply to affected area tid-qid. Use applicator for anal administration w/ ProctoFoam-HC.	C >
Hydrocortisone Acetate/ Pramoxine HCl (ProctoFoam-HC)	**Aer:** 1%-1%; **Cre:** 1%-1%, 1%-2.5%; **Lot:** 1%-2.5%	**Anal Dermatoses: Adults & Peds:** Apply to affected area tid-qid. Use applicator for anal administration w/ ProctoFoam-HC.	C >

NAME	FORM/STRENGTH	DOSAGE	COMMENTS
MISCELLANEOUS			
Pimecrolimus (Elidel)	**Cre:** 1%	**Moderate-Severe Atopic Dermatitis: ≥2 yo:** Apply bid. D/C upon resolution.	C v
Tacrolimus (Protopic)	**Oint:** 0.03%, 0.1%	**Moderate-Severe Atopic Dermatitis: Adults: ≥16 yo:** Apply bid. **Peds: 2-15 yo:** Apply 0.03% oint bid. Continue x 1 wk after symptoms clear.	C v

Psoriasis

NAME	FORM/STRENGTH	DOSAGE	COMMENTS
ANTIMETABOLITES			
Methotrexate	**Inj:** 20 mg, 1 gm, 25 mg/ml; **Tab:** 2.5 mg, 5 mg, 7.5 mg, 10 mg,15 mg	**Adults: Usual:** 10-25 mg/wk PO/IV/IM until adequate response achieved or use 2.5 mg q12h x 3 doses. **Titrate:** May increase gradually. **Max:** 30 mg/wk.	X v **W** 19
IMMUNOSUPPRESSIVES			
Alefacept (Amevive)	**Inj:** (IV) 7.5 mg, (IM) 15 mg	**Adults:** 7.5 mg IV bolus or 15 mg IM once wkly x 12 wks. May retreat x 12 wks if >12 wk interval since 1st course. Adjust dose, d/c, and/or retreat, based on CD4+ T-lymphocyte counts.	B v CI w/ HIV.
Cyclosporine (Neoral)	**Cap:** 25 mg, 100 mg; **Sol:** 100 mg/ml	**Adults: Initial:** 1.25 mg/kg bid x 4 wks. **Maint:** If no improvement, increase q2wks by 0.5 mg/kg/d. **Max:** 4 mg/kg/d.	C v **W** 90

MONOCLONAL ANTIBODY

Infliximab (Remicade)	**Inj:** 100 mg	**Plaque Psoriasis: Adults:** 5 mg/kg IV infusion; repeat at 2 & 6 wks. **Maint:** 5 mg/kg q8wks.	B v **W** 86

PSORALENS

Methoxsalen (Oxsoralen-Ultra)	**Cap:** 10 mg	**Adults: Initial: <30 kg:** 10 mg. **30-50 kg:** 20 mg. **51-65 kg:** 30 mg. **66-80 kg:** 40 mg. **81-90 kg:** 50 mg. **91-115 kg:** 60 mg. **>115 kg:** 70 mg. Take 1.5-2h before UVA exposure w/ a low fat meal or milk. **Titrate:** May increase by 10 mg after 15th treatment under certain conditions. **Max:** Do not treat more often than qod.	C v **W** 21

RETINOIDS

Tazarotene (Tazorac)	**Cre:** 0.05%, 0.1%; **Gel:** 0.05%, 0.1%	**Adults & Peds: ≥12 yo:** Apply to lesions qpm. Apply gel to no more than 20% of BSA.	X >

STEROIDS, TOPICAL

Clobetasol Propionate (Clobex)	**Lot:** 0.05%; **Shampoo:** 0.05%; **Spr:** 0.05%	**Adults: ≥18 yo: Lot:** Apply bid for up to 2 consecutive wks. Reassess after 2 wks; may repeat for additional 2 wks. Limit treatment to 4 wks. **Max:** 50 gm/wk or 50 ml/wk. **Shampoo:** Apply thin film daily to dry scalp for up to 4 consecutive wks. Leave in place for 15 min before lathering & rinsing. **Spr:** Spr on affected area(s) bid. Rub in gently &	C >

Continued on Next Page

NAME	FORM/STRENGTH	DOSAGE	COMMENTS
Clobetasol Propionate (Clobex) *Continued*		completely. Reassess after 2 wks. Limit treatment to 4 wks. **Max:** 50 gm/wk.	
Fluocinonide (Vanos)	**Cre:** 0.1%	**Adults:** Apply qd-bid. **Max:** 60 gm/wk. Do not exceed 2 wks.	C v

TUMOR NECROSIS FACTOR RECEPTOR BLOCKER

NAME	FORM/STRENGTH	DOSAGE	COMMENTS
Etanercept (Enbrel)	**Inj:** 25 mg, 50 mg/ml	**Plaque Psoriasis: Adults: Initial:** 50 mg SC twice wkly given 3-4 days apart x 3 mths. May begin w/ 25-50 mg/wk. **Maint:** 50 mg/wk.	B v **W** [86]

Miscellaneous

ALPHA-REDUCTASE INHIBITORS

NAME	FORM/STRENGTH	DOSAGE	COMMENTS
Finasteride (Propecia)	**Tab:** 1 mg	**Androgenetic Alopecia: Adults:** 1 mg qd.	X v

VASODILATORS (PERIPHERAL)

NAME	FORM/STRENGTH	DOSAGE	COMMENTS
Minoxidil (Rogaine Extra Strength)	**Sol:** 5%	**Adults:** ≥**18 yo:** Apply 1 ml bid directly onto scalp in hair loss area.	N >

Anticholinergics

Ipratropium Bromide (Atrovent Nasal)	**Spr:** (0.03%) 21 mcg/spr, (0.06%) 42 mcg/spr	**Rhinorrhea w/ Common Cold: Adults & Peds: ≥12 yo:** (0.06%) 2 spr/nostril tid-qid. **5-11 yo:** (0.06%) 2 spr/nostril tid. **Rhinorrhea w/ Seasonal Allergic Rhinitis: Adults & Peds: ≥5 yo:** (0.06%) 2 spr/nostril qid. **Rhinorrhea w/ Allergic/Nonallergic Perennial Rhinitis: Adults & Peds: ≥6 yo:** (0.03%) 2 spr/nostril bid-tid.	B >

Antihistamines

Azelastine HCl (Astelin)	**Spr:** 137 mcg/spr	**Seasonal Allergic/Vasomotor Rhinitis: Adults & Peds: ≥12 yo:** 2 sprays per nostril bid. **5-11 yo: Seasonal Allergic Rhinitis:** 1 spray per nostril bid.	C >
Azelastine HCl (Astepro)	**Spr:** 137 mcg	**Seasonal Allergic Rhinitis: Adults & Peds: ≥12 yo:** 1 or 2 spr/nostril bid.	C >
Olopatadine HCl (Patanase)	**Spray:** 665 mcg (0.6%)	**Seasonal Allergic Rhinitis: Adults & Peds: ≥12 yo:** 2 spr/nostril bid.	C >

Corticosteroids

NAME	FORM/STRENGTH	DOSAGE	COMMENTS
Beclomethasone (Beconase, Beconase AQ)	**Spr:** 42 mcg/spr	**Allergic/Nonallergic (Vasomotor) Rhinitis: Beconase AQ: Adults & Peds: ≥6 yo:** 1-2 spr per nostril bid. **Beconase: Adults & Peds: ≥12 yo:** 1 spr per nostril bid-qid. **6-12 yo:** 1 spr per nostril tid.	C v
Budesonide (Rhinocort Aqua)	**Spr:** 32 mcg/spr	**Seasonal/Perennial Rhinitis: Adults & Peds: ≥6 yo: Initial:** 1 spr per nostril qd. **Max: ≥12 yo:** 4 spr/nostril/d. **6-12 yo:** 2 spr/nostril/d.	B >
Ciclesonide (Omnaris)	**Spr:** 50 mcg/spr	**Seasonal Allergic Rhinitis: Adults & Peds: ≥6 yo:** 2 spr each nostril qd. **Perennial Allergic Rhinitis: Adults & Peds: ≥12 yo:** 2 spr each nostril qd. **Max:** 2 spr/nostril/d (200 mcg/d).	C >
Flunisolide (Nasarel)	**Spr:** 29 mcg/spr	**Seasonal/Perennial Rhinitis: Adults: Initial:** 2 spr per nostril bid. **Titrate:** Increase to 2 spr per nostril tid. **Max:** 16 spr/d. **6-14 yo:** 1 spr per nostril tid or 2 spr per nostril bid. **Max:** 8 spr/d.	C >
Fluticasone Furoate (Veramyst)	**Spr:** 27.5 mcg/spr	**Seasonal/Perennial Allergic Rhinitis: Adults & Peds: ≥12 yo: Initial:** 2 spr/nostril qd. **Maint:** 1 spr/nostril qd. **2-11 yo: Initial:** 1 spr/nostril qd. **Titrate:** If inadequate response, may increase to 2 spr/nostril.	C >

Fluticasone Propionate (Flonase)	**Spr:** 50 mcg/spr	**Seasonal & Perennial Allergic/Nonallergic Rhinitis: Adults: Initial:** 2 spr per nostril qd or 1 spr per nostril bid. **Maint:** 1 spr per nostril qd. **≥4 yo: Initial:** 1-2 spr per nostril qd. **Maint:** 1 spr per nostril qd. **Max:** 2 spr per nostril/d. **Seasonal Allergic Rhinitis: ≥12 yo:** May also dose as 2 spr per nostril qd prn.	◉C ✿>
Mometasone Furoate Monohydrate (Nasonex)	**Spr:** 50 mcg/spr	**Treatment & Prevention of Seasonal Allergic Rhinitis/ Treatment of Perennial Allergic Rhinitis: Adults & Peds: ≥12 yo:** 2 spr per nostril qd. **Treatment of Seasonal/ Perennial Allergic Rhinitis: Peds: 2-11 yo:** 1 spr per nostril qd. **Nasal Polyps: Adults: ≥18 yo:** 2 spr per nostril bid.	◉C ✿>
Triamcinolone Acetonide (Nasacort AQ)	**Spr:** 55 mcg/spr	**Allergic/Nonallergic Rhinitis: Nasacort AQ: Adults & Peds: ≥12 yo: Initial/Max:** 2 spr/nostril qd. **Maint:** 1 spr/ nostril qd. **6-12 yo: Initial:** 1 spr/nostril qd. **Max:** 2 spr/ nostril qd. **2-5 yo: Initial/Max:** 1 spr/nostril qd.	◉C ✿>

EENT/OPHTHALMOLOGY

Antibiotic Agents

Azithromycin (Azasite)	**Sol:** 1%	**Bacterial Conjunctivitis: Adults & Peds: ≥1 yo: Initial:** 1 gtt bid, 8-12 hrs apart x first 2d. **Maint:** 1 gtt qd x next 5d.	◉B ✿>

NAME	FORM/STRENGTH	DOSAGE	COMMENTS
Ciprofloxacin HCl (Ciloxan)	**Oint, Sol:** 0.3%	**Bacterial Conjunctivitis: Sol: Adults & Peds: ≥1 yo:** 1-2 gtts q2h w/a x 2d, then 1-2 gtts q4h w/a x 5d. **Oint: Adults & Peds: ≥2 yo:** 1/2 in tid x 2d, then bid x 5d. **Corneal Ulcers: Sol: Adults & Peds: ≥2 yo:** 2 gtts q15 min x 6h, then 2 gtts q30min on Day 1, then 2 gtts q1h on Day 2, then 2 gtts q4h on Days 3-14.	C >
Gentamicin Sulfate (Genoptic, Genoptic S.O.P.)	**Oint, Sol:** 0.3%	**Adults & Peds: Usual:** 1/2 inch bid-tid or 1-2 gtts q4h. **Severe Infection:** 2 gtts q1h.	C >
Levofloxacin (Iquix)	**Sol:** 1.5%	**Adults & Peds: ≥6 yo: Corneal Ulcer: Days 1-3:** 1-2 gtts q30min-2h while awake & 4-6 hrs after retiring. **Days 4-Completion:** 1-2 gtts q1-4h while awake.	C >
Levofloxacin (Quixin)	**Sol:** 0.5%	**Bacterial Conjunctivitis: Adults & Peds: ≥1 yo: Days 1-2:** 1-2 gtts q2h w/a up to 8x/d. **Days 3-7:** 1-2 gtts q4h w/a up to qid.	C >
Moxifloxacin HCl (Vigamox)	**Sol:** 0.5%	**Adults & Peds:** 1 gtt tid x 7d.	C >
Ofloxacin (Ocuflox)	**Sol:** 0.3%	**Adults & Peds: ≥1 yo: Bacterial Conjunctivitis:** 1-2 gtts q2-4h x 2d, then 1-2 gtts qid x 5d. **Bacterial Corneal Ulcer:** 1-2 gtts q30min w/a & 1-2 gtts 4-6h after retiring x 2d, then 1-2 gtts q1h w/a x 5-7d, then 1-2 gtts qid x 2d.	C v
Polymyxin B Sulfate/ Bacitracin Zinc/Neomycin (Neosporin Ointment)	**Oint:** 400 U-3.5 mg-10,000 U/gm	**Adults:** Apply q3-4h x 7-10d.	C >

Sulfacetamide Sodium (Bleph-10, AK-Sulf)	**Oint:** (AK-Sulf) 10%; **Sol:** (Bleph-10) 10%	**Adults: Initial:** Apply 1/2 inch qid & qhs or 1-2 gtts q2-3h w/a x 7-10d. **Maint:** Increase dose interval as condition responds. **Trachoma:** 2 gtts q2h w/ systemic administration.	◙C ❋v
Tobramycin (Tobrex)	**Oint:** 0.3%; **Sol:** 0.3%	**Adults: Usual:** 1/2 inch bid-tid or 1-2 gtts q4h. **Severe Infection:** 1/2 inch q3-4h or 2 gtts q1h until improvement.	◙B ❋v

Antibiotic/Corticosteroid Combinations

Dexamethasone/Tobramycin (TobraDex)	**Oint:** 0.1%-0.3%; **Susp:** 0.1%-0.3%	**Adults & Peds: ≥2 yo: Oint:** Apply 1/2 inch up to tid-qid. **Susp:** 1-2 gtts q2h x 24-48h, then 1-2 gtts q4-6h thereafter.	◙C ❋>
Fluorometholone/ Sulfacetamide Sodium (FML-S)	**Susp:** 0.1%-10%	**Adults:** 1 gtt qid.	◙C ❋v
Polymyxin B Sulfate/ Neomycin Sulfate/ Bacitracin Zinc/ Hydrocortisone (Cortisporin Ophthalmic)	**Oint:** 400 U-1%-3.5 mg-10,000 U/gm	**Adults:** Apply q3-4h, depending on severity.	◙C ❋v
Prednisolone Acetate/ Sulfacetamide Sodium (Blephamide, Blephamide S.O.P.)	**Oint, Susp:** 0.2%-10%	**Adults & Peds: ≥6 yo: Initial:** Apply 1/2 inch 3-4x/d & 1-2x/qpm or instill 2 gtts q4h & qhs. Reduce dose when condition improves.	◙C ❋v

NAME	FORM/STRENGTH	DOSAGE	COMMENTS
Corticosteroids			
Dexamethasone Sodium Phosphate (Decadron Ophthalmic)	**Oint:** 0.05%; **Sol:** 0.1%	**Adults: Initial:** Apply oint tid-qid or instill 1-2 gtts q1h w/a & q2h during night. With improvement, apply oint qd-bid or instill 1 gtt 3-6x/d. **Ear:** 3-4 gtts bid-tid w/ gradual dose reduction.	C v
Loteprednol Etabonate (Alrex)	**Susp:** 0.5%	**Adults:** 1-2 gtts qid, may increase to 1 gtt q1h during 1st wk. **Post-Op:** 1-2 gtts qid starting 24h post-op. Continue x 2 wks.	C v
Prednisolone Acetate (Pred Forte)	**Susp:** 0.12%, 0.125%, 1%	**Adults:** 1-2 gtts bid-qid. May increase frequency during 1st 24-48h.	C v
Prednisolone Acetate (Pred Mild)	**Susp:** 0.12%, 0.125%, 1%	**Adults:** 1-2 gtts bid-qid. May increase frequency during 1st 24-48h.	C v
Glaucoma			
ADRENERGIC AGONISTS			
Dipivefrin HCl (Propine)	**Sol:** 0.1%	**Adults: Usual:** 1 gtt q12h.	B >
BETA BLOCKERS			
Betaxolol (Betoptic S)	**Susp:** 0.25%	**Adults:** 1-2 gtts bid.	C >

Carteolol HCl (Ocupress)	**Sol:** 1%	**Adults:** 1 gtt bid.	C >
Levobunolol HCl (Betagan, Betagan C Cap)	**Sol:** (Betagan C Cap) 0.25%, (Betagan) 0.5%	**Adults: Usual:** (0.5%) 1-2 gtts qd. (0.25%) 1-2 gtts bid. **Severe/Uncontrolled:** (0.5%) 1-2 gtts bid.	C >
Metipranolol (Optipranolol)	**Sol:** 0.3%	**Adults:** 1 gtt bid.	C v
Timolol Maleate (Timoptic, Timoptic Ocudose, Timoptic-XE)	**Sol:** 0.25%, 0.5%; **Sol,Gel-Forming:** (XE) 0.25%, 0.5%	**Adults: Timoptic/Timoptic Ocudose:** 1 gtt 0.25% bid, may increase to 1 gtt 0.5% bid. **Maint:** 1 gtt 0.25%/0.5% qd. **Timoptic-XE:** 1 gtt 0.25%/0.5% qd. **Max:** 1 gtt 0.5% qd.	C v

CARBONIC ANHYDRASE INHIBITOR/BETA BLOCKER

Dorzolamide HCl/ Timolol Maleate (Cosopt)	**Sol:** 2%-0.5%	**Adults:** 1 gtt bid.	C v

CARBONIC ANHYDRASE INHIBITORS

Brinzolamide (Azopt)	**Susp:** 1%	**Adults:** 1 gtt tid.	C v
Dorzolamide (Trusopt)	**Sol:** 2%	**Adults & Peds:** 1 gtt tid.	C v

NAME	FORM/STRENGTH	DOSAGE	COMMENTS
CHOLINERGIC AGONISTS			
Pilocarpine HCl (Isopto Carpine)	**Sol:** (Generic) 0.5%, 1%, 2%, 3%, 4%, 6%, (Isopto Carpine) 1%, 2%, 4%	**Usual: Sol:** 2 gtts tid-qid.	◙C ❁>
Pilocarpine HCl (Pilopine HS)	**Gel:** (Pilopine HS) 4%	**Usual:** Apply 1/2 inch ribbon qhs.	◙C ❁>
PROSTAGLANDIN ANALOGUES			
Bimatoprost (Lumigan)	**Sol:** 0.03%	**Adults: Usual/Max:** 1 gtt qpm.	◙C ❁>
Latanoprost (Xalatan)	**Sol:** 0.005%	**Adults: Usual/ Max:** 1 gtt qpm.	◙C ❁>
Travoprost (Travatan, Travatan Z)	**Sol:** 0.004%	**Adults:** 1 gtt qpm.	◙C ❁>
SYMPATHOMIMETIC/BETA-BLOCKER			
Brimonidine Tartrate/ Timolol Maleate (Combigan)	**Sol:** 2 mg-5 mg/ml	**Adults & Peds: ≥2 yo:** 1 gtt in affected eye(s) bid approximately 12h apart. Instill other topical ophthalmic products ≥5 min apart.	◙C ❁v

SYMPATHOMIMETICS

Brimonidine Tartrate (Alphagan P)	**Sol:** 0.1%, 0.15%	**Adults & Peds: ≥2 yo:** 1 gtt tid (q8h). Separate other topical products that lower IOP by at least 5 min.	B v

Mydriatics/Cycloplegics

ANTICHOLINERGICS

Atropine Sulfate	**Oint:** 1%; **Sol:** 1%	1-2 gtts tid or small amt of oint qd-bid.	C >

NSAIDs

Bromfenac (Xibrom)	**Sol:** 0.09%	**Adults: Cataract Extraction:** 1 gtt bid, begin 24h post-op x 2wks.	C >
Flurbiprofen Sodium (Ocufen)	**Sol:** 0.03%	**Inhibit Intraoperative Miosis: Adults:** 1 gtts q30min x 4 doses, beginning 2h prior to surgery.	C v
Ketorolac Tromethamine (Acular)	**Sol:** 0.5%	**Adults & Peds: ≥3 yo: Acular: Ocular Itching:** 1 gtt qid. **Post-Op Inflammation:** 1 gtt qid. Begin 24h post-op & continue x 2wks. **Acular PF: Pain/Photophobia:** 1 gtt post-op qid prn up to 3d.	C >
Nepafenac (Nevanac)	**Susp:** 0.1%	**Cataract Surgery: Adults:** 1 gtt tid, start 24 h prior to surgery, continue on day of surgery & for 2 wks post-op.	C >

NAME	FORM/STRENGTH	DOSAGE	COMMENTS

Ocular Decongestant/Allergic Conjunctivitis

H_1 RECEPTOR ANTAGONISTS

NAME	FORM/STRENGTH	DOSAGE	COMMENTS
Azelastine HCl (Optivar)	**Sol:** 0.05%	**Adults & Peds: ≥3 yo:** 1 gtt bid.	C >
Epinastine HCl (Elestat)	**Sol:** 0.05%	**Adults & Peds: ≥3 yo:** 1 gtt in each eye bid.	C >

H_1 ANTAGONIST/MAST CELL STABILIZERS

NAME	FORM/STRENGTH	DOSAGE	COMMENTS
Ketotifen Fumarate (Zaditor)	**Sol:** 0.025%	**Adults & Peds: ≥3 yo:** 1 gtt bid, q8-12h.	C >
Olopatadine HCl (Patanol)	**Sol:** 0.1%	**Adults & Peds: ≥3 yo:** 1-2 gtts bid, q6-8h.	C >

MAST CELL STABILIZERS

NAME	FORM/STRENGTH	DOSAGE	COMMENTS
Cromolyn Sodium (Crolom)	**Sol:** 4%	**Adults & Peds: ≥4 yo:** 1-2 gtts 4-6x/d.	B >
Pemirolast Potassium (Alamast)	**Sol:** 0.1%	**Adults & Peds: ≥3 yo:** 1-2 gtts in affected eye qid.	C >

SYMPATHOMIMETICS

NAME	FORM/STRENGTH	DOSAGE	COMMENTS
Naphazoline (Albalon)	**Sol:** 0.1%	**Adults:** 1-2 gtts q3-4h prn.	C >

Miscellaneous

Cyclosporine (Restasis)	**Emul:** 0.05%	**Keratoconjunctivitis Sicca: Adults:** 1 gtt bid, q12h.	C >
Pegaptanib Sodium (Macugen)	**Inj:** 0.3 mg	**Macular Degeneration: Adults:** Administer 0.3 mg by intravitreous inj once q6wks.	B >
Ranibizumab (Lucentis)	**Inj:** 10 mg/ml	**Macular Degeneration: Adults:** Administer 0.5 mg (0.05 ml) by intravitreal inj once a mth. May reduce to 1 inj q3mths after first 4 inj, if mthly inj not feasible.	C >

EENT/OTIC PREPARATIONS

Antibacterial/Corticosteroid Combinations

Ciprofloxacin HCl/ Dexamethasone (Ciprodex)	**Susp:** 0.3%-0.1%	**Adults & Peds: ≥6 mths:** 4 gtts bid x 7d.	C v
Ciprofloxacin HCl/ Hydrocortisone (Cipro HC)	**Susp:** 0.2%-1%	**Adults & Peds: ≥1 yo:** 3 gtts bid x 7d.	C v
Hydrocortisone Acetate/ Thonzonium Bromide/ Neomycin Sulfate/ Colistin Sulfate (Cortisporin-TC Otic)	**Susp:** 3-10-3.3-0.5 mg/ml	**Adults:** 4-5 gtts tid-qid. **Peds:** 3-4 gtts tid-qid.	N >

NAME	FORM/STRENGTH	DOSAGE	COMMENTS
Neomycin Sulfate/ Polymyxin B Sulfate/ Hydrocortisone	**Sol, Susp:** 1%-0.35%-10,000 U/ml	**Adults:** 4 gtts tid-qid up to 10d. **Peds:** 3 gtts tid-qid up to 10d.	◙C ❋>

Antibiotic Agents

NAME	FORM/STRENGTH	DOSAGE	COMMENTS
Ofloxacin (Floxin Otic, Floxin Otic Singles)	**Sol:** 0.3%	**Otitis Externa: Peds: 6 mths-13 yo:** 5 gtts or 1 single-dispensing container (SDC) qd x 7d. ≥**13 yo:** 10 gtts or 2 SDCs qd x 7d. **Acute Otitis Media w/ Tympanostomy Tubes: Peds: 1-12 yo:** 5 gtts or 1 SDC bid x 10d. **Chronic Suppurative Otitis Media w/ Perforated Tympanic Membranes: Adults & Peds: ≥12 yo:** 10 gtts or 2 SDCs bid x 14d.	◙C ❋v

ENDOCRINE/METABOLIC

Androgens

NAME	FORM/STRENGTH	DOSAGE	COMMENTS
Methyltestosterone CIII (Testred)	**Cap:** 10 mg	**Adults: Androgen-Deficient Males:** 10-50 mg/d. **Breast Cancer in Females:** 50-200 mg/d. **Peds: Delayed Puberty:** Use lower range of 10-50 mg/d x 4-6 mths.	◙X ❋v
Testosterone CIII (Androderm)	**Patch:** 2.5 mg/24 h, 5 mg/24 h	**Adults & Peds: ≥15 yo: Initial:** 5 mg qhs x 24h on back, abdomen, upper arm, or thigh. **Maint:** 2.5-7.5 mg/d.	◙X ❋v
Testosterone CIII (Androgel)	**Gel:** 1%	**Adults: Gel: Initial:** Apply 5 gm qd on shoulders & upper arms and/or abdomen. **Titrate:** May increase to 7.5 gm qd, then 10 gm qd.	◙X ❋v

Testosterone CIII (Striant)	**Tab,Buccal:** 30 mg	**Adults:** 30 mg q12h to gum region above incisor tooth on either side of mouth. Rotate sites w/ each application. Hold in place for 30 sec.	⦿X ❁v

Antidiabetic Agents

BIGUANIDE/MEGLITINIDE

Metformin HCl/Repaglinide (Prandimet)	**Tab:** (Repaglinide/ Metformin) 1-500 mg, 2-500 mg	**Adults:** Individualize dose. (repaglinide-metformin) Give 2-3x/d up to 4-1000 mg/meal . **Max: Daily Dose:** 10 mg repaglinide-2500 mg metformin. **Patient Inadequately Controlled w/ Metformin Monotherapy: Initial:** 1-500 mg bid w/ meals. **Titrate:** Gradually escalate dose to reduce risk of hypoglycemia. **Patient Inadequately Controlled w/ Meglitinide Monotherapy: Initial:** 500 mg of metformin bid. **Titrate:** Gradually escalate dose to reduce GI side effects. **Concomitant use of Repaglinide/Metformin:** Initiate at dose of repaglinide & metformin similar to (not exceeding) current doses. Titrate to max daily dose as necessary.	⦿C ❁v May cause lactic acidosis.

NAME	FORM/STRENGTH	DOSAGE	COMMENTS
BIGUANIDES			
Metformin HCl (Glucophage, Glucophage XR, Riomet)	**Sol:** (Riomet) 500 mg/ 5 ml; **Tab:** (Glucophage) 500 mg, 850 mg, 1000 mg; **Tab,ER:** (Glucophage XR) 500 mg, 750 mg	**Adults: Sol/Tab: Initial:** 500 mg bid or 850 mg qd w/ meals. **Titrate:** Increase by 500 mg qwk, or 850 mg q2wks, or from 500 mg bid to 850 mg bid after 2 wks. **Max:** 2550 mg/d. **With Insulin: Initial:** 500 mg qd. **Titrate:** 500 mg qwk. **Max:** 2500 mg/d. Decrease insulin dose by 10-25% when FPG <120 mg/dl. **Tab,ER: Glucophage XR: With/Without Insulin: Initial:** 500 mg qd w/ evening meal. **Titrate:** Increase by 500 mg qwk. **Max:** 2000 mg/d. **Peds: 10-16 yo: Sol/Tab: Initial:** 500 mg bid w/ meals. **Titrate:** Increase by 500 mg qwk. **Max:** 2000 mg/d in divided doses.	●B ❉v **H R** Lactic acidosis reported (rare).
Metformin HCl (Fortamet)	**Tab,ER:** 500 mg, 1000 mg	**Adults: Initial:** 500-1000 mg qd w/ evening meal. **With Insulin: Initial:** 500 mg qd. **Titrate:** May increase by 500 mg/wk. **Max:** 2500 mg/d. Decrease insulin dose by 10-25% when FPG <120 mg/dl.	●B ❉v **H R** Lactic acidosis reported (rare).
Metformin HCl (Glumetza)	**Tab,ER:** 500 mg, 1000 mg	**Adults: Initial:** 1000 mg qd w/ evening meal. **With Insulin: Initial:** 500 mg qd. **Titrate:** May increase by 500 mg/wk. **Max:** 2000 mg/d. Decrease insulin dose by 10-25% if FPG <120 mg/dl. **Peds: 10-16 yo: Sol/Tab: Initial:** 500 mg bid w/ meals. **Titrate:** Increase by 500 mg qwk. **Max:** 2000 mg/d in divided doses.	●B ❉v **H R** Lactic acidosis reported (rare).

BILE ACID SEQUESTRANTS

Colesevelam HCl (WelChol)	**Tab:** 625 mg	**Improve Glycemic Control: Adults:** 3 tabs bid or 6 tabs qd. Take w/ a meal & liquid.	B >

DIPEPTIDYL PEPTIDASE-4 INHIBITOR

Sitagliptin Phosphate (Januvia)	**Tab:** 25 mg, 50 mg, 100 mg	**Monotherapy/Combination Therapy: Adults:** 100 mg qd. **CrCl 30-<50 ml/min:** 50 mg qd. **CrCl <30 ml/min:** 25 mg qd.	B > **R**

DIPEPTIDYL PEPTIDASE-4 INHIBITOR/BIGUANIDE

Sitagliptin/Metformin HCl (Janumet)	**Tab:** 50-500 mg, 50-1000 mg	**Adults:** Individualize dosing. **Patient Not Controlled on Metformin Monotherapy: Initial:** 100 mg/d (50 mg bid) of sitagliptin + metformin dose. **Patient on Metformin 850 mg BID: Initial:** 50-1000 mg tab bid. **Patient Not Controlled on Sitagliptin Monotherapy: Initial:** 50-500 mg tab bid. **Titrate:** Gradual increase to 50-1000 mg tab bid. **Max:** 100 mg of sitagliptin & 2000 mg of metformin. Take w/ meals.	B > **R** Lactic acidosis reported (rare).

GLUCOSIDASE INHIBITORS

Acarbose (Precose)	**Tab:** 25 mg, 50 mg, 100 mg	**Adults: Initial:** 25 mg tid w/ meals. **Titrate:** Adjust at 4-8 wk intervals. **Maint:** 50-100 mg tid. **Max:** **≤60 kg:** 50 mg tid. **>60 kg:** 100 mg tid.	B v **R**

NAME	FORM/STRENGTH	DOSAGE	COMMENTS
Miglitol (Glyset)	**Tab:** 25 mg, 50 mg, 100 mg	**Adults: Initial:** 25 mg tid w/ meals. **Titrate:** Increase after 4-8 wks to 50 mg tid x approx. 3 mths, then may further increase to 100 mg tid. **Maint:** 50-100 mg tid. **Max:** 100 mg tid.	B v **R**
INCRETIN MIMETIC			
Exenatide (Byetta)	**Inj:** 250 mcg/ml	**Adults:** 5 mcg SC bid, 60 min before qam & qpm meals. **Titrate/Max:** 10 mcg bid after 1 mth. Reduction of sulfonylurea dose may be considered to reduce risk of hypoglycemia.	C > **R**
INSULIN			
Insulin Glargine, Human (Lantus)	**Inj:** 100 U/ml, (OptiClik) 100 U/ml	**Adults & Peds: ≥6 yo:** Dose per requirement. Give same time qd.	C >
Insulin Glulisine, rDNA (Apidra)	**Inj:** 100 U/ml	**Adults & Peds: ≥4 yo:** Individualize dose. Inject SC within 15 min before a meal or within 20 min after starting a meal. Rotate inj site (abdomen, thigh, or deltoid).	C >
MEGLITINIDES			
Nateglinide (Starlix)	**Tab:** 60 mg, 120 mg	**Adults:** 120 mg tid 1-30 min ac. May use 60 mg tid for near goal HbA_{1c}. Skip dose if meal is skipped.	C v

Repaglinide (Prandin)	**Tab:** 0.5 mg, 1 mg, 2 mg	**Adults: Initial: Treatment-Naive or HbA1c <8%:** 0.5 mg w/ each meal. **Previous Oral Antidiabetic Therapy/ Combination Therapy & HbA1c ≥8%:** 1-2 mg w/ meals. **Titrate:** May adjust wkly by doubling preprandial dose up to 4 mg (bid-qid). **Maint:** 0.5-4 mg w/ meals. **Max:** 16 mg/d. Take within 15-30 min ac. Skip dose if skip meal & add dose if add meal.	C v **H R**

SULFONYLUREA/BIGUANIDE

Glipizide/Metformin HCl (Metaglip)	**Tab:** 2.5/250 mg, 2.5/500 mg, 5/500 mg	**Adults: Initial:** 2.5/250 mg qd w/ meals. If FBG 280-320 mg/dl, give 2.5/500 mg bid. **Titrate:** Increase by 1 tab/d q2wks. **Max:** 10/2000 mg/d. **2nd-Line Therapy: Initial:** 2.5/500 mg or 5/500 mg bid w/ meals. **Titrate:** Increase by ≤5/500 mg/d. **Max:** 20/2000 mg/d.	C v Lactic acidosis reported (rare). **H R**
Glyburide/Metformin HCl (Glucovance)	**Tab:** 1.25-250 mg, 2.5-500 mg, 5-500 mg	**Adults: Initial:** 1.25-250 mg qd-bid w/ meals. **Titrate:** Increase by 1.25-250 mg/d q2wks. **Max:** 10-2000 mg/d. **2nd-Line Therapy: Initial:** 2.5-500 mg or 5-500 mg bid w/ meals. **Titrate:** Increase by ≤5-500 mg/d. **Max:** 20-2000 mg/d.	B v Lactic acidosis reported (rare). **H R**

SULFONYLUREAS-2ND GENERATION

Glimepiride (Amaryl)	**Tab:** 1 mg, 2 mg, 4 mg	**Adults: Initial:** 1-2 mg qd w/ breakfast. **Titrate:** Increase ≤2 mg at 1-2 wk intervals. **Maint:** 1-4 mg qd. **Max:** 8 mg/d.	C v **H R**

NAME	FORM/STRENGTH	DOSAGE	COMMENTS
Glipizide (Glucotrol, Glucotrol XL)	**Tab:** 5 mg, 10 mg; **Tab,ER:** 2.5 mg, 5 mg, 10 mg	**Adults: Glucotrol XL: Initial/Combination Therapy:** 5 mg qd w/ breakfast. **Usual:** 5-10 mg qd. **Max:** 20 mg/d. **Glucotrol: Initial:** 5 mg qd 30 min ac. **Titrate:** Increase by 2.5-5 mg; divide if above 15 mg. **Max:** 40 mg/d.	C v **H R**
Glyburide (Glynase PresTab)	**Tab:** 1.5 mg, 3 mg, 4.5 mg, 6 mg	**Adults: Initial:** 1.5-3 mg qd w/ breakfast. **Titrate:** Increase by no more than 1.5 mg at wkly intervals; >6 mg may give bid. **Maint:** 0.75-12 mg/d. **Max:** 12 mg/d.	B v **H R**
Glyburide (Diabeta)	**Tab:** 1.25 mg, 2.5 mg, 5 mg	**Adults: Initial:** 2.5-5 mg qd w/ breakfast. **Titrate:** Increase by no more than 2.5 mg at wkly intervals. **Maint:** 1.25-20 mg given qd or in divided doses. **Max:** 20 mg/d. May give bid if dose >10 mg/d.	C v **H R**
THIAZOLIDINEDIONE/BIGUANIDE			
Pioglitazone HCl/ Metformin HCl (Actoplus Met)	**Tab:** (Actoplus Met) 15-500 mg, 15-850 mg; (Actoplus Met XR) 15-1000 mg, 30-1000 mg	**Adults: Prior Pioglitazone/Metformin:** Based on current regimen. **Actoplus Met: Initial:** 15-500 mg or 15-850 mg qd-bid with food. **Titrate:** Gradually increase after assessing adequacy of therapeutic response. **Max:** 45-2550 mg. **Actoplus Met XR: Initial:** 15-1000 mg or 30-1000 mg qd with evening meal. **Max:** 45-2000 mg qd. **Elderly/Debilitated/Malnourished:** Conservative dosing; do not titrate to max dose.	C v **H R** Lactic acidosis reported (rare). **W** [79]

Rosiglitazone Maleate/ Metformin HCl (Avandamet)	**Tab:** 2-500 mg, 4-500 mg, 2-1000 mg, 4-1000 mg	**Adults: Prior Metformin Therapy of 1000 mg/d: Initial:** 2 mg-500 mg tab bid. **Prior Metformin Therapy of 2000 mg/d: Initial:** 2 mg-1000 mg tab bid. **Prior Rosiglitazone Therapy of 4 mg/d: Initial:** 2 mg-500 mg tab bid. **Prior Rosiglitazone Therapy of 8 mg/d:** 4 mg-500 mg tab bid. **Titrate:** May increase by increments of 4 mg rosiglitazone and/or 500 mg metformin. **Max:** 8 mg-2000 mg/d. **Drug-Naive Patients: Initial:** 2 mg-500 mg qd-bid. **If HbA1c >11% & FPG >270mg/dl: Initial:** 2 mg-500 mg bid. **Titrate:** After 4 wks, may increase by increments of 2 mg-500 mg per day. **Max:** 8 mg-2000 mg per day. **Elderly/Debilitated/Malnourished:** Conservative dosing; do not titrate to max dose. Take w/ meals.	C v Lactic acidosis reported (rare). **H R W** [82]

THIAZOLIDINEDIONE/SULFONYLUREA

Pioglitazone HCl/Glimepiride (Duetact)	**Tab:** 30-2 mg, 30-4 mg	**Adults:** Base recommended starting dose on current regimen of pioglitazone and/or sulfonylurea. Give w/ 1st meal of day. **Current Glimepiride Monotherapy or Prior Therapy of Pioglitazone plus Glimepiride Separately: Initial:** 30 mg-2 mg or 30 mg-4 mg qd. **Current Pioglitazone or Different Sulfonylurea Monotherapy or Combination of Both: Initial:** 30 mg-2 mg qd. Adjust dose based on response. **Max:** Once-daily at any dosage	C v **H R W** [79]

Continued on Next Page

NAME	FORM/STRENGTH	DOSAGE	COMMENTS
Pioglitazone HCl/Glimepiride (Duetact) *Continued*		strength. **Elderly/Debilitated/Malnourished/Renal or Hepatic Insufficiency (ALT=2.5x ULN): Initial:** 1 mg glimepiride prior to prescribing Duetact. **Systolic Dysfunction: Initial:** 15-30 mg of pioglitazone; titrate carefully to lowest Duetact dose.	
Rosiglitazone Maleate/ Glimepiride (Avandaryl)	**Tab:** 4-1 mg, 4-2 mg, 4-4 mg	**Adults: Prior Sulfonylurea Monotherapy or Inital Response To Rosiglitazone Alone Requiring Additional Control:** 4-1 mg or 4-2 mg qd w/ 1st meal of day. **Switching From Prior Combination Therapy:** Same dose already taken of each component. **Prior Thiazolidinedione Monotherapy:** Titrate dose. After 1-2 wks w/ inadequate control, increase glimepiride component in no more than 2 mg increments at 1-2 wk intervals. **Max:** 8-4 mg qd. **Prior Sulfonylurea Monotherapy:** May take 2-3 mths for full effect of rosiglitazone; do not exceed 8 mg of rosiglitazone daily. **Titrate:** May increase glimepiride component. **Elderly/Debilitated/Malnourished/Renal, Hepatic or Adrenal Insufficiency: Initial:** 4-1 mg qd. Titrate carefully.	C ❁v **H R W** 82

THIAZOLIDINEDIONES

NAME	FORM/STRENGTH	DOSAGE	COMMENTS
Pioglitazone (Actos)	**Tab:** 15 mg, 30 mg, 45 mg	**Adults: Initial:** 15-30 mg qd. **Max:** 45 mg/d. **Combination Therapy w/ Insulin:** Decrease insulin by 10-25% if hypoglycemic or FPG <100 mg/dl; individualize further adjustments based on glucose-lowering response.	C ❁v **H W** 79

Rosiglitazone Maleate (Avandia)	**Tab:** 2 mg, 4 mg, 8 mg	**Adults: ≥18 yo: Initial:** 2 mg bid or 4 mg qd. **Titrate:** May increase after 8-12 wks to 4 mg bid or 8 mg qd. **Max:** 8 mg/d as monotherapy or w/ metformin, sulfonylureas, or sulfonylureas plus metformin; 4 mg/d w/ insulin. **Combination Therapy w/ Insulin:** Decrease insulin by 10-25% if hypoglycemic or FPG <100 mg/dl; individualize further adjustments based on glucose-lowering response.	C v **H W** [82]

Antithyroid Agents

Methimazole (Tapazole)	**Tab:** 5 mg, 10 mg	**Adults: Initial:** 5 mg q8h for mild hyperthyroidism; 30-40 mg/d given q8h for moderately severe hyperthyroidism, 20 mg q8h for severe hyperthyroidism. **Maint:** 5-15 mg/d. **Peds: Initial:** 0.4 mg/kg/d divided q8h. **Maint:** 1/2 of initial dose.	D v CI in nursing.
Propylthiouracil	**Tab:** 50 mg	**Adults:** 100 mg q8h, 400 mg/d as q8h for severe hyperthyroidism/large goiters, up to 600-900 mg/d if needed. **Maint:** 100-150 mg/d. **Peds: 6-10 yo: Initial:** 50-150 mg/d. ≥**10 yo:** 150-300 mg/d. **Maint:** Determine dose by response.	D v CI in nursing.

Gout

NAME	FORM/STRENGTH	DOSAGE	COMMENTS
URICOSURICS			
Probenecid	**Tab:** 500 mg	**Adults:** 250 mg bid x 1 wk. **Titrate:** Increase by 500 mg q4wks. **Maint:** 500 mg bid. **Max:** 2 gm/d.	N > **R**
XANTHINE OXIDASE INHIBITORS			
Allopurinol (Zyloprim)	**Tab:** 100 mg, 300 mg	**Adults: Usual:** 200-300 mg/d. **Prevention of Uric Acid Nephropathy w/ Chemo: Usual:** 600-800 mg/d for 2-3d w/ high fluid intake.	C > **R**
Febuxostat (Uloric)	**Tab:** 40 mg, 80 mg	**Hyperuricemia w/ Gout: Adults: Initial:** 40 mg qd. **Range:** 40-80 mg qd. **Serum Uric Acid <6mg/dl After 2 Wks at 40mg:** 80mg qd.	C >
MISCELLANEOUS			
Colchicine	**Inj:** 0.5 mg/ml; **Tab:** 0.5 mg, 0.6 mg	**Adults: Acute Gouty Arthritis:** 1-1.2 mg, then 0.5-0.6 mg/h or 1-1.2 mg q2h until pain relieved or diarrhea ensues up to 4-8 mg; wait 3d between courses to avoid toxicity. **Prophylaxis:** (<1 attack/yr) 0.5-0.6 mg/d 3-4x/wk; (>1 attack/wk) 0.5-0.6 mg/d, severe cases may need 2-3 tabs/d.	C > **H R**

		Adults: Initial: 1 tab qd x 1 wk, then 1 tab bid. **Titrate:** May increase by 1 tab/d q4wks. **Max:** 4 tabs/d. Not for acute gouty attacks. May reduce dose by 1 tab q6mths if acute attacks absent ≥6 mths.	◙N ❊> CI in pregnancy. **R**

Osteoporosis

BISPHOSPHONATES AND COMBINATIONS

Alendronate Sodium/ Cholecalciferol (Fosamax Plus D)	**Tab:** 70 mg/2800 IU, 70 mg/5600 IU	**Adults: Treatment in Females/Bone Mass Increase in Men:** 1 tab qwk. Take at least 30 min before 1st food, beverage or med of day. Take tab w/ 6-8 oz water, followed by 2 oz water. Do not lie down x 30 min after dose & until after 1st food of day.	◙C ❊> **R**
Alendronate Sodium (Fosamax)	**Sol:** 70 mg/75 ml; **Tab:** 5 mg, 10 mg, 35 mg, 40 mg, 70 mg	**Adults: Treatment in Females/Bone Mass Increase in Men:** 10 mg qd or 70 mg qwk. **Prevention: Females:** 5 mg qd or 35 mg qwk. **Glucocorticoid-Induced: Men/Women:** 5 mg qd. **Postmenopausal Women Not Receiving Estrogen:** 10 mg qd. Take at least 30 min before 1st food, beverage, or med of day. Take tab w/ 6-8 oz water, followed by 2 oz water. Do not lie down x 30 min after dose & until after 1st food of day.	◙C ❊> **R**
Ibandronate Sodium (Boniva)	**Inj:** 3 mg/3 ml; **Tab:** 2.5 mg, 150 mg	**Treatment/Prevention: Female: PO:** 2.5 mg qd or 150 mg once mthly. Take at least 60 min before 1st food, beverage, or med. Do not lie down x 60 min after dose. **Treatment: Inj:** 3 mg IV over 15-30 sec q3mths.	◙C ❊> **R**

NAME	FORM/STRENGTH	DOSAGE	COMMENTS
Risedronate Sodium (Actonel)	**Tab:** 5 mg, 30 mg, 35 mg, 75 mg, 150 mg	**Adults: Treatment/Prevention: Postmenopausal:** 5 mg qd or 35 mg qwk or 75 mg on 2 consecutive days each mth or 150 mg once mthly. **Glucocorticoid-Induced: Men/Women:** 5 mg qd. **Increase Bone Mass in Men w/ Osteoporosis:** 35 mg qwk. **Paget's Disease: Men/Women:** 30 mg qd x 2 mths. May retreat after 2 mths. Take at least 30 min before 1st food or drink of day other than water. Swallow in upright position w/ 6-8 oz water. Do not lie down for 30 min after dose.	C v **R**
Risedronate Sodium/ Calcium Carbonate (Actonel with Calcium)	**Tab:** (Risedronate) 35 mg; **Tab:** (Calcium): 1250 mg	**Adults: Treatment/Prevention: Postmenopausal: Actonel:** 35 mg qwk on Day 1 of 7-day treatment cycle. Take at least 30 min before 1st food or drink of day other than water. Swallow in upright position w/ 6-8 oz water. Do not lie down for 30 min after dose. **Calcium:** 1250 mg qd on Days 2-7 of 7-day treatment cycle.	C v **R**

CALCITONIN

NAME	FORM/STRENGTH	DOSAGE	COMMENTS
Calcitonin-Salmon (Miacalcin)	**Inj:** 200 IU/ml; **Nasal Spr:** 200 IU/spr	**Treatment: Adults: Female: Spr:** 200 IU (1 spr) qd intranasally, alternate nostrils daily. **Inj:** 100 IU IM/SC qod.	C v

ESTROGEN/PROGESTIN COMBINATION

NAME	FORM/STRENGTH	DOSAGE	COMMENTS
Estradiol/Levonorgestrel (Climara Pro)	**Patch:** 0.045-0.015 mg/d	**Prevention: Adults:** Apply 1 patch qwk to lower abdomen (avoid breasts/waistline). Rotate application site; allow 1 wk between same site.	X > **W** 4, 10, 28

Estradiol/Norethindrone (Activella)	**Tab:** 1-0.5 mg	**Prevention: Adults: Female:** 1 tab qd.	X > **W**[28]
Medroxyprogesterone Acetate/Conjugated Estrogens (Premphase)	**Tab:** 0.625 mg (estrogens, conj.) & 0.625-5 mg	**Prevention: Adults: Female:** 0.625 mg tab qd on Days 1-14 & 0.625-5 mg tab qd on Days 15-28. Re-evaluate after 3-6 mths.	X > **W**[4, 10, 28]
Medroxyprogesterone Acetate/Conjugated Estrogens (Prempro)	**Tab:** 0.3-1.5 mg, 0.45-1.5 mg, 0.625-2.5 mg, 0.625-5 mg	**Prevention: Adults: Female:** 0.3-1.5 mg qd. Adjust dose based on response. Re-evaluate after 3-6 mths.	X > **W**[4, 10, 28]
Norethindrone Acetate/ Ethinyl Estradiol (femhrt)	**Tab:** 2.5 mcg-0.5 mg, 5 mcg-1 mg	**Prevention: Female: Usual:** 1 tab qd.	X > **W**[4]

ESTROGENS

Conjugated Estrogens (Premarin Tablets)	**Tab:** 0.3 mg, 0.45 mg, 0.625 mg, 0.9 mg, 1.25 mg	**Prevention: Adults: Female: Initial:** 0.3 mg qd given continuously or cyclically (eg, 25d on, 5d off).	X > **W**[4, 28]
Estradiol (Alora)	**Patch:** 0.025 mg/d, 0.05 mg/d, 0.075 mg/d, 0.1 mg/d	**Prevention: Adults: Female:** Apply 0.025 mg/d patch twice wkly. **Titrate:** May increase depending on bone mineral density & adverse events.	X > **W**[4, 10, 28]
Estradiol (Climara)	**Patch:** 0.025 mg/d, 0.0375 mg/d, 0.05 mg/d, 0.06 mg/d, 0.075 mg/d, 0.1 mg/d	**Prevention: Adults: Female:** Apply 0.025 mg/d patch qwk (minimum effective dose).	X > **W**[4, 10, 28]

NAME	FORM/STRENGTH	DOSAGE	COMMENTS
Estradiol (Estrace)	**Tab:** 0.5 mg, 1 mg, 2 mg	**Prevention: Adults: Female:** 0.5 mg qd (23 days on & 5 days off).	X v **W** [4, 10, 28]
Estradiol (Menostar)	**Patch:** 14 mcg/d	**Prevention: Adults: Female:** Apply 1 patch (14 mcg/d) qwk.	X > **W** [4, 28]
Estropipate (Ogen)	**Tab:** 0.625 mg (0.75 mg estropipate), 1.25 mg (1.5 mg estropipate), 2.5 mg (3 mg estropipate)	**Prevention: Adults: Female:** 0.625 mg (0.75 mg estropipate) qd x 25d of 31d cycle per mth.	X > **W** [4, 10, 28]

SERM (SELECTIVE ESTROGEN RECEPTOR MODULATOR)

NAME	FORM/STRENGTH	DOSAGE	COMMENTS
Raloxifene HCl (Evista)	**Tab:** 60 mg	**Treatment/Prevention: Adults: Female:** 60 mg qd.	X v

Thyroid Agents

THYROID HORMONES

NAME	FORM/STRENGTH	DOSAGE	COMMENTS
Levothyroxine Sodium, T4 (Levothroid)	**Tab:** 0.025 mg, 0.05 mg, 0.075 mg, 0.088 mg, 0.1 mg, 0.112 mg, 0.125 mg, 0.137 mg, 0.15 mg, 0.175 mg, 0.2 mg, 0.3 mg	**Hypothyroidism: Adults <50 yo or >50 yo & Recently Treated for Hyperthyroidism or Hypothyroid for Short Time & Peds >12 yo (Growth/Puberty Complete):** 1.7 mcg/kg/d. >200 mcg/d seldom required. **>50 yo or <50 yo w/ Underlying Cardiac Disease: Initial:** 25-50 mcg/d until TSH normalized. **Severe Hypothyroidism/Elderly w/ Cardiac Disease: Initial:**	A >

		12.5-25 mcg/d until TSH normalized. **Peds: >12 yo (Growth/Puberty Incomplete):** 2-3 mcg/kg/d. **6-12 yo:** 4-5 mcg/kg/d. **1-5 yo:** 5-6 mcg/kg/d. **6-12 mths:** 6-8 mcg/kg/d. **3-6 mths:** 8-10 mcg/kg/d. **0-3 mths:** 10-15 mcg/kg/d. **Adults: Pituitary TSH Suppression: Thyroid Cancer, Well-Differentiated: Adjunct:** TSH suppression to <0.1 mU/L usually requires >2 mcg/kg/d. **High-Risk Tumors:** Target TSH suppression may be <0.01 mU/L. **Benign Nodules/Nontoxic Multinodular Goiter:** Target TSH suppression of 0.1-1 mU/L.	
Levothyroxine Sodium, T4 (Levoxyl)	**Tab:** 0.025 mg, 0.05 mg, 0.075 mg, 0.088 mg, 0.1 mg, 0.112 mg, 0.125 mg, 0.137 mg, 0.15 mg, 0.175 mg, 0.2 mg, 0.3 mg	**Hypothyroidism: Adults <50 yo or >50 yo & Recently Treated for Hyperthyroidism or Hypothyroid for Short Time & Peds >12 yo (Growth/Puberty Complete):** 1.7 mcg/kg/d. >200 mcg/d seldom required. **>50 yo or <50 yo w/ Underlying Cardiac Disease: Initial:** 25-50 mcg/d until TSH normalized. **Peds: >12 yo (Growth/Puberty Incomplete):** 2-3 mcg/kg/d. **6-12 yo:** 4-5 mcg/kg/d. **1-5 yo:** 5-6 mcg/kg/d. **6-12 mths:** 6-8 mcg/kg/d. **3-6 mths:** 8-10 mcg/kg/d. **0-3 mths:** 10-15 mcg/kg/d. **Adults: Pituitary TSH Suppression: Thyroid Cancer, Well-Differentiated: Adjunct:** TSH suppression to <0.1 mU/L usually requires >2 mcg/kg/d. **High-Risk Tumors:** Target TSH suppression	A >

Continued on Next Page

NAME	FORM/STRENGTH	DOSAGE	COMMENTS
Levothyroxine Sodium, T4 (Levoxyl) *Continued*		may be <0.01 mU/L. **Benign Nodules/Nontoxic Multinodular Goiter:** Target TSH suppression of 0.1-1 mU/L.	
Levothyroxine Sodium, T4 (Synthroid)	**Tab:** 0.025 mg, 0.05 mg, 0.075 mg, 0.088 mg, 0.1 mg, 0.112 mg, 0.125 mg, 0.137 mg, 0.15 mg, 0.175 mg, 0.2 mg, 0.3 mg	**Hypothyroidism: Adults <50 yo or >50 yo & Recently Treated for Hyperthyroidism or Hypothyroid for Short Time & Peds >12 yo (Growth/Puberty Complete):** 1.7 mcg/kg/d. >200 mcg/d seldom required. **>50 yo or <50 yo w/ Underlying Cardiac Disease: Initial:** 25-50 mcg/d until TSH normalized. **Peds: >12 yo (Growth/Puberty Incomplete):** 2-3 mcg/kg/d. **6-12 yo:** 4-5 mcg/kg/d. **1-5 yo:** 5-6 mcg/kg/d. **6-12 mths:** 6-8 mcg/kg/d. **3-6 mths:** 8-10 mcg/kg/d. **0-3 mths:** 10-15 mcg/kg/d. **Adults: Pituitary TSH Suppression: Thyroid Cancer, Well-Differentiated: Adjunct:** TSH suppression to <0.1 mU/L usually requires >2 mcg/kg/d. **High-Risk Tumors:** Target TSH supression may be <0.01 mU/L. **Benign Nodules/Nontoxic Multinodular Goiter:** Target TSH suppression of 0.1-1 mU/L.	A ❋>
Liothyronine, T3 (Cytomel)	**Tab:** 0.005 mg, 0.025 mg, 0.05 mg	**Adults: Initial:** 25 mcg qd. **Titrate:** Increase up to 25 mcg q1-2wks. **Maint:** 25-75 mcg qd. **Peds: Initial:** 5 mcg qd. **Titrate:** Increase by 5 mcg qd q3-4d until desired response. **Maint: >3 yo:** 25-75 mcg/d. **1-3 yo:** 50 mcg qd. **<1 yo:** 20 mcg qd.	A ❋>

Thyroid, Desiccated (Armour Thyroid)	**Tab:** 15 mg, 30 mg, 60 mg, 90 mg, 120 mg, 180 mg, 240 mg, 300 mg	**Adults: Initial:** 30 mg qd (15 mg qd w/ long-standing myxedema). **Titrate:** Increase by 15 mg q2-3wks. **Maint:** 60-120 mg/d. **Peds: >12 yo:** 1.2-1.8 mg/kg/d. **6-12 yo:** 2.4-3 mg/kg/d. **1-5 yo:** 3-3.6 mg/kg/d. **6-12 mths:** 3.6-4.8 mg/kg/d. **0-6 mths:** 4.8-6 mg/kg/d.	A >

Miscellaneous

CALCIMIMETIC AGENT

Cinacalcet HCl (Sensipar)	**Tab:** 30 mg, 60 mg, 90 mg	**Hypercalcemia in Parathyroid Carcinoma: Initial:** 30 mg bid. **Titrate:** Increase q 2-4 wks through sequential doses of 30 mg bid, 60 mg bid, 90 mg bid, & 90 mg tid-qid prn to normalize serum Ca levels.	C v

GASTROINTESTINAL AGENTS

Antidiarrheal Agents

Atropine Sulfate/ Diphenoxylate HCl CV (Lomotil, Lonox)	**Liq:** 0.025-2.5 mg/5 ml; **Tab:** 0.025-2.5 mg	**Adults: Initial:** 2 tabs or 10 ml qid. **Maint:** 2 tabs or 10 ml tid. **Max:** 20 mg diphenoxylate/d. **13-16 yo: Initial:** 2 tabs or 10 ml qd. **2-12 yo: Initial:** 0.3-0.4 mg/kg/d given qid. **Maint:** 1/4 of initial daily dose.	C >

NAME	FORM/STRENGTH	DOSAGE	COMMENTS
Loperamide (Imodium A-D)	**Liq:** 1 mg/5 ml; **Tab:** 2 mg	**Adults & Peds: ≥12 yo:** 4 mg after 1st loose BM, then 2 mg after loose BM. **Max:** 8 mg/d. **9-11 yo (60-95 lbs):** 2 mg after 1st loose BM, then 1 mg after loose BM. **Max:** 6 mg/d. **6-8 yo (48-59 lbs):** 2 mg after 1st loose BM, then 1 mg after loose BM. **Max:** 4 mg/d. **2-5 yo (24-47 lbs):** 1 mg after 1st loose BM, then 1 mg after loose BM. **Max:** 3 mg/d.	N >
Rifaximin (Xifaxan)	**Tab:** 200 mg	**Adults & Peds: ≥12 yo:** 1 tab tid x 3d.	C v

Antiemetics

5-HT$_3$ ANTAGONISTS

NAME	FORM/STRENGTH	DOSAGE	COMMENTS
Dolasetron Mesylate (Anzemet)	**Inj:** 20 mg/ml; **Tab:** 50 mg, 100 mg	**Prevent Chemo N/V: Adults:** 1.8 mg/kg IV or 100 mg IV/PO. **Peds: 2-16 yo:** 1.8 mg/kg IV/PO, up to 100 mg IV/PO. Give IV 30 min before or PO within 1h before chemo. **Prevent Post-Op N/V: Adults:** 12.5 mg IV or 100 mg PO. **Peds: 2-16 yo:** 0.35 mg/kg IV, up to 12.5 mg IV; or 1.2 mg/kg PO, up to 100 mg PO. Give PO within 2h pre-op, IV 15 min before anesthesia cessation or at start of n/v. **Treat Post-op N/V: Adults:** 12.5 mg IV. **Peds: 2-16 yo:** 0.35 mg/kg IV up to 12.5 mg IV.	B >

Granisetron HCl (Kytril)	**Inj:** 1 mg/ml; **Sol:** 2 mg/ 10 ml; **Tab:** 1 mg	**Prevent Chemo N/V: Adults & Peds: 2-16 yo: IV:** 10 mcg/ kg within 30 min before chemo. **Adults: PO:** 2 mg qd up to 1h before chemo or 1 mg bid (up to 1h before chemo & 12h later). **Prevent Radiation N/V: Adults: PO:** 2 mg qd within 1h of radiation. **Prevent Post-Op N/V: Adults: IV:** 1 mg over 30 sec before anesthesia induction or immediately before anesthesia reversal. **Treat Post-Op N/V: Adults: IV:** 1 mg over 30 sec.	B >
Granisetron (Sancuso)	**Patch:** 3.1 mg/24h	**Adults:** Apply single patch to upper outer arm a minimum of 24h before chemo. May be applied up to max of 48h before chemo. Remove patch minimum of 24h after completion of chemo. Patch may be worn for up to 7d depending on duration of chemo regimen.	B >
Ondansetron HCl (Zofran)	**Inj:** 2 mg/ml, 32 mg/ 50 ml; **Sol:** 4 mg/5 ml; **Tab:** 4 mg, 8 mg, 24 mg; **Tab,Dissolve:** (ODT) 4 mg, 8 mg	**Prevent Chemo-Induced N/V: Adults (>18 yo):** Single 32 mg dose IV over 15 min, 30 min before chemo or three 0.15 mg/kg doses IV over 15 min, 1st dose 30 min before chemo w/ subsequent doses given 4 & 8h after 1st dose. **Peds: 6 mths-18 yo:** Three 0.15 mg/kg doses IV over 15 min, 1st dose 30 min before chemo w/ subsequent doses given 4 & 8h after 1st dose. **Prevent Highly Emetogenic Chemo N/V: Adults:** 24 mg tab PO 30 min before chemo. **Prevent Moderately Emetogenic Chemo N/V: Adults & Peds: ≥12 yo:** 8 mg PO 30 min before chemo, then 8h after 1st dose, then 8 mg bid x 1-2d.	B > **H**

Continued on Next Page

NAME	FORM/STRENGTH	DOSAGE	COMMENTS
Ondansetron HCl (Zofran) *Continued*		**4-11 yo:** 4 mg PO 30 min before chemo, then 4 & 8h after 1st dose, then 4 mg tid x 1-2d. **Prevent Post-Op N/V: Adults:** 16 mg PO 1h before anesthesia. **Peds: >12 yo:** 4 mg IV/IM immediately before anesthesia or post-op. **1mth-12 yo: ≤40 kg:** 0.1 mg/kg IV single dose; **>40 kg:** 4 mg IV single dose. **Prevent Radiation N/V: Adults: Usual:** 8 mg PO tid. **Total Body Irradiation:** 8 mg PO 1-2h before therapy daily. **Single High-Dose Therapy To Abdomen:** 8 mg PO 1-2h before therapy then q8h after 1st dose x 1-2d after complete therapy. **Daily Fractionated Therapy To Abdomen:** 8 mg PO 1-2h before therapy then q8h after 1st dose. **Severe Hepatic Dysfunction: Max:** 8 mg/d IV single dose 30 min before chemo or 8 mg/d PO.	
Palonosetron HCl (Aloxi)	**Cap:** 0.5 mg; **Inj:** 0.25 mg/5 ml, 0.075 mg/1.5 ml	**Adults: Chemo-Induced-N/V: Inj:** 0.25 mg IV single dose 30 min before start of chemo. Repeated dosing within 7d interval not recommended. **Cap:** 0.5 mg 1h prior to chemo. **Post-Op N/V:** 0.075 mg IV single dose 10 sec before induction of anesthesia.	B v

ANTICHOLINERGICS

NAME	FORM/STRENGTH	DOSAGE	COMMENTS
Scopolamine (Transderm Scop)	**Patch:** 0.33 mg/24 h	**Adults: Motion Sickness:** 1 patch behind ear 4h prior to event. Replace after 3d. **Prevent Post-Op N/V:** 1 patch x 24h post-op.	C >

Trimethobenzamide (Tigan)	**Cap:** 300 mg; **Inj:** 100 mg/ml	**Nausea in Gastroenteritis/Post-Op N/V: Adults: Cap:** 300 mg tid-qid. **Inj:** 200 mg IM tid-qid.	◉N ✽>
ANTIHISTAMINES			
Hydroxyzine HCl	**Inj:** 25 mg/ml, 50 mg/ml	**N/V: Adults:** 25-100 mg IM. **Peds:** 0.5 mg/lb IM.	◉N ✽v CI in early pregnancy.
Meclizine HCl (Antivert)	**Tab:** 12.5 mg, 25 mg, 50 mg	**Adults & Peds: ≥12 yo: Vertigo: Usual:** 25-100 mg/d in divided doses. **Motion Sickness:** 25-50 mg 1h before trip/departure; repeat q24h prn.	◉B ✽>
Prochlorperazine	**Inj:** (edisylate) 5 mg/ml; **Sup:** 5 mg, 25 mg; **Tab:** (maleate) 5 mg, 10 mg	**Severe N/V: Adults: PO:** 5-10 mg tab tid-qid; 10 mg cap q12h; 15 mg cap on arising. **PR:** 25 mg sup bid. **IM:** 5-10 mg 3-4h prn. **IV:** 2.5-10 mg (slow push). **Max:** 10 mg/IV single dose; 40 mg/d PO/IM/IV. **Peds: >2 yo & >20lbs: PO/PR: 20-29 lbs:** 2.5 mg qd-bid. **Max:** 7.5 mg/d. **30-39 lbs:** 2.5 mg bid-tid. **Max:** 10 mg/d. **40-85 lbs:** 2.5 mg tid or 5 mg bid. **Max:** 15 mg/d. **IM:** 0.06 mg/lb. **N/V w/ Surgery: Adults: IM/IV:** 5-10 mg IM 1-2h or 5-10 mg IV 15-30 min before anesthesia, or during or after surgery; repeat once if needed.	◉N ✽>

NAME	FORM/STRENGTH	DOSAGE	COMMENTS
Promethazine (Phenergan)	(Generic) **Inj:** 25 mg/ml, 50 mg/ml; **Sup:** 12.5 mg, 25 mg, 50 mg; **Syr:** 6.25 mg/5 ml; **Tab:** 12.5 mg, 25 mg, 50 mg; (Phenergan) **Inj:** 25 mg/ml, 50 mg/ml; **Sup:** 12.5 mg, 25 mg, 50 mg; **Tab:** 12.5 mg, 25 mg, 50 mg	**Prevent N/V & Post-Op N/V: Adults:** 12.5-25 mg IM/IV q4h; 25 mg PO/PR initially, then 12.5-25 mg q4-6h prn. **Peds: ≥2 yo:** 0.5 mg/lb PO/PR/IM/IV q4-6h prn.	C v
DOPAMINE ANTAGONIST/PROKINETIC			
Metoclopramide (Reglan)	(Generic) **Inj:** 5 mg/ml; **Syr:** 5 mg/5 ml; **Tab:** 5 mg, 10 mg; (Reglan) **Inj:** 5 mg/ml; **Tab:** 5 mg, 10 mg	**Adults: Prevent Chemo N/V:** 1-2 mg/kg 30 min before chemo, then q2h x 2 doses, then q3h x 3 doses. **Prevent Post-Op N/V:** 10-20 mg IM near end of surgery.	B >R
SUBSTANCE P/NEUROKININ 1 RECEPTOR ANTAGONIST			
Aprepitant (Emend)	**Cap:** 40 mg, 80 mg, 125 mg; Tri-Pak (one 125 mg & two 80 mg caps)	**Adults: Prevention of Chemo-Induced N/V: Day 1:** 125 mg 1h prior to chemo. **Days 2 & 3:** 80 mg qam. Regimen should include a corticosteroid & 5-HT_3 antagonist. **Concomitant Corticosteroid:** Reduce dexamethasone PO or methylprednisolone PO by 50% & methylprednisolone	B >

		IV by 25%. **Prevention of Post-Op N/V:** 40 mg within 3 hrs prior to induction on anesthesia.	
MISCELLANEOUS			
Dronabinol CIII (Marinol)	**Cap:** 2.5 mg, 5 mg, 10 mg	**Adults & Peds: Prevent Chemo N/V:** 5 mg/m^2 1-3 h before chemo, then 2-4h after chemo, up to 4-6 doses/d. **Titrate:** May increase by 2.5 mg/m^2 increments. **Max:** 15 mg/m^2/dose.	C v
Nabilone CII (Cesamet)	**Cap:** 1 mg	**Adults: Initial:** 1 or 2 mg bid; given 1-3 hrs before chemo. Dose of 1 or 2 mg night before may be useful. **Max:** 6 mg/d given in divided doses tid.	C v

Antispasmodics

Clidinium/ Chlordiazepoxide CIV (Librax)	**Cap:** 5-2.5 mg	**Adults: Usual:** 1-2 caps tid-qid ac & qhs.	N >
Dicyclomine HCl (Bentyl)	**Cap:** 10 mg; **Inj:** 10 mg/ml; **Syr:** 10 mg/5 ml; **Tab:** 20 mg	**Adults: Initial: PO:** 20 mg qid. **Maint:** 40 mg qid if tolerated. D/C if no improvement after 2 wks or if doses ≥80 mg/d not tolerated. **IM:** 20 mg qid x 1-2d, followed by PO dose. Not for IV use.	B v

NAME	FORM/STRENGTH	DOSAGE	COMMENTS
Hyoscyamine Sulfate (Levbid, Levsin, Levsinex)	(Levbid) **Tab,ER:** 0.375 mg. (Levsin) **Drops:** 0.125 mg/ml; **Eli:** 0.125 mg/5 ml; **Inj:** 0.5 mg/ml; **Tab:** 0.125 mg; **Tab,SL:** 0.125 mg. (Levsinex) **Cap,ER:** 0.375 mg	**Adults & Peds: ≥12 yo: Drops/Eli/Tab/Tab,SL:** 0.125-0.25 mg q4h or prn. **Max:** 1.5 mg/24h. **Cap,ER/Tab,ER:** 0.375-0.75 mg q12h; or 1 cap q8h. **Max:** 1.5 mg/24h. **2 to <12 yo: Tab/Tab,SL:** 0.0625-0.125 mg q4h or prn. **Max:** 0.75 mg/24h. **Eli:** Give q4h or prn. **10 kg:** 1.25 ml. **20 kg:** 2.5 ml. **40 kg:** 3.75 ml. **50 kg:** 5 ml. **Max:** 30 ml/24h. **Drops:** 0.25-1 ml q4h or prn. **Max:** 6 ml/24h. **<2 yo: Drops:** Give q4h or prn. **3.4 kg:** 4 gtts. **Max:** 24 gtts/24h. **5 kg:** 5 gtts. **Max:** 30 gtts/24h. **7 kg:** 6 gtts. **Max:** 36 gtts/24h. **10 kg:** 8 gtts. **Max:** 48 gtts/24h.	C >
Scopolamine Hydrobromide/ Hyoscyamine Sulfate/ Atropine Sulfate/ Phenobarbital (Donnatal)	**Tab/Eli (per 5 ml):** 0.0194-0.1037-16.2-0.0065 mg	**Adults:** 1-2 tabs or 5-10 ml tid-qid. **Peds: 100 lbs:** 5 ml q4h or 7.5 ml q6h. **75 lbs:** 3.75 ml q4h or 5 ml q6h. **50 lbs:** 2.5 ml q4h or 3.75 ml q6h. **30 lbs:** 1.5 ml q4h or 2 ml q6h. **20 lbs:** 1 ml q4h or 1.5 ml q6h. **10 lbs:** 0.5 ml q4h or 0.75 ml q6h.	C > H

Antiulcer Agents

DUODENAL ULCER ADHERENT COMPLEX

NAME	FORM/STRENGTH	DOSAGE	COMMENTS
Sucralfate (Carafate)	**Susp:** 1 gm/10 ml; **Tab:** 1 gm	**Active Ulcer: Adults: Sus/Tab:** 1 gm qid x 4-8 wks. **Maint: Tab:** 1 gm bid.	B >

Cimetidine (Tagamet)	(Generic) **Cap:** 150 mg, 300 mg; **Inj:** 150 mg/ml, 300 mg/50 ml; **Sol:** 300 mg/5 ml; **Tab:** 200 mg, 300 mg, 400 mg, 800 mg; (Tagamet) **Tab:** 200 mg, 300 mg, 400 mg	**Adults & Peds: ≥16 yo: PO: Active DU:** 800 mg qhs or 300 mg qid or 400 mg bid x 4-8 wks. **Maint:** 400 mg qhs. **Active Benign GU:** 800 mg qhs or 300 mg qid x 6 wks. **IM/IV:** 300 mg q6-8h. **Max:** 2400 mg/d.	B v **R**
Famotidine (Pepcid, Pepcid RPD)	**Inj:** 0.4 mg/ml, 10 mg/ml; **Susp:** 40 mg/5 ml; **Tab:** 20 mg, 40 mg; **Tab,Dissolve:** 20 mg, 40 mg	**Adults: DU: PO:** 20 mg bid or 40 mg qhs x 4-8 wks. **Maint:** 20 mg qhs. **IV:** 20 mg q12h. **GU: PO:** 20 mg bid up to 6 wks. **Peds 1-16 yo: DU/GU:** 0.25 mg/kg IV/PO q12h or 0.5 mg/kg/d PO qhs. **Max:** 40 mg/d.	B v **R**
Nizatidine (Axid, Axid Oral Solution)	**Cap:** 150 mg, 300 mg; **Sol:** 15 mg/ml	**Adults:** 150 mg bid or 300 mg qhs up to 8 wks. **Maint:** 150 mg qhs up to 1 yr.	B v **R**
Ranitidine HCl (Zantac)	**Inj:** 1 mg/ml, 25 mg/ml; **Syr:** 15 mg/ml; **Tab:** 150 mg, 300 mg; **Tab,Eff:** 25 mg, 150 mg	**Adults: GU/DU: PO:** 150 mg bid, or (DU) 300 mg after evening meal or qhs. **Maint:** 150 mg qhs. **IV/IM:** 50 mg q6-8h. **Continuous IV:** 6.25 mg/h. **Max:** 400 mg/d. **1 mth-16 yo: GU/DU: PO:** 2-4 mg/kg bid. **Max:** 300 mg/d. **Maint:** 2-4 mg/kg qd. **Max:** 150 mg/d. **DU: IV:** 2-4 mg/kg/d given q6-8h. **Max:** 50 mg q6-8h.	B > **R**

NAME	FORM/STRENGTH	DOSAGE	COMMENTS
PROSTAGLANDIN E_1 ANALOG			
Misoprostol (Cytotec)	**Tab:** 100 mcg, 200 mcg	**NSAID Ulcer Prevention: Adults:** 200 mcg qid w/ food. May use 100 mcg dose if 200 mcg not tolerated.	X; v Abortifacient.
PROTON PUMP INHIBITORS AND COMBINATIONS			
Esomeprazole Magnesium (Nexium)	**Cap,Delay:** 20 mg, 40 mg; **Sus,Delay:** 20 mg, 40 mg (granules/pkt)	**Risk Reduction of NSAID-Associated Gastric Ulcer: Adults:** 20 mg or 40 mg qd x up to 6 mths. **Severe Hepatic Dysfunction: Max:** 20 mg/d. Take 1h before meals. Swallow cap whole.	B; v **H**
Lansoprazole/Naproxen (Prevacid NapraPAC)	**Cap, Delay**: (Lansoprazole) 15 mg; **Tab:** (Naproxen) 500 mg	**NSAID-Associated GU: Risk Reduction: Adults:** Take AM dose before eating. Lansoprazole 15 mg qam + naproxen 500 mg bid in AM & PM. **Max:** 1000 mg naproxen/day. Take naproxen w/ glass of water. Swallow lansoprazole whole.	C; v **H R**
Lansoprazole (Prevacid, Prevacid SoluTab)	**Cap, Delay:** 15 mg, 30 mg; **Sus, Delay:** 15 mg, 30 mg (granules/pkt); **Tab, Delay, Dissolve:** (SoluTab) 15 mg, 30 mg	**Adults: DU:** 15 mg qd x 4 wks. **Maint:** 15 mg qd. **Benign GU:** 30 mg qd x up to 8 wks. **NSAID-Associated GU: Healing:** 30 mg qd x 8 wks. **Risk Reduction:** 15 mg qd x up to 12 wks.	B; v **H**

Omeprazole/ Sodium Bicarbonate (Zegerid)	**Cap:** 20-1100 mg, 40-1100 mg; **Pow:** 20-1680 mg/pkt, 40-1680 mg/pkt	**Adults: Cap/Pow: DU:** 20 mg qd x 4-8 wks. **GU:** 40 mg qd x 4-8 wks. **Pow (40-1680 mg): Risk Reduction of Upper GI Bleeding in Critically Ill Patients: Initial:** 40 mg, followed by 40 mg 6-8 h later. **Maint:** 40 mg qd x 14d.	C v
Omeprazole (Prilosec)	**Cap,Delay:** 10 mg, 20 mg, 40 mg	**Adults: DU:** 20 mg qd x 4-8 wks. **GU:** 40 mg qd x 4-8 wks. Swallow whole. Take before eating.	C v
Rabeprazole Sodium (Aciphex)	**Tab, Delay:** 20 mg	**DU Treatment: Adults:** 20 mg qd up to 4 wks.	B v

GERD

DOPAMINE ANTAGONIST/PROKINETIC

Metoclopramide (Reglan)	(Generic) **Syr:** 5 mg/5 ml; **Tab:** 5 mg, 10 mg; (Reglan) **Tab:** 5 mg, 10 mg	**Adults:** 10-15 mg qid 30 min ac & qhs. **Max:** 12 wks of therapy. **Intermittent Symptoms:** Up to 20 mg single dose prior to provoking situation.	B > **R**

H_2 ANTAGONISTS

Cimetidine (Tagamet)	(Generic) **Sol:** 300 mg/5 ml; **Tab:** 200 mg, 300 mg, 400 mg, 800 mg; (Tagamet) **Tab:** 200 mg, 300 mg, 400 mg	**Adults & Peds: ≥16 yo: PO:** 400 mg qid or 800 mg bid x 12 wks.	B v **R**

NAME	FORM/STRENGTH	DOSAGE	COMMENTS
Famotidine (Pepcid, Pepcid RPD)	**Inj:** 0.4 mg/ml, 10 mg/ml; **Susp:** 40 mg/5 ml; **Tab:** 20 mg, 40 mg; **Tab,Dissolve:** 20 mg, 40 mg.	**Adults: PO:** 20 mg bid up to 6 wks. **Peds: 1-16 yo: IV/PO:** 0.25 mg/kg IV q12h (up to 40 mg/d) or 0.5 mg/kg PO bid (up to 40 mg bid). **3 mths-1 yo: PO:** 0.5 mg/kg bid x up to 8 wks. **<3 mths: PO:** 0.5 mg/kg qd x up to 8 wks. **Esophagitis: Adults: PO:** 20-40 mg bid x up to 12 wks.	B v **R**
Nizatidine (Axid, Axid Oral Solution)	**Cap:** 150 mg, 300 mg; **Sol:** 15 mg/ml	**Adults:** 150 mg bid up to 12 wks. **Peds: ≥12 yo: Erosive Esophagitis/GERD: Sol:** 150 mg bid up to 8 wks. **Max:** 300 mg/d.	B v **R**
Ranitidine HCl (Zantac)	**Inj:** 1 mg/ml, 25 mg/ml; **Syr:** 15 mg/ml; **Tab:** 150 mg, 300 mg; **Tab,Eff:** 25 mg, 150 mg	**Adults: PO: Symptomatic:** 150 mg bid. **Erosive Esophagitis:** 150 mg qid. **Maint:** 150 mg bid. **IV/IM:** 50 mg q6-8h. **Continuous IV:** 6.25 mg/h. **Max:** 400 mg/d. **1 mth-16 yo: Symptomatic/Erosive Esophagitis:** 2.5-5 mg/kg PO bid.	B > **R**

PROTON PUMP INHIBITORS AND COMBINATIONS

NAME	FORM/STRENGTH	DOSAGE	COMMENTS
Amoxicillin/Clarithromycin/ Lansoprazole (Prevpac)	**Cap:** (Amoxicillin) 500 mg, **Tab:** (Clarithromycin) 500 mg, **Cap,Delay:** (Lansoprazole) 30 mg	**Adults:** 1 gm amoxicillin, 500 mg clarithromycin & 30 mg lansoprazole, all bid (am & pm) before meals x 10 or 14 days. Swallow each pill whole. **Renal Impairment (with or w/o hepatic impairment):** Decrease clarithromycin dose or prolong intervals. Avoid w/ CrCl <30 ml/min.	C v **H**

Dexlansoprazole (Kapidex)	**Cap,DR:** 30 mg, 60 mg	**Adults: Erosive Esophagitis:** 60 mg qd x up to 8 wks. **Maint:** 30 mg qd x up to 6 mths. **Symptomatic Nonerosive GERD:** 30 mg qd x 4 wks. Swallow whole. May open cap & sprinkle intact granules on 1 tbsp of applesauce; swallow immediately.	B v **H**
Esomeprazole Magnesium (Nexium)	**Cap,Delay:** 20 mg, 40 mg; **Sus,Delay:** 20 mg, 40 mg (granules/pkt)	**Adults: PO: Symptomatic GERD:** 20 mg qd x 4 wks; additional 4 wks w/ continued symptoms. **Erosive Esophagitis: Healing:** 20 mg or 40 mg qd x 4-8 wks; additional 4-8 wks if not healed. **Maint:** 20 mg qd x up to 6 mths. **Peds: PO: Symptomatic GERD: 12-17 yo:** 20 mg or 40 mg qd x up to 8 wks. **1-11 yo:** 10 mg qd x up to 8 wks. **Erosive Esophagitis: 1-11 yo: ≥20 kg:** 10 mg or 20 mg qd x 8 wks. **<20 kg:** 10 mg qd x 8 wks. **Severe Hepatic Dysfunction: Max:** 20 mg/d. Take 1h before meals. Swallow cap whole.	B v **H**
Esomeprazole Sodium (Nexium IV)	**Inj:** 20 mg, 40 mg	**Adults: GERD w/ history of Erosive Esophagitis:** 20-40 mg IV qd x up to 10d. Change to PO ASAP.	B v **H**
Lansoprazole (Prevacid, Prevacid IV, Prevacid Solutab)	**Cap, Delay:** 15 mg, 30 mg; **Inj:** 30 mg; **Sus, Delay:** 15 mg, 30 mg (granules/pkt); **Tab, Delay, Dissolve:** (SoluTab) 15 mg, 30 mg	**Adults: PO: Symptomatic GERD:** 15 mg qd x up to 8 wks. **Erosive Esophagitis:** 30 mg qd x up to 8 wks. May repeat x 8 wks, if needed. If recurrence, may consider additional 8 wks. **Maint:** 15 mg qd. **IV: Erosive Esophagitis:** 30 mg/d x up to 7d. Switch to PO when possible. **Peds: PO: 12-17 yo: Symptomatic GERD/Nonerosive:** 15 mg qd x up	B v **H**

Continued on Next Page

NAME	FORM/STRENGTH	DOSAGE	COMMENTS
Lansoprazole (Prevacid, Prevacid IV, Prevacid Solutab) *Continued*		to 8 wks. **Symptomatic GERD/Erosive Esophagitis:** 30 mg qd x up to 8 wks. **1-11 yo: Symptomatic GERD/Erosive Esophagitis: ≤30 kg:** 15 mg qd x up to 12 wks. **>30 kg:** 30 mg qd x up to 12 wks. **Titrate:** May increase up to 30 mg bid after 2 wks if still symptomatic.	
Omeprazole/ Sodium Bicarbonate (Zegerid)	**Cap:** 20-1100 mg, 40-1100 mg; **Pow:** 20-1680 mg/pkt, 40-1680 mg/pkt	**Adults: Cap/Pow: Symptomatic GERD:** 20 mg qd x up to 4 wks. **Erosive Esophagitis:** 20 mg qd x 4-8 wks. **Maint:** 20 mg qd.	C v
Omeprazole (Prilosec)	**Cap,Delay:** 10 mg, 20 mg, 40 mg	**Adults: Symptomatic GERD:** 20 mg qd x up to 4 wks. **Erosive Esophagitis:** 20 mg qd x 4-8 wks. **Maint:** 20 mg qd. **Peds: 1-16 yo: GERD/Erosive Esophagitis: ≥20 kg:** 20 mg qd. **10 to <20 kg:** 10 mg qd. **5 to <10 kg:** 5 mg qd. Swallow whole. Take before eating. May add contents of caps to applesauce if difficulty swallowing; swallow immediately w/o chewing.	C v
Pantoprazole Sodium (Protonix, Protonix IV)	**Inj:** 40 mg; **Sus, Delay:** 40 mg (granules/pkt); **Tab, Delay:** 20 mg, 40 mg	**Adults: Erosive Esophagitis: PO:** 40 mg qd x up to 8 wks. May repeat course. **Maint:** 40 mg qd. **GERD: IV:** 40 mg qd x 7-10d.	B v

Rabeprazole Sodium (Aciphex)	**Tab, Delay:** 20 mg	**Adults: Erosive/Ulcerative GERD: Healing:** 20 mg qd x 4-8 wks. May repeat x 8 wks if needed. **Maint:** 20 mg qd. **Symptomatic GERD:** 20 mg qd x 4 wks. May repeat x 4 wks if needed. **Peds:** **≥12 yo: Symptomatic GERD:** 20 mg qd x up to 8 wks.	◙B ❁V

Laxatives

BOWEL EVACUANTS

Polyethylene Glycol 3350/ Potassium Chloride/ Sodium Sulfate/ Sodium Chloride/ Sodium Bicarbonate (Colyte, Colyte w/ Flavor Packs, Colyte-Flavored)	**Pow for Sol:** 240-2.98-6.72-5.84-22.72 gm/4 L	**Adults: GI Exam Prep: PO:** 240 ml q10min until fecal discharge is clear. **NG-Tube:** 20-30 ml/min (1.2-1.8 L/h).	◙C ❁>
Polyethylene Glycol 3350/ Potassium Chloride/ Sodium Sulfate/ Sodium Chloride/ Sodium Bicarbonate (GoLYTELY)	**Pow for Sol:** 236-2.97-6.74-5.86-22.74 gm/4 L	**Adults: PO:** 240 ml q10min until fecal discharge is clear or 4 L consumed. **NG-Tube:** 20-30 ml/min (1.2-1.8 L/h).	◙C ❁>

NAME	FORM/STRENGTH	DOSAGE	COMMENTS
BULK-FORMING AGENTS			
Psyllium (Metamucil)	**Pow:** 3.4 gm psyllium husk/dose	**Adults & Peds: ≥12 yo:** 1 tsp, 1 tbs, or 1 pkt (depending on product). **6-12 yo:** 1/2 adult dose. May take qd-tid. Mix w/ 8 oz of liquid.	N ❋>
COLONIC ACIDIFIER			
Lactulose (Constilac, Constulose, Enulose, Generlac, Lactulose)	**Sol:** 10 gm/15 ml	**Adults:** 15-30 ml qd. **Max:** 60 ml/d.	B ❋>
OSMOTIC AGENT			
Polyethylene Glycol 3350 (MiraLax)	**Pow:** 17 gm/dose	**Adults & Peds: ≥17 yo:** Dissolve 17 gm in 4-8 oz of beverage & drink qd. Use no more than 7d.	N ❋>
STIMULANT/STOOL SOFTENERS			
Docusate Sodium/Senna (Peri-Colace)	**Tab:** 50-8.6 mg	**Adults:** 2-4 tabs daily. **Peds: ≥12 yo:** 2-4 tabs daily. **6-<12 yo:** 1-2 tabs daily. **2-<6 yo: Max:** 1 tab daily.	N ❋>
STIMULANTS			
Bisacodyl (Dulcolax)	**Sup:** 10 mg; **Tab, Delay:** 5 mg	**Adults & Peds: ≥12 yo:** 2-3 tabs or 1 sup qd as single dose. **6-12 yo:** 1 tab or 1/2 sup qd.	N ❋>

Senna (Senokot)	**Granules:** 15 mg/tsp; **Tab:** 8.6 mg, 17 mg	**Adults & Peds:** ≥**12 yo:** 2 tabs or 1 tsp qd. **Max**: 4 tabs or 2 tsp bid. **6-12 yo:** 1 tab or 1/2 tsp qd. **Max:** 2 tabs or 1 tsp bid. **2-6 yo:** 1/2 tab or 1/4 tsp qd. **Max:** 1 tab or 1/2 tsp bid. SenokotXTRA dose is 1/2 of reg strength tab.	◙N ❁>

STOOL SOFTENERS

Docusate Sodium (Colace)	**Cap:** 50 mg, 100 mg; **Liq:** 10 mg/ml; **Syr:** 20 mg/5 ml	**Adults & Peds:** ≥**12 yo:** 50-200 mg qd. **6-12 yo:** 40-120 mg/d liq. **3-6 yo:** 2 ml liq tid. Mix liq/syr w/ 6-8 oz of milk, juice or formula. **Retention/Flushing Enemas:** Add 5-10 ml liq to enema fluid.	◙N ❁>
Glycerin (Fleet Glycerin Laxatives)	**Enema:** (Babylax) 2.3 gm, (Liquid Glycerin) 5.6 gm; **Sup:** 1 gm, 2 gm, 3 gm	**Adults & Peds:** ≥**6 yo:** 1 enema (5.6 gm) or 1 sup (2 gm or 3 gm) PR. **2-5 yo:** 1 enema (2.3 gm) or 1 sup (1 gm) PR.	◙N ❁>

Ulcerative Colitis

ANTI-INFLAMMATORY/IMMUNOMODULATORY AGENTS

Sulfasalazine (Azulfidine)	**Tab:** 500 mg	**Adults: Initial:** 1-4 gm/d in divided doses. **Maint:** 2 gm/d. **Peds:** ≥**2 yo:** 40-60 mg/kg/24h divided in 3-6 doses. **Maint:** 7.5 mg/kg qid.	◙B ❁>

NAME	FORM/STRENGTH	DOSAGE	COMMENTS
SALICYLATES			
Mesalamine (Asacol)	**Tab, Delay:** 400 mg	**Active Mild-to-Moderate Active Ulcerative Colitis: Adults:** 800 mg tid x 6 wks. **Remission Maint:** 1.6 gm/d in divided doses.	◙B ❋>
Mesalamine (Lialda)	**Tab, Delay:** 1.2 gm	**Active Mild-to-Moderate Active Ulcerative Colitis: Adults:** 2-4 tabs qd w/ meals x up to 8 wks. **Max:** 2.4 gm/d or 4.8 gm/d.	◙B ❋>
Mesalamine (Pentasa)	**Cap, ER:** 250 mg, 500 mg	**Mild-to-Moderate Active Ulcerative Colitis: Adults:** 1 gm qid x up to 8 wks.	◙B ❋>

Zollinger-Ellison Agents

NAME	FORM/STRENGTH	DOSAGE	COMMENTS
H_2 ANTAGONISTS			
Cimetidine (Tagamet)	(Generic) **Inj:** 150 mg/ml, 300 mg/50 ml; **Sol:** 300 mg/5 ml; **Tab:** 200 mg, 300 mg, 400 mg, 800 mg; (Tagamet) **Tab:** 200 mg, 300 mg, 400 mg	**Adults: PO:** 300 mg qid. **Max:** 2400 mg/d. **IM/IV:** 300 mg q6-8h. **Max:** 2400 mg/d.	◙B ❋v **R**

Famotidine (Pepcid, Pepcid RPD)	**Inj:** 0.4 mg/ml, 10 mg/ml; **Susp:** 40 mg/5 ml; **Tab:** 20 mg, 40 mg; **Tab,Dissolve:** 20 mg, 40 mg	**Adults: PO: Initial:** 20 mg q6h. **Max:** 160 mg q6h. **IV:** 20 mg q12h or greater if required.	B v **R**
Ranitidine HCl (Zantac)	**Inj:** 1 mg/ml, 25 mg/ml; **Syr:** 15 mg/ml; **Tab:** 150 mg, 300 mg; **Tab,Eff:** 25 mg, 150 mg	**Adults: PO:** 150 mg bid. May give up to 6 gm/d w/ severe disease. **IM/IV (Intermittent):** 50 mg q6-8h. **IV (Continuous):** 1 mg/kg/h IV. **Titrate:** May increase after 4 h by 0.5 mg/kg/h increments. **Max:** 2.5 mg/kg/h or 220 mg/h.	B > **R**

PROTON PUMP INHIBITORS AND COMBINATIONS

Esomeprazole Magnesium (Nexium)	**Cap,Delay:** 20 mg, 40 mg; **Sus,Delay:** 20 mg, 40 mg (granules/pkt)	**Adults:** 40 mg bid. **Severe Hepatic Dysfunction: Max:** 20 mg/d. Take 1h before meals. Swallow cap whole.	B v **H**
Lansoprazole (Prevacid, Prevacid SoluTab)	**Cap, Delay:** 15 mg, 30 mg; **Sus, Delay:** 15 mg, 30 mg (granules/pkt); **Tab, Delay, Dissolve:** (SoluTab) 15 mg, 30 mg.	**Adults:** 60 mg qd. **Max:** 90 mg bid. Divide dose if >120 mg/d.	B v **H**

NAME	FORM/STRENGTH	DOSAGE	COMMENTS
Omeprazole (Prilosec)	**Cap,Delay:** 10 mg, 20 mg, 40 mg	**Adults:** 60 mg qd, then adjust as needed. Divide dose if >80 mg/d. Doses up to 120 mg tid have been given. Swallow whole. Take before eating.	C v
Pantoprazole Sodium (Protonix, Protonix IV)	**Inj:** 40 mg; **Sus, Delay:** 40 mg (granules/pkt); **Tab, Delay:** 20 mg, 40 mg	**Adults: PO:** 40 mg bid. **Max:** 240 mg/d. **IV:** 80 mg q12h, adjust based on acid output. **Max:** 240 mg/d or 6 days.	B v

Miscellaneous

NAME	FORM/STRENGTH	DOSAGE	COMMENTS
Adalimumab (Humira)	**Inj:** 40 mg/0.8 ml	**Crohn's Disease: Adults: Initial:** 160 mg (may be given as 4 inj on Day 1 or 2 inj/d x 2 consecutive days); 80 mg at Wk 2. **Maint:** 40 mg every other wk beginning Wk 4.	B v **W** [86]
Alosetron HCl (Lotronex)	**Tab:** 0.5 mg, 1 mg	**Diarrhea-Predominant Irritable Bowel Syndrome (Women): Adults: Initial:** 1 mg qd x 4 wks. **Titrate:** May increase to 1 mg bid. D/C after 4 wks if symptoms uncontrolled on 1 mg bid.	B > **W** [43]
Celecoxib (Celebrex)	**Cap:** 50 mg, 100 mg, 200 mg, 400 mg	**Familial Adenomatous Polyposis: Adults: ≥18 yo:** 400 mg bid w/ food. **Poor Metabolizers of CYP2C9 Substrates:** Half the lowest recommended dose.	C D (≥30 wks gestation) > **H W** [66,67]
Certolizumab pegol (Cimzia)	**Inj:** 200 mg	**Crohn's Disease: Adults: Initial:** 400 mg SC at Weeks 2 & 4. **Maint:** 400 mg SC q4wks.	B v **W** [86]

Infliximab (Remicade)	**Inj:** 100 mg	**Adults: Crohn's Disease/Fistulizing Crohn's Disease: Induction:** 5 mg/kg IV at 0, 2, & 6 wks. **Maint:** 5 mg/kg q8wks. For patients who respond then lose response, may increase to 10 mg/kg. Consider d/c if no response by Wk 14. **Ulcerative Colitis: Induction:** 5 mg/kg IV at 0, 2, & 6 wks. **Maint:** 5 mg/kg q8wks. **Peds: ≥6 yo: Crohn's Disease: Induction:** 5 mg/kg IV at 0, 2, & 6 wks. **Maint:** 5 mg/kg q8wks.	B v **W** [86]
Lubiprostone (Amitiza)	**Cap:** 8 mcg, 24 mcg	**Adults: Chronic Idiopathic Constipation:** 24 mcg bid w/ food. **Irritable Bowel Syndrome w/ Constipation:** (Females) 8 mcg bid w/ food.	C v
Methylnaltrexone Bromide (Relistor)	**Inj:** 12 mg/0.6 ml	**Opioid-Induced Constipation: Adults:** Inject SC in upper arm, abdomen, or thigh. **Usual:** 1 dose qod prn. **Max:** 1 dose/24h. **Patient Wt: 38 to <62 kg (84 to <136 lbs):** 8 mg. **62-114 kg (136-251 lbs):** 12 mg. **Patients Outside These Ranges:** 0.15 mg/kg. To calculate inj volume for these patients, multiply wt in lbs by 0.0034 or wt in kg by 0.0075 & round up volume to nearest 0.1ml.	B > **R**
Ursodiol (Actigall)	**Cap:** 300 mg	**Adults: Gallstone Dissolution:** 8-10 mg/kg/d in 2-3 divided doses. **Prevention:** 300 mg bid.	B >

GYNECOLOGY

Anti-Infective Agents

ANTIBACTERIALS

NAME	FORM/STRENGTH	DOSAGE	COMMENTS
Clindamycin Phosphate (Clindesse)	**Cre:** 2%	**Bacterial Vaginosis: Adults:** 1 applicatorful intravaginally any time of day.	B v
Clindamycin Phosphate (Cleocin Vaginal, Cleocin Vaginal Ovules, Clindamax Vaginal)	**Cre:** 2%; **Sup, Vaginal:** (Ovules) 100 mg	**Bacterial Vaginosis: Adults:** (Cre) 1 applicatorful intravaginally qhs. Treat non-pregnant females x 3-7d (non-pregnant) or 7d (2nd/3rd trimester). (Sup) 1 sup intravaginally qhs x 3d. **Peds: Post-Menarchal:** (Sup) 1 sup intravaginally qhs x 3d.	B v
Metronidazole (Flagyl)	**Cap:** 375 mg; **Tab:** 250 mg, 500 mg	**Adults: Flagyl: Trichomoniasis:** 375 mg (cap) bid or 250 mg (tab) tid x 7d. **Alternate Regimen:** If non-pregnant, 2 gm (tab) as single or divided dose.	B v CI in 1st trimester. **H W** 83
Metronidazole (Flagyl ER)	**Tab,ER:** 750 mg	**Adults: Bacterial Vaginosis:** 750 mg qd x 7d on empty stomach.	B v **H** CI in 1st trimester. **W** 83
Metronidazole (MetroGel-Vaginal)	**Gel:** 0.75%	**Bacterial Vaginosis: Adults:** Insert 1 applicatorful intravaginally qd-bid x 5d. For qd dosing, give hs.	B v

ANTIFUNGALS

NAME	FORM/STRENGTH	DOSAGE	COMMENTS
Butoconazole Nitrate (Mycelex-3)	**Cre:** 2%	**Vulvovaginal Candidiasis: Adults:** 1 applicatorful intravaginally qhs x 3d.	C >

Clotrimazole (Gyne-Lotrimin 3, Gyne-Lotrimin Combination Pack)	**Cre-Sup:** (Gyne-Lotrimin Combination) 1%-100 mg, (Gyne-Lotrimin 3) 2%-200 mg	**Vulvovaginal Candidiasis: Adults & Peds: ≥12 yo:** (Gyne-Lotrimin 3) 1 applicatorful or 1 insert intravaginally qhs x 3d. (Gyne-Lotrimin Combination) 1 sup intravaginally qhs for 7d. Apply cre prn.	N >
Clotrimazole (Mycelex-7)	**Cre:** 1%	**Vulvovaginal Candidiasis: Adults & Peds: ≥12 yo:** 1 applicatorful intravaginally qhs x 7d.	N >
Fluconazole (Diflucan)	**Tab:** 150 mg	**Vaginal Candidiasis: Adults:** 150 mg single dose.	C v
Miconazole Nitrate (Monistat 3, Monistat 7)	**Cre-Sup:** (Monistat-3) 4%-200 mg, (Monistat-7) 2%-100 mg	**Vulvovaginal Candidiasis: Adults & Peds: ≥12 yo:** (Monistat 3) 200 mg sup or 4% cre intravaginally qhs x 3d. (Monistat 7) 100 mg sup or 2% cre intravaginally x 7d.	C >
Terconazole (Terazol 3)	**Cre-Sup:** 0.8%-80 mg	**Vulvovaginal Candidiasis: Adults:** 1 applicatorful of 0.8% or 80 mg sup intravaginally qhs x 3d.	C >
Terconazole (Terazol 7)	**Cre:** 0.4%	**Vulvovaginal Candidiasis: Adults:** 1 applicatorful of 0.4% intravaginally qhs x 7d.	C >
Tioconazole (Vagistat-1)	**Oint:** 6.5%	**Vulvovaginal Candidiasis: Adults & Peds: ≥12 yo:** Insert contents of applicator intravaginally once hs.	N >

Contraceptives

NAME	FORM/STRENGTH	DOSAGE	COMMENTS
PROGESTOGEN			
Levonorgestrel (Norplant II)	**Implant:** 75 mg	**Adults:** Implant 150 mg (2 implants) in midportion of upper arm during 1st 7d of onset of menses. Place in a "V" shape 30° apart. Replace by end of 5th yr.	N >
Levonorgestrel (Mirena)	**IUD:** 52 mg	**Adults:** Insert intravaginally initially within 7d of menses onset. May replace any time in the cycle. May insert 6 wks postpartum or until involution of uterus is complete & immediately after 1st trimester abortion. Replace q5yrs.	X v
Levonorgestrel (Plan B)	**Tab:** 0.75 mg	**Adults:** 1 tab as soon as possible, within 72h after unprotected intercourse, then 1 tab 12h after 1st dose. May use during menstrual cycle.	N >
Medroxyprogesterone Acetate (Depo-Provera Contraceptive)	**Inj:** 150 mg/ml	**Adults:** 150 mg IM q3mths. Give 1st inj during 1st 5d of menses; within 1st 5d postpartum if not nursing; or 6 wks postpartum if nursing.	X >
MISCELLANEOUS			
Ethinyl Estradiol/ Levonorgestrel (Lybrel)	**Tab:** 0.02-0.09 mg	**Adults:** 1 tab qd. **Start Day: No Current Contraceptive Therapy:** Day 1 of menstrual cycle. **21- or 28-day Regimen:** Day 1 of withdrawal bleed (at latest 7d after last active tab). **Progestin-Only Pill:** Day after taking progestin-only pill. **Implant:** Day of implant removal. **Inj:** Day next inj due. Use nonhormonal back-up method of	X v

		birth control for 1st 7d of Lybrel therapy when initiating after progestin-only pill, implant, or inj.	
Ethinyl Estradiol/ Levonorgestrel (Seasonale)	**Tab:** 0.03-0.15 mg	**Adults:** 1 tab qd x 91d, then repeat. Start 1st Sunday after menses begin.	X v

Dysmenorrhea

NSAIDS

Celecoxib (Celebrex)	**Cap:** 50 mg, 100 mg, 200 mg, 400 mg	**Adults: Day 1:** 400 mg, then 200 mg if needed. **Maint:** 200 mg bid prn. **Poor Metabolizers of CYP2C9 Substrates:** Half lowest recommended dose.	C D (≥30 wks gestation) v **H W** [66, 67]
Ibuprofen (Motrin)	**Susp:** 100 mg/5 ml; **Tab:** 400 mg, 600 mg, 800 mg	**Adults:** 400 mg q4h prn.	C v **R W** [66, 67]
Naproxen Sodium (Anaprox, Anaprox DS)	**Tab:** (Anaprox) 275 mg, (Anaprox DS) 550 mg	**Adults: Tab: Initial:** 550 mg, then 550 mg q12h or 275 mg q6-8h prn. **Max:** 1100 mg/d for maint.	C v **W** [66, 67]
Naproxen (Naprosyn)	**Susp:** 25 mg/ml; **Tab:** 250 mg, 375 mg, 500 mg	**Adults: Initial:** 500 mg, then 250 mg q6-8h prn.	C v **W** [66, 67]

NAME	FORM/STRENGTH	DOSAGE	COMMENTS

Endometriosis

GONADOTROPINS

NAME	FORM/STRENGTH	DOSAGE	COMMENTS
Nafarelin Acetate (Synarel)	**Spr:** 200 mcg/inh	**Adults:** ≥**18 yo:** 1 spr into one nostril qam & 1 spr into other nostril qpm. Initiate b/w Days 2-4 of menstrual cycle. Increase to 1 spr/nostril qam & qpm after 2 mths if amenorrhea has not occurred. Treat x 6 mths.	X v

PROGESTOGEN

NAME	FORM/STRENGTH	DOSAGE	COMMENTS
Norethindrone Acetate (Aygestin)	**Tab:** 5 mg	**Adults:** Assume interval between menses is 28d. **Initial:** 5 mg qd x 2 wks. **Titrate:** Increase by 2.5 mg/d q2wks until 15 mg/d. Continue x 6-9 mths or until breakthrough bleeding demands temporary termination.	X > **H**

Hormone Therapy

NAME	FORM/STRENGTH	DOSAGE	COMMENTS
Conjugated Estrogens (Cenestin)	**Tab:** 0.3 mg, 0.45 mg, 0.625 mg, 0.9 mg, 1.25 mg	**Adults: Vasomotor Symptoms: Initial:** 0.45 mg qd. Adjust dose based on response. **Vulvar/Vaginal Atrophy:** 0.3 mg qd.	N > CI in pregnancy. **W** 4, 10, 28
Conjugated Estrogens (Enjuvia)	**Tab:** 0.3 mg, 0.45 mg, 0.625 mg, 0.9 mg, 1.25 mg	**Vasomotor Symptoms/Vulvar & Vaginal Atrophy/Vaginal Dryness & Pain w/ Intercourse: Adults:** Individualize dose. **Initial:** 0.3 mg qd. Adjust dose based on response.	X > **W** 4, 10, 28

Conjugated Estrogens (Premarin Tablets)	**Tab:** 0.3 mg, 0.45 mg, 0.625 mg, 0.9 mg, 1.25 mg	**Adults: Tab: Vasomotor Symptoms/Vulvar & Vaginal Atrophy: Initial:** 0.3 mg continuous or cyclically (eg, 25d on, 5d off). **Female Hypogonadism: Initial:** 0.3-0.625 mg qd cyclically. **Female Castration/Primary Ovarian Failure: Initial:** 1.25 mg qd cyclically.	X > **W** 4, 10, 28
Conjugated Estrogens (Premarin Vaginal)	**Cre:** 0.625 mg/gm	**Adults: Atrophic Vaginitis/Kraurosis Vulvae: Usual:** 0.5 gm intravaginally qd cyclically (3 wks on, 1 wk off). **Titrate:** 0.5-2 gm based on individual response. **Moderate to Severe Dyspareunia:** 0.5 gm intravaginally BIW (eg, Mon & Thurs) continuous regimen or qd cyclically (3 wks on, 1 wk off).	X > **W** 4, 10, 28
Drospirenone/Estradiol (Angeliq)	**Tab:** 0.5-1 mg	**Vasomotor Symptoms, Vulvar/Vaginal Atrophy: Adults:** 1 tab qd. Re-evaluate after 3-6 mths.	X > **W** 28
Esterified Estrogens (Menest)	**Tab:** 0.3 mg, 0.625 mg, 1.25 mg, 2.5 mg	**Adults: Vasomotor Symptoms:** 1.25 mg qd cyclically (3 wks on, 1 wk off). **Atrophic Vaginitis/Kraurosis Vulvae:** 0.3-1.25 mg qd cyclically. **Female Hypogonadism:** 2.5-7.5 mg/d in divided doses x 20d, then 10d off therapy; repeat until menses occurs. **Female Castration/Primary Ovarian Failure:** 1.25 mg qd cyclically. **Maint:** Lowest effective dose.	X v **W** 4, 10, 28
Estradiol Acetate (Femring, Femtrace)	**Vaginal Ring:** (Femring) 0.05 mg/d, 0.1 mg/d **Tab:** (Femtrace) 0.45 mg, 0.9 mg, 1.8 mg	**Adults: Femring: Initial:** Use lowest effective dose. Insert ring vaginally. Replace q3mths. Re-evaluate periodically. **Femtrace:** 1 tab qd. Use lowest effective dose. Re-evaluate periodically.	X > **W** 4, 28

NAME	FORM/STRENGTH	DOSAGE	COMMENTS
Estradiol/Levonorgestrel (Climara Pro)	**Patch:** 0.045-0.015 mg/d	**Vasomotor Symptoms: Adults:** Apply 1 patch qwk to lower abdomen (avoid breasts/waistline). Rotate application site; allow 1 wk between same site.	X > **W** 4, 10, 28
Estradiol/Norethindrone (Activella)	**Tab:** 1-0.5 mg	**Vulval/Vaginal Atrophy, Vasomotor Symptoms: Adults: Intact Uterus:** 1-0.5 mg qd.	X > **W** 28
Estradiol/Norgestimate (Prefest)	**Tab:** 1 mg-none, 1 mg-0.09 mg	**Vasomotor Symptoms, Vulvar/Vaginal Atrophy: Adults: Intact Uterus:** 1 mg estradiol x3d alternating w/ 1-0.09 mg x 3d on continuous schedule.	X v **W** 28
Estradiol (Climara)	**Patch:** 0.025 mg/d, 0.0375 mg/d, 0.05 mg/d, 0.06 mg/d, 0.075 mg/d, 0.1 mg/d	**Vasomotor Symptoms, Vulval/Vaginal Atrophy, Hypoestrogenism: Adults: Initial:** Apply 0.025 mg/d qwk. **Titrate:** Adjust dose prn. Wait 1 wk after withdrawal of PO therapy before initiating patch.	X > **W** 4, 10, 28
Estradiol (Divigel)	**Gel:** 0.1%	**Adults:** Initial: 0.25 gm qd applied on skin of right or left upper thigh. Adjust dose based on response.	X > **W** 4, 10, 28
Estradiol (Estrace)	**Cre:** 0.1 mg/gm; **Tab:** 0.5 mg, 1 mg, 2 mg	**Adults: Vulval/Vaginal Atrophy: Cre:** 2-4 gm/d x 1-2 wks, then 1-2 gm/d x 1-2 wks. **Maint:** 1 gm 1-3 times/wk. **Menopause/Vulval/Vaginal Atrophy: Tab:** 1-2 mg/d (3 wks on, 1 wk off). D/C or taper at 3-6 mth intervals. **Maint:** Minimum effective dose. **Hypoestrogenism:** 1-2 mg/d. **Maint:** Minimum effective dose.	X v **W** 4, 10, 28
Estradiol (Estrasorb)	**Emul:** 2.5 mg/gm	**Vasomotor Symptoms: Adults:** 2 pouches (0.05 mg/d) qam. Apply 1 pouch to each leg from the upper thigh to the calf. Rub in for 3 min.	X > **W** 4, 10, 28

Estradiol (Estring)	Vag Ring: 2 mg/ring	**Postmenopausal Urogenital Symptoms: Adults:** Insert ring into upper 1/3 of vaginal vault, remove & replace after 90d.	X v **W** 4, 10
Estradiol (Evamist)	**Spr:** 1.53 mg/spr	**Adults:** 1 spr qd on inner surface of forearm. Adjust dose based on response.	X > **W** 4, 10, 28
Estradiol (Gynodiol)	**Tab:** 0.5 mg, 1 mg, 1.5 mg, 2 mg	**Menopause/Vulval/Vaginal Atrophy:** 1-2 mg/d (3 wks on, 1 wk off). **Maint:** Minimum effective dose. **Hypoestrogenism:** 1-2 mg/d. **Maint:** Minimum effective dose.	X v **W** 4, 10, 28
Estrogens, Esterified/ Methyltestosterone (Estratest, Estratest H.S.)	**Tab:** 1.25-2.5 mg, (H.S.) 0.625-1.25 mg	**Vasomotor Symptoms: Adults:** 0.625-1.25 mg or 1.25-2.5 mg qd cyclically (3 wks on, 1 wk off).	X v **W** 4, 10, 28
Estropipate (Ogen)	**Tab:** 0.625 mg (0.75 mg estropipate), 1.25 mg (1.5 mg estropipate), 2.5 mg (3 mg estropipate)	**Adults: Vasomotor Symptoms:** 0.75-6 mg/d (as estropipate). **Vulval/Vaginal Atrophy:** 0.75-6 mg/d (as estropipate), cyclically. **Female Hypoestrogenism:** 1.5-9 mg/d (as estropipate) for 1st 3 wks of cycle, then 8-10d off. **Maint:** Lowest effective dose.	X > **W** 4, 10, 28
Ethinyl Estradiol/ Norethindrone Acetate (femhrt)	**Tab:** 2.5 mcg-0.5 mg, 5 mcg-1 mg	**Vasomotor Symptoms: Adults:** 1 tab qd.	X > **W** 10, 28
Medroxyprogesterone Acetate/Conjugated Estrogens (Premphase)	**Tab:** 0.625 mg (estrogens, conj.) & 0.625-5 mg	**Vasomotor Symptoms, Vulvar/Vaginal Atrophy: Adults:** 0.625 mg tab qd on Days 1-14 & 0.625-5 mg tab qd on Days 15-28. Re-evaluate after 3-6 mths.	X > **W** 4, 10, 28

NAME	FORM/STRENGTH	DOSAGE	COMMENTS
Medroxyprogesterone Acetate/Conjugated Estrogens (Prempro)	**Tab:** 0.3-1.5 mg, 0.45-1.5 mg, 0.625-2.5 mg, 0.625-5 mg	**Menopause/Atrophy: Adults: Initial:** 0.3-1.5 mg qd. Adjust dose based on response. Re-evaluate after 3-6 mths.	X > **W** [4, 10, 28]

Premenstrual Dysphoric Disorder

ESTROGEN/PROGESTIN COMBINATION

NAME	FORM/STRENGTH	DOSAGE	COMMENTS
Ethinyl Estradiol/ Drospirenone (YAZ)	**Tab:** 0.02-3 mg	**Adults:** 1 tab qd x 28d, then repeat. Start 1st Sunday after menses begin or 1st day of menses.	X v

SSRIS & COMBINATIONS

NAME	FORM/STRENGTH	DOSAGE	COMMENTS
Fluoxetine (Sarafem)	**Cap:** 10 mg, 20 mg	**Adults: Continuous: Initial:** 20 mg qd. **Maint:** 20 mg/d up to 6 mths. **Max:** 60 mg/d. **Intermittent: Initial:** 20 mg qd; start 14d before menses onset through 1st full day of menses. **Maint:** 20 mg/d up to 3 mths. **Max:** 60 mg/d.	C v **H W** [29]
Paroxetine HCl (Paxil CR)	**Tab, CR:** 12.5 mg, 25 mg, 37.5 mg	**Adults: Initial:** 12.5 mg qd continuous or limited to luteal phase. **Titrate:** Wait at least 1 wk between dose changes.	D > **H R W** [29]
Sertraline (Zoloft)	**Sol:** 20 mg/ml; **Tab:** 25 mg, 50 mg, 100 mg	**Initial:** 50 mg qd continuous or limit to luteal cycle phase. **Titrate:** Increase by 50 mg/cycle up to 150 mg/d for continuous or 100 mg/d for luteal phase dosing. If 100 mg/d is established for luteal phase dosing, then titrate by 50 mg/d x 3d at beginning of each luteal phase dosing period.	C > **H W** [29]

Anemia

IRON/VITAMINS

Ferrous Sulfate (Feosol)	**Tab:** 200 mg (65 mg iron)	**Adults & Peds:** **≥12 yo:** 1 tab qd w/ food.	◙N ❋> **W** [22]
Folic Acid	**Inj:** 5 mg/ml; **Tab:** 0.4 mg, 0.8 mg, 1 mg	**Adults & Peds:** Up to 1 mg/d. **Maint:** 0.1-0.8 mg qd.	◙A ❋^
Iron Carbonyl (Feosol)	**Tab:** 50 mg (45 mg iron)	**Adults & Peds:** **≥12 yo:** 1 tab qd w/ food.	◙N ❋> **W** [22]
Iron Dextran (INFeD)	**Inj:** 50 mg/ml	**Iron-Deficiency Anemia: Adults & Peds: ≥4 mths & >15 kg:** Dose (ml) = 0.0442 (desired Hgb-observed Hgb) x LBW + (0.26 x LBW); LBW = lean body wt (kg). **Peds: 5-15 kg:** Use calculation above w/ wt in place of LBW.	◙C ❋> Anaphylactic reactions.
Iron Sucrose (Venofer)	**Sol:** 20 mg/ml	**Adults: Hemodialysis-Dependent Chronic Kidney Disease:** 100 mg IV inj over 2-5 min or 100 mg IV infusion over ≥15 min per consecutive hemodialysis session for a total cumulative dose of 1000 mg. **Non-Dialysis Dependent Chronic Kidney Disease:** 1000 mg over 14 day period as 200 mg slow IV inj undiluted over 2-5 min on 5 different occasions within the 14 day period.	◙B ❋>

NAME	FORM/STRENGTH	DOSAGE	COMMENTS
Sodium Ferric Gluconate Complex (Ferrlecit)	**Inj:** 62.5 mg elemental iron/5 ml	**Iron-Deficiency Anemia: Adults:** 10 ml (125 mg) as IV infusion (diluted) or as slow IV inj (undiluted). **Minimum Cumulative Dose:** 1 gm elemental iron over 8 sequential dialysis sessions. **Peds: ≥6 yo:** 0.12 ml/kg (1.5 mg/kg) as IV infusion over 1h at 8 sequential dialysis sessions. **Max:** 125 mg/dose.	◙B ❊>

Hematopoietic Agents

NAME	FORM/STRENGTH	DOSAGE	COMMENTS
Darbepoetin Alfa (Aranesp)	**Inj:** (Syr) 0.025 mg/0.42 ml, 0.04 mg/0.4 ml, 0.06 mg/0.3 ml, 0.1 mg/0.5 ml, 0.15 mg/0.3 ml, 0.2 mg/0.4 ml, 0.3 mg/0.6 ml, 0.5 mg/ml; **SDV:** 0.025 mg/ml, 0.04 mg/ml, 0.06 mg/ml, 0.1 mg/ml, 0.15 mg/0.75 ml, 0.2 mg/ml, 0.3 mg/ml	**Adults: CRF: Initial:** 0.45 mcg/kg IV/SC wkly. **Conversion from Epoetin Alfa:** Base dose on wkly epoetin dose. Give once wkly if receiving epoetin 2-3x/wk. Give q2wks if receiving epoetin once wkly. (See PI for more info). **Titrate:** Adjust to target Hgb <12 gm/dl. If Hgb increases >1 gm/dl in a 2-wk period or is approaching 12 gm/dl, decrease dose by 25%. If Hgb continues to increase, hold dose until Hgb begins to decrease & reinitiate at 25% below previous dose. Do not increase more than once monthly. **Malignancy: Initial:** 2.25 mcg/kg SC wkly. **Titrate:** Increase to 4.5 mcg/kg if Hgb increase is <1 gm/dl after 6 wks of therapy. If Hgb increases >1 gm/dl in a 2-wk period or if Hgb >12 gm/dl, decrease dose by 25%. If Hgb >13 gm/dl, hold dose until Hgb falls to 12 gm/dl & reinitiate at 25% below previous dose.	◙C ❊> **W** 76

Epoetin Alfa (Epogen)	**Inj:** 2000 U/ml, 3000 U/ml, 4000 U/ml, 10,000 U/ml, 20,000 U/ml, 40,000 U/ml	**CRF: Adults: Initial:** 50-100 U/kg IV/SC TIW. **Maint:** Adjust based on Hgb. **Peds: Initial:** 50 U/kg TIW IV/SC. **Maint:** Adjust based on Hgb. **Zidovudine-Treated HIV Patients: Initial:** 100 U/kg IV/SC TIW x 8 wks. **Titrate:** After 8 wks of therapy, may increase by 50-100 U/kg TIW up to 300 U/kg TIW. **Maint:** Adjust based on AZT dose & Hgb. **Chemo-Induced Anemia: Adults: Initial:** 150 U/kg SC TIW or 40,000 U SC wkly x up to 8 wks. **Titrate:** May increase to 300 U/kg TIW or 60,000 U wkly after 4 wks of therapy. **Maint:** Adjust based on Hgb. **Peds: Initial:** 600 U/kg IV wkly. **Max:** 40,000 U. **Titrate:** May increase to 900 U/kg IV after 4 wks of therapy. **Max:** 60,000 U. **Surgery Patients:** 300 U/kg/d SC x 10d prior to surgery, on day of, & 4d after surgery; or 600 U/kg SC wkly on Days 21, 14, & 7 prior to surgery & a 4th dose on day of surgery.	C > **W** 75
Epoetin Alfa (Procrit)	**Inj:** 2000 U/ml, 3000 U/ml, 4000 U/ml, 10,000 U/ml, 20,000 U/ml, 40,000 U/ml	**CRF: Adults: Initial:** 50-100 U/kg IV/SC TIW. **Maint:** Adjust based on Hgb. **Peds: Initial:** 50 U/kg TIW IV/SC. **Maint:** Adjust based on Hgb. **Zidovudine-Treated HIV Patients: Initial:** 100 U/kg IV/SC TIW x 8 wks. **Titrate:** After 8 wks of therapy, may increase by 50-100 U/kg TIW up to 300 U/kg TIW. **Maint:** Adjust based on AZT dose & Hgb. **Chemo-Induced Anemia: Adults: Initial:** 150 U/kg SC TIW or 40,000 U SC wkly x up to 8 wks. **Titrate:** May increase to 300 U/kg TIW or 60,000 U wkly after 4 wks of therapy.	C > **W** 75

Continued on Next Page

NAME	FORM/STRENGTH	DOSAGE	COMMENTS
Epoetin Alfa (Procrit) *Continued*		**Maint:** Adjust based on Hgb. **Peds: Initial:** 600 U/kg IV wkly. **Max:** 40,000 U. **Titrate:** May increase to 900 U/kg IV after 4 wks of therapy. **Max:** 60,000 U. **Surgery Patients:** 300 U/kg/d SC x 10d prior to surgery, on day of & 4d after surgery; or 600 U/kg SC wkly on Days 21, 14, & 7 prior to surgery, & a 4th dose on day of surgery.	
Filgrastim (Neupogen)	**Inj:** 300 mcg/0.5 ml, 300 mcg/ml, 480 mcg/0.8 ml, 480 mcg/1.6 ml	**Adults:** Adjust dose based on ANC. **Myelosuppressive Chemo: Initial:** 5 mcg/kg/d IV/SC. **Bone Marrow Transplant: Initial:** 10 mcg/kg/d IV/SC. **Peripheral Blood Progenitor Cell Collection: Initial:** 10 mcg/kg/d SC 4d before & x 6-7d w/ leukapheresis on Days 5, 6 & 7. **Congenital Neutropenia: Initial:** 6 mcg/kg SC bid. **Idiopathic/Cyclic Neutropenia: Initial:** 5 mcg/kg SC qd.	C >
Oprelvekin (Neumega)	**Inj:** 5 mg	**Severe Thrombocytopenia Prevention: Adults:** 50 mcg/kg SC qd. Initiate 6-24h after chemo completion. Continue therapy until post-nadir platelets ≥50,000 cells/mcl. D/C at least 2d before next chemo cycle. **Max:** 21d of therapy.	C v
Pegfilgrastim (Neulasta)	**Inj:** 6 mg/0.6 ml	**Infection/Febrile Neutropenia w/ Non-Myeloid Malignancies: Adults:** 6 mg SC, once per chemo cycle. Do not administer in period 14d before & 24h after chemo.	C >

Immunosuppressives

Azathioprine (Imuran)	**Tab:** 50 mg	**Adults: Prevention of Renal Homotransplantation Rejection: Initial:** 3-5 mg/kg/d. **Maint:** 1-3 mg/kg/d.	◙D ❀v **R** Risk of neoplasia, mutagenesis & hematologic toxicities.

Vaccines/Toxoids/Immunoglobulins

Anthrax Vaccine Adsorbed (Biothrax)	**Inj:** 5 ml	**Pre-exposure Prophylaxis: Adults: 18-65 yo:** 0.5 ml IM at 0 & 4 wks, then at 6, 12, & 18 mths. **Booster:** 0.5 ml yearly.	◙D ❀>
Diphtheria Toxoid/ Pertussis Vaccine, Acellular/ Tetanus Toxoid (Infanrix)	**Inj:** 0.5 ml	**Peds: ≥6 wks up to 7 yo:** 3 doses of 0.5 ml IM at 4-8 wk intervals. **Booster Doses:** Give at 15-20 mths & at 4-6 yo.	◙C ❀>
Diphtheria Toxoid/ Tetanus Toxoid	**Inj:** 2-5 LFU/0.5 ml, 6.6-5 LFU/0.5 ml,10-5 LFU/0.5 ml	**>7 yo:** 0.5 ml IM in the vastus lateralis or deltoid. Repeat 4-8 wks later. Give 3rd dose 6-12 mths after 2nd dose. **Booster:** 0.5 ml IM every 10 yrs. **6 wks-12 mths:** 0.5 ml IM x 3 doses 4-8 wks apart. 4th dose 6-12 mths after 3rd dose. **1-6 yo:** 0.5 ml IM x 2 doses 4-8 wks apart. 3rd dose 6-12 mths after 2nd dose. **Booster: If Received 4 Doses:** 0.5 ml IM before entering school.	◙C ❀>

NAME	FORM/STRENGTH	DOSAGE	COMMENTS
Diphtheria Toxoid/ Tetanus Toxoid/ Pertussis Vaccine, Acellular (Tripedia)	**Inj:** 0.5 ml	**Peds: ≥6 wks up to 7 yo:** 3 doses of 0.5 ml IM at 4-8 wk intervals. **Booster Doses:** Give at 15-18 mths & at 4-6 yo.	C >
***Haemophilus B* Conjugate Vaccine** (ActHIB)	**Inj:** 10 mcg	**Peds: Reconstituted w/ DTP or Saline:** 0.5 ml IM at 2, 4, & 6 mths old; 4th dose at 15-18 mths; 5th dose at 4-6 yo. **Reconstituted w/ Tripedia (as 4th dose in series):** 0.5 ml IM at 15-18 mths; 5th dose at 4-6 yo. **Unvaccinated: 7-11 mths:** 2 doses at 8 wk intervals w/ a booster at 15-18 mths. **12-14 mths:** 1 dose followed by a booster 2 mths later.	C >
Hepatitis B (Recombinant) (Engerix-B, Engerix-B Pediatric/ Adolescent)	**Inj:** (Adult) 20 mcg/ml, (Ped) 10 mcg/0.5 ml	**Adults: >19 yo:** 20 mcg/ml IM at 0, 1, & 6 mths. **Peds: ≤19 yo:** 10 mcg/0.5 ml IM at 0, 1, & 6 mths. **Booster: Adults & Peds: ≥11 yo:** 20 mcg IM. **≤10 yo:** 10 mcg IM.	C >
Hepatitis B (Recombinant) (Recombivax HB Adult, Recombivax HB Dialysis, Recombivax HB Pediatric/ Adolescent)	**Inj:** (Adult) 10 mcg/ml, (Dialysis) 40 mcg/ml, (Ped) 5 mcg/0.5 ml	**Adults: ≥20 yo:** 10 mcg IM at 0, 1, & 6 mths. **Peds: 0-19 yo: 3-Dose Regimen:** 5 mcg IM at 0, 1, & 6 mths. **11-15 yo: 2-Dose Regimen:** 10 mcg 1st dose, then 10 mcg 4-6 mths later.	C >
Hepatitis B (Recombinant)/ *Haemophilus B* Conjugate (Comvax)	**Inj:** 7.5-5-125 mcg/ 0.5 ml	**Peds: ≥6 wks:** 0.5 ml IM at 2, 4, & 12-15 mths of age. If cannot follow schedule, wait at least 6 wks between 1st 2 doses. 2nd & 3rd dose should be close to 8-11 mths apart.	C >

Hepatitis B (Recombinant)/ Hepatitis A Vaccine (Inactivated) (Twinrix)	**Inj:** 720 U-20 mcg	**Adults: 3-Dose Schedule:** 1 ml IM at 0-, 1- & 6-mths. **Alternative 4-Dose Schedule:** 1 ml IM on Days 0, 7 & 21-30 followed by booster dose at 12 mths. Inject into deltoid region.	C >
Hepatitis B Immune Globulin (Vaqta)	**Inj:** 25 U/0.5 ml, 50 U/ml	**Adults:** 50 U IM, repeat 6-18 mths later. **Peds: 1-18 yo:** 25 U IM, repeat 6-18 mths later.	C >
Hepatitis B Immune Globulin (Nabi-HB)	**Inj:** 1 ml, 5 ml	**Adults: Acute Exposure to Blood Containing HBsAg:** 0.06 ml/kg IM after exposure & within 24 hrs. Sexual exposure to HBsAg-Positive Person(s): 0.06mL/kg IM (single dose) & start hepatitis B vaccine series within 14d of last sexual contact or if sexual contact w/ infected person will continue. Refer to PI for recommendations for hepatitis B prophylaxis following percutaneous or permucosal exposure. **Peds: Prophylaxis of Infant to HBsAg-Positive Mother:** 0.5 ml IM within 12h. **Prophylaxis of Infant (<12 mths) Exposed to Mother or Caregiver w/ Acute HBV-Infection:** 0.5 ml IM. Refer to PI for recommended schedule of hepatitis B immunoprophylaxis to prevent perinatal transmission.	C >
Human Papillomavirus Recombinant Vaccine, Quadrivalent (Gardasil)	**Inj:** 0.5 ml	**Genital Warts/Cervical/Vulvar/Vaginal Cancer Prevention: Adults & Peds: ≥9 yo:** Give 3 separate 0.5 ml IM doses in deltoid region of upper arm or higher anterolateral area of thigh. 1st dose: at elected date; 2nd dose: 2 mths after 1st dose; 3rd dose: 6 mths after 1st dose.	B >

NAME	FORM/STRENGTH	DOSAGE	COMMENTS
Influenza Virus Vaccine Live, Intranasal (FluMist)	**Nasal Spr:** 0.2 ml/spr	**Adults & Peds: 9-49 yo:** One 0.2 ml (0.1 ml per nostril) dose. **2-8 yo: Not Previously Vaccinated w/ Influenza Vaccine:** 0.2 ml (0.1 ml per nostril) x 2 doses at least 1 month apart. **Previously Vaccinated w/ Influenza Vaccine:** One 0.2 ml (0.1 ml per nostril) dose.	◙C ❁>
Influenza Virus Vaccine, Subvirion (Fluvirin)	**Inj:** 45 mcg/0.5 ml	**Adults & Peds: ≥4 yo:** 0.5 ml IM. **Peds: <9 yo (Not Previously Vaccinated):** Repeat dose min 1 mth apart. Administer in deltoid muscle to older children & thigh muscle in young children.	◙C ❁>
Influenza Virus Vaccine (Afluria)	**Inj:** (Syringe) 0.5 ml, (MDV) 5ml	**Adults: ≥18 yo:** 0.5 ml IM in deltoid region of upper arm.	◙C ❁>
Influenza Virus Vaccine (Fluzone)	**Inj:** 0.25 ml, 0.5 ml, 5 ml	**Adults & Peds: ≥9 yo:** 0.5 ml IM in deltoid muscle. **Peds: 6-35 mths:** 0.25 ml IM. **3-8 yo:** 0.5 ml IM. Children <9 yo who have not previously been vaccinated should receive two doses of vaccine ≥1 mth apart. Administer in deltoid muscle for children >36 mths & anterolateral aspect of thigh for children ≤36 mths.	◙C ❁>
Measles Vaccine Live (Attenuvax)	**Inj:** 1000 $TCID_{50}$	**Peds: 12-15 mths:** 0.5 ml SC in upper arm. If vaccinated <12 mths old, revaccinate at 12-15 mths old. Revaccinate prior to school entry.	◙C ❁>

Rubella Vaccine Live/ Mumps Vaccine Live (M-M-R II)		Recommended primary vaccination is at 12-15 mths; repeat before elementary school entry. If vaccinated at 6-12 mths due to outbreak, give another dose at 12-15 mths & before elementary school entry.	◉C ❃>
Meningococcal Polysaccharide Diptheria Toxoid Conjugate Vaccine (Menactra)	**Inj:** 0.5 ml	**Adults ≤55 yo & Peds ≥2 yo:** 0.5 ml IM into deltoid region.	◉C ❃>
Mumps Virus Vaccine Live (Mumpsvax)	**Inj:** 20,000 $TCID_{50}$	**Adults & Peds: ≥12 mths:** 0.5 ml SC in outer aspect of upper arm. Give primary vaccine at 12-15 mths. Revaccinate prior to elementary school.	◉C ❃>
Pneumococcal Vaccine (Pneumovax 23)	**Inj:** 0.5 ml/dose	**Adults & Peds: ≥2 yo:** Usual: 0.5 ml SC/IM in deltoid muscle or lateral mid-thigh.	◉C ❃>
Pneumococcal Vaccine, Diphtheria Conjugate (Prevnar)	**Inj:** 16 mcg/0.5 ml	**Peds: *S.pneumoniae*/Otitis Media:** 0.5 ml IM. 1st dose at 6 wks-2 mths old, then q2mths x 2 more doses. 4th dose given at 12-15 mths. **Unvaccinated: ≥24 mths-9 yo:** 0.5 ml IM single dose. **12-23 mths:** 0.5 ml IM x 2 doses given at least 2 mths apart. **7-11 mths:** 0.5 ml IM. 1st 2 doses at least 4 wks apart, then 3rd dose after 1 yo birthday at least 2 mths after 2nd dose.	◉C ❃v
Rabies Immune Globulin, Human (Imogam Rabies-HT)	**Inj:** 150 IU/ml	**Adults/Peds:** 20 IU/kg infiltrated in area around wound & rest IM in gluteal area.	◉C ❃>

NAME	FORM/STRENGTH	DOSAGE	COMMENTS
Rabies Vaccine (RabAvert)	**Inj:** 2.5 IU	**Adults/Peds: Pre-exposure:** 1 ml IM on Days 0, 7 & either 21 or 28 (3 total doses), booster shots as needed based on titers. **Post-exposure:** 1 ml IM on Days 0, 3, 7, 14 & 28.	◙C ❀>
Rubella Vaccine Live (Meruvax II)	**Inj:** 1000 $TCID_{50}$	**Adults:** 0.5 ml SC in outer aspect of upper arm. **Peds: 12-15 mths:** 0.5 ml SC in outer aspect of upper arm. Revaccinate w/ MMR II prior to elementary school entry.	◙C ❀>
Tetanus Immunoglobulin (BayTet)	**Inj:** 250 U	**Prophylactic: Adults & Peds: ≥7 yo:** 750 U IM. **Peds: <7 yo:** 4 U/kg or 250 U. **Active Case:** Adjust dose to severity of infection.	◙C ❀>
Tetanus Toxoid	**Inj:** 0.5 ml/dose	**Adults & Peds: ≥1 yo:** 0.5 ml IM. Repeat at 4-8 wks then 6-12 mths after 2nd dose. **Booster:** 0.5 ml IM q10yrs. **<1 yo:** 3 doses of 0.5 ml IM 4-8 wks apart, then 4th dose (0.5 ml) 6-12 mths after 3rd dose. Last dose before 4 yo. **Booster:** 0.5 ml at 4-6 yo.	◙C ❀>
Tetanus Toxoid/ Pertussis Vaccine Acellular, Adsorbed/Diphtheria Toxoid, Reduced (Adacel)	**Inj:** 0.5 ml	**Adults & Peds: 11-64 yo:** 0.5 ml IM (deltoid).	◙C ❀>
Varicella Virus Vaccine Live (Varivax)	**Inj:** 1350 PFU/vial	**Adults & Peds: ≥13 yo:** 0.5 ml SC, repeat in 4-8 wks. **1-12 yo:** 0.5 ml SC x 1 dose.	◙C ❀> CI in pregnancy.

Zoster Vaccine Live (Zostavax)	**Inj:** 19,400 PFU/0.65 ml	**Adults: ≥60 yo:** Inject SC immediately after reconstitution w/ supplied diluent.	◙C ✻>

NEUROLOGY/PSYCHOTHERAPEUTICS

ADHD/Narcolepsy Agents

NOREPINEPHRINE REUPTAKE INHIBITOR

Atomoxetine HCl (Strattera)	**Cap:** 10 mg, 18 mg, 25 mg, 40 mg, 60 mg, 80 mg, 100 mg	**ADHD: Adults & Peds: ≥6 yo & >70 kg: Initial:** 40 mg/d given qam or evenly divided doses in am & late afternoon/ early evening. **Titrate:** Increase after minimum of 3d to target dose of about 80 mg/d. After 2-4 wks, may increase to max of 100 mg/d. **Max:** 100 mg/d. **≥6 yo & ≤70 kg: Initial:** 0.5 mg/kg/d given qam or evenly divided doses in am & late afternoon/early evening. **Titrate:** Increase after minimum of 3d to target dose of about 1.2 mg/kg/d. **Max:** 1.4 mg/kg/d or 100 mg, whichever is less. Adjust w/ CYP2D6 inhibitors.	◙C ✻> **H** Increased risk of suicidal ideation in children or adolescents.

SYMPATHOMIMETICS

Amphetamine Salt Combo CII (Adderall XR)	**Cap,ER:** 5 mg, 10 mg, 15 mg, 20 mg, 25 mg, 30 mg	**ADHD: Adults: Initial:** 20 mg qam. **Peds: 13-17 yo: Initial:** 10 mg/d. **Titrate:** May increase to 20 mg/d after 1 wk. **≥6 yo: Initial:** 10 mg qam. **Titrate:** May increase qwk by 5-10 mg/d. **Max:** 30 mg/d. **Currently Using Adderall:** May switch to Adderall XR at same total daily dose taken qd. Titrate at wkly intervals prn.	◙C ✻v **W** [49]

NAME	FORM/STRENGTH	DOSAGE	COMMENTS
Amphetamine Salt Combo CII (Adderall)	**Tab:** 5 mg, 7.5 mg, 10 mg, 12.5 mg, 15 mg, 20 mg, 30 mg	**ADHD: Peds: ≥6 yo:** 5 mg qd-bid. **Titrate:** May increase qwk by 5 mg. **Max:** 40 mg/d. **3-5 yo:** 2.5 mg qd. **Titrate:** May increase qwk by 2.5 mg until optimal response. **Narcolepsy: Adults & Peds: ≥12 yo: Initial:** 10 mg/d. **Titrate:** May increase by 10 mg qwk. **Usual:** 5-60 mg/d. **6-12 yo: Initial:** 5 mg/d. **Titrate:** May increase by 5 mg qwk. Give 1st dose upon awakening & additional doses q4-6h.	C v **W** 49
Dexmethylphenidate HCl CII (Focalin XR)	**Cap,ER:** 5 mg, 10 mg, 15 mg, 20 mg	**ADHD: Methylphenidate-Naive: Adults: Initial:** 10 mg/d. **Titrate:** May adjust wkly by 10 mg/d. **Max:** 20 mg/d. **Peds: ≥6 yo:** 5 mg/d. **Titrate:** May adjust wkly by 5 mg/d. **Max:** 20 mg/d. **Adults & Peds: ≥6 yo: Currently on Methylphenidate: Initial:** Take 1/2 methylphenidate dose. **Max:** 20 mg/d. D/C if no improvement after 1 mth. **Currently on Dexmethylphenidate IR:** Switch to same daily dose of XR. **Max:** 20 mg/d. Reduce or d/c if paradoxical aggravation of symptoms. D/C if no improvement after dose adjustments over 1 mth. Swallow whole or sprinkle on applesauce.	C > **W** 102
Dexmethylphenidate HCl CII (Focalin)	**Tab:** 2.5 mg, 5 mg, 10 mg	**ADHD: Methylphenidate-Naive: Initial: Adults & Peds: ≥6 yo:** 2.5 mg bid at least 4 h apart. **Titrate:** May adjust wkly by 2.5-5 mg/d. **Max:** 20 mg/d. **Currently on Methylphenidate: Initial:** Take 1/2 methylphenidate dose. **Max:** 20 mg/d. D/C if no improvement after 1 mth.	C > **W** 102

Dextroamphetamine Sulfate CII (DextroStat)	**Tab:** 5 mg, 10 mg	**ADHD: Peds: ≥6 yo: Initial:** 5 mg qd-bid. **Titrate:** Increase qwk by 5 mg. **Max:** 40 mg/d. **3-5 yo: Initial:** 2.5 mg qd. **Titrate:** Increase qwk by 2.5 mg. **Narcolepsy: Adults & Peds: ≥12 yo: Initial:** 10 mg qd. **Titrate:** Increase qwk by 10 mg/d. **Usual:** 5-60 mg/d. **6-12 yo: Initial:** 5 mg/d. **Titrate:** Increase qwk by 5 mg.	C v **W** 49
Lisdexamfetamine Dimesylate CII (Vyvanse)	**Cap:** 20 mg, 30 mg, 40 mg, 50 mg, 60 mg, 70 mg	**ADHD: Adults & Peds: 6-12 yo:** Individualize dose. **Usual:** 30 mg qam. **Titrate:** If needed, may increase in increments of 10 mg or 20 mg at wkly intervals. **Max:** 70 mg/d. Re-evaluate periodically.	C v High potential for abuse.
Methylphenidate CII (Daytrana)	**Patch:** 10 mg/9h, 15 mg/9h, 20 mg/9h, 30 mg/9h	**ADHD: Adults & Peds ≥6 yo:** Individualize dose. Apply to hip area 2h before effect needed & remove 9h after application. **Recommended Titration Schedule: Wk 1:** 10 mg/9h. **Wk 2:** 15 mg/9h. **Wk 3:** 20 mg/9h. **Wk 4:** 30 mg/9h.	C > **W** 102
Methylphenidate HCl CII (Concerta)	**Tab,ER:** 18 mg, 27 mg, 36 mg, 54 mg	**Adults & Peds: ≥6 yo: Methylphenidate-Naive or Receiving Other Stimulant: Initial:** 18 mg qam. **Titrate:** Adjust dose at wkly intervals. **Max: 6-12 yo:** 54 mg/d; **13-17 yo:** 72 mg/d not to exceed 2 mg/kg/d. **Previous Methylphenidate Use: Initial:** 18 mg qam if previous dose 10-15 mg/d; 36 mg qam if previous dose 20-30 mg/d; 54 mg qam if previous dose 30-45 mg/d. Initial conversion should not exceed 54 mg/d. **Titrate:** Adjust dose at wkly	C > **W** 102

Continued on Next Page

NAME	FORM/STRENGTH	DOSAGE	COMMENTS
Methylphenidate HCl CII (Concerta) *Continued*		intervals. **Max:** 72 mg/d. Reduce dose or d/c if paradoxical aggravation of symptoms occurs. D/C if no improvement after appropriate dosage adjustments over 1 mth. Swallow whole w/ liquids.	
Methylphenidate HCl CII (Metadate CD)	**Cap,ER:** 10 mg, 20 mg, 30 mg, 40 mg, 50 mg, 60 mg	**Peds: ≥6 yo: Usual:** 20 mg qam before breakfast. **Titrate:** Increase wkly by 20 mg depending on tolerability/ efficacy. **Max:** 60 mg/d. Reduce dose or d/c if paradoxical aggravation of symptoms occur. D/C if no improvement after appropriate dose adjustments over 1 mth. Swallow whole w/ liquids or open & sprinkle on 1 tbsp applesauce followed by water.	C > **W** 102
Methylphenidate HCl CII (Metadate ER)	**Tab,ER:** 10 mg, 20 mg	**ADHD: Adults:** (Immediate-Release Methylphenidate) 10-60 mg/d given bid-tid 30-45 min ac. **Peds: ≥6 yo: Initial:** (Immediate-Release Methylphenidate) 5 mg bid before breakfast & lunch. **Titrate:** Increase gradually by 5-10 mg wkly. **Max:** 60 mg/d. (Tab,ER) May use in place of immediate-release tabs when 8h dose corresponds to titrated 8h immediate-release dose. Swallow whole. Reduce dose or d/c if paradoxical aggravation of symptoms occur. D/C if no improvement after appropriate dose adjustment over 1 mth.	C > **W** 102

Methylphenidate HCl CII (Methylin, Methylin ER)	**Sol:** (Methylin) 5 mg/5 ml, 10 mg/5 ml; **Tab:** (Methylin) 5 mg, 10 mg, 20 mg; **Tab, Chew:** (Methylin) 2.5 mg, 5 mg, 10 mg; **Tab, ER:** (Methylin ER) 10 mg, 20 mg	**ADHD: Adults: Methylin:** 10-60 mg/d divided bid-tid 30-45 min ac. **Peds: ≥6 yo: Methylin:** 5 mg bid. **Titrate:** May increase by 5-10 mg qwk. **Max:** 60 mg/d. May use Methylin ER when 8h extended-release dose corresponds to titrated 8h immediate-release dose.	C > W [102]
Methylphenidate HCl CII (Ritalin, Ritalin LA, Ritalin SR)	**Cap, ER:** (Ritalin LA) 10 mg, 20 mg, 30 mg, 40 mg; **Tab:** (Ritalin) 5 mg, 10 mg, 20 mg; **Tab, ER:** (Ritalin-SR) 20 mg	**ADHD: Adults: Ritalin:** 10-60 mg/d divided bid-tid 30-45 min ac. **Peds: ≥6 yo: Ritalin:** 5 mg bid. **Titrate:** May increase by 5-10 mg qwk. **Max:** 60 mg/d. **Ritalin LA: Initial:** 10-20 mg qam. **Titrate:** May adjust wkly by 10 mg increments. **Max:** 60 mg/d. May use Ritalin-SR when 8h extended-release dose corresponds to titrated 8h immediate-release dose.	C > W [102]

MISCELLANEOUS

Armodafinil CIV (Nuvigil)	**Tab:** 50 mg, 150 mg, 250 mg	**Adults: Narcolepsy/Obstructive Sleep Apnea/Hypopnea Syndrome:** 150 mg or 250 mg qd in AM. **Shiftwork Sleep Disorder:** 150 mg qd 1h prior to work shift. **Elderly:** Consider dose reduction.	C > H

NAME	FORM/STRENGTH	DOSAGE	COMMENTS
Modafinil CIV (Provigil)	**Tab:** 100 mg, 200 mg	**Adults & Peds: ≥ 16 yo:** 200 mg qd. **Narcolepsy/ Obstructive Sleep Apnea/Hypopnea Syndrome:** Take in AM. **Shiftwork Sleep Disorder:** Take 1h prior to start of work shift.	C > H

Alzheimer's Therapy

CHOLINESTERASE INHIBITORS

NAME	FORM/STRENGTH	DOSAGE	COMMENTS
Donepezil HCl (Aricept, Aricept ODT)	**Tab:** 5 mg, 10 mg; **Tab,Dissolve:** (ODT) 5 mg, 10 mg	**Adults: Mild-to-Moderate Alzheimer's Disease: Initial:** 5 mg qhs. **Titrate:** May increase to 10 mg after 4-6 wks. **Severe Alzheimer's Disease:** 10 mg qhs. Start w/ 5 mg qhs & increase to 10 mg after 4-6 wks.	C v
Galantamine Hydrobromide (Razadyne, Razadyne ER)	**Sol:** 4 mg/ml; **Tab:** 4 mg, 8 mg, 12 mg; **Tab,ER:** 8 mg, 16 mg, 24 mg	**Adults: Sol/Tab: Initial:** 4 mg bid w/ am & pm meals. **Titrate:** Increase to 8 mg bid after 4 wks if tolerated, then increase to 12 mg bid after 4 wks if tolerated. **Usual:** 16-24 mg/d. **Max:** 24 mg/d. **Tab,ER: Initial:** 8 mg qd w/ am meal. **Titrate:** Increase to 16 mg qd after 4 wks, then increase to 24 mg/d after 4 wks if tolerated. **Usual:** 16-24 mg/d. **Max:** 24 mg/d.	B v **H R**
Rivastigmine Tartrate (Exelon)	**Cap:** 1.5 mg, 3 mg, 4.5 mg, 6 mg; **Sol:** 2 mg/ml; **Patch:** 4.6 mg/ 24h, 9.5 mg/24h	**Alzheimer's Dementia: Adults: PO: Initial:** 1.5 mg bid. **Titrate:** May increase by 1.5 mg bid q2wks. **Max:** 12 mg/d. If not tolerating, suspend therapy for several doses & restart at same or next lower dose. If interrupted longer than several days, reinitiate w/ lowest daily dose & titrate as above. **Patch: Initial:** Apply 4.6 mg/24h patch qd to clean,	B v

		dry, hairless intact skin. **Maint:** May increase dose after 4 wks. **Max:** 9.5 mg/24h if well tolerated. **Switching from PO: Total PO Daily Dose <6 mg:** Switch to 4.6 mg/24h patch. **Total PO Daily Dose 6-12 mg:** Switch to 9.5 mg/24h patch. Apply 1st patch on day following last PO dose.	

NMDA-RECEPTOR ANTAGONIST

Memantine HCl (Namenda)	**Sol:** 2 mg/ml; **Tab:** 5 mg, 10 mg	**Adults: Initial:** 5 mg qd. **Maint:** 10 mg bid. **Titrate:** Increase at intervals no less than 1 wk to 10 mg/d (5 mg bid), 15 mg/d (5 mg & 10 mg as separate doses), then 20 mg/d (10 mg bid).	B > **R**

Antianxiety/Hypnotic Agents

BARBITURATES

Secobarbital CII (Seconal Sodium)	**Cap:** 100 mg	**Adults: Hypnotic:** 100 mg qhs. **Peds: Pre-op:** 2-6 mg/kg. **Max:** 100 mg.	D > **H R**

BENZODIAZEPINES

Alprazolam CIV (Xanax XR)	**Tab, ER:** 0.5 mg, 1 mg, 2 mg, 3 mg	**Adults: Panic Disorder: Initial:** 0.5-1 mg qd, preferably in am. **Titrate:** Increase by no more than1 mg/d q3-4d. **Maint:** 1-10 mg/d. **Usual:** 3-6 mg/d. Decrease dose slowly (no more than 0.5 mg q3d). **Elderly/Advanced Liver Disease/Debilitated: Initial:** 0.5 mg qd.	D v **H**

NAME	FORM/STRENGTH	DOSAGE	COMMENTS
Alprazolam CIV (Xanax)	**Tab:** 0.25 mg, 0.5 mg, 1 mg, 2 mg	**Adults: Anxiety: Initial:** 0.25-0.5 mg tid. **Titrate:** May increase q3-4d. **Max:** 4 mg/d. **Panic Disorder: Initial:** 0.5 mg tid. **Titrate:** Increase by no more than 1 mg/d q3-4d; slower titration if ≥4 mg/d. **Usual:** 1-10 mg/d. Decrease dose slowly (no more than 0.5 mg q3d). **Elderly/Advanced Liver Disease/Debilitated: Initial:** 0.25 mg bid-tid. **Titrate:** Increase gradually as tolerated.	D v **H**
Chlordiazepoxide HCl CIV (Librium)	**Cap:** 5 mg, 10 mg, 25 mg	**Adults: Mild-Moderate Anxiety:** 5-10 mg tid-qid. **Severe Anxiety:** 20-25 mg tid-qid. **Alcohol Withdrawal:** 50-100 mg; repeat until agitation controlled. **Max:** 300 mg/d. **Preoperative Anxiety:** 5-10 mg PO tid-qid on days prior to surgery. **Peds: ≥ 6 yo:** 5 mg bid-qid. May increase to 10 mg bid-tid. **Elderly/Debilitated:** 5 mg bid-qid.	N >
Clorazepate CIV (Tranxene T-Tab, Tranxene-SD, Tranxene-SD Half Strength)	**Tab:** (T-Tab) 3.75 mg, 7.5 mg, 15 mg; **Tab, ER:** (SD) 11.25 mg, 22.5 mg	**Anxiety: Adults & Peds: >9 yo: Tab: Initial:** 15 mg qhs. **Usual:** 30 mg/d in divided doses. **Max:** 60 mg/d. **Tab,ER:** 22.5 mg qd if controlled on 7.5 mg tid or 11.25 mg qd if controlled on 3.75 mg tid.	N v
Diazepam CIV (Valium)	**Inj:** 5 mg/ml; **Tab:** 2 mg, 5 mg, 10 mg	**Anxiety: Adults: PO:** 2-10 mg bid-qid. **IM/IV:** (moderate) 2-5 mg or (severe) 5-10 mg, repeat in 3-4h if needed. **Peds: ≥6 mths: Initial:** 1-2.5 mg PO tid-qid.	N >
Lorazepam CIV (Ativan)	**Tab:** 0.5 mg, 1 mg, 2 mg	**Adults & Peds: >12 yo: Anxiety: Initial:** 2-3 mg/d given bid-tid. **Usual:** 2-6 mg/d. **Insomnia:** 2-4 mg qhs.	N v

Midazolam HCl CIV	**Syr:** 2 mg/ml	**Sedation & Anxiolysis: Pre-Op: Peds: PO:** 0.25-1 mg/kg single dose. **Max:** 20 mg/dose. **IM:** 0.1-0.15 mg/kg, up to 0.5 mg/kg. **Max:** 10 mg/dose. **6-15 yo or Cooperative Patients:** 0.25 mg/kg. **Max:** 20 mg. **Cardiac/Respiratory Compromised, Higher Risk Surgical Patients, or Patients who have Received Concomitant Narcotics or Other CNS Depressants:** 0.25 mg/kg. **Max:** 20 mg.	D > Associated w/ respiratory depression & respiratory arrest.
Temazepam CIV (Restoril)	**Cap:** 7.5 mg, 15 mg, 22.5 mg, 30 mg	**Adults: ≥18 yo: Insomnia:** 7.5-30 mg qhs. **Transient Insomnia:** 7.5 mg qhs.	X >
Triazolam CIV (Halcion)	**Tab:** 0.125 mg, 0.25 mg	**Insomnia: Adults: ≥18 yo: Usual:** 0.25 mg qhs. **Max:** 0.25 mg qhs. **Low-Wt Patients:** 0.125 mg qhs. **Max:** 0.25 mg qhs.	X v

SEROTONIN/NOREPINEPHRINE REUPTAKE INHIBITORS

Duloxetine (Cymbalta)	**Cap,Delay:** 20 mg, 30 mg, 60 mg	**Generalized Anxiety Disorder: Adults: Initial:** 60 mg qd or 30 mg qd x 1 wk to adjust before increasing to 60 mg qd. **Titrate:** May increase by increments of 30 mg qd if needed. **Max:** 120 mg qd. Do not chew or crush.	C v **H R W** [29]
Venlafaxine (Effexor XR)	**Cap, ER:** 37.5 mg, 75 mg, 150 mg	**Generalized Anxiety Disorder/Social Anxiety Disorder: Adults: Initial:** 75 mg/d, or 37.5 mg/d increase to 75 mg/d after 4-7d. **Titrate:** Increase by 75 mg/d at intervals of no less than 4 d. **Max:** 225 mg/d. **Panic Disorder: Initial:** 37.5 mg/d x 7d. **Titrate:** Increase by 75 mg/d at intervals of no less than 7d. **Max:** 225 mg/d.	C v **H R W** [29]

NAME	FORM/STRENGTH	DOSAGE	COMMENTS
SSRIS & COMBINATIONS			
Escitalopram Oxalate (Lexapro)	**Sol:** 5 mg/5 ml; **Tab:** 5 mg, 10 mg, 20 mg	**Generalized Anxiety Disorder: Adults: Initial:** 10 mg qd, in am or pm. **Titrate:** May increase to 20 mg after at least 1 wk. **Elderly/Hepatic Impairment:** 10 mg qd. Re-evaluate periodically.	C v **H R W** [29]
Fluoxetine (Prozac)	**Cap:** 10 mg, 20 mg, 40 mg; **Sol:** 20 mg/5ml; **Tab:** 10 mg	**Panic Disorder: Adults: Initial:** 10 mg/d. May increase to 20 mg/d after 1 wk. May increase further after several wks if needed. **Max:** 60 mg/d.	C v **H W** [29]
Paroxetine HCl (Paxil CR)	**Tab, CR:** 12.5 mg, 25 mg, 37.5 mg	**Adults: Panic Disorder: Initial:** 12.5 mg/d. **Titrate:** May increase wkly by 12.5 mg/d. **Max:** 75 mg/d. **SAD: Initial:** 12.5 mg/d. **Titrate:** May increase weekly by 12.5 mg/d. **Max:** 37.5 mg/d.	D > **H R W** [29]
Paroxetine HCl (Paxil)	**Susp:** 10 mg/5 ml; **Tab:** 10 mg, 20 mg, 30 mg, 40 mg	**Adults: Panic Disorder: Susp/Tab: Initial:** 10 mg qam. **Usual:** 40 mg/d. **Max:** 60 mg/d. **Social Anxiety Disorder: Susp/Tab: Initial/Usual:** 20 mg qam. **GAD/PTSD: Susp/Tab: Initial:** 20 mg qam. **Usual:** 20-50 mg qam. May increase wkly by 10 mg/d.	D > **H R W** [29]
Paroxetine Mesylate (Pexeva)	**Tab:** 10 mg, 20 mg, 30 mg, 40 mg	**Panic Disorder: Adults: Initial:** 10 mg/d. **Titrate:** 10 mg/d wkly. **Max:** 40 mg/d.	C > **H R W** [29]
Sertraline (Zoloft)	**Sol:** 20 mg/ml; **Tab:** 25 mg, 50 mg, 100 mg	**Panic Disorder/Social Anxiety Disorder/PTSD: Adults: Initial:** 25 mg qd. **Titrate:** Increase to 50 mg qd after 1 wk. Adjust wkly. **Max:** 200 mg/d.	C > **H W** [29]

Buspirone (BuSpar)	**Tab:** (BuSpar) 5 mg, 10 mg, 15 mg, 30 mg	**Anxiety: Adults: ≥18 yo: Initial:** 7.5 mg bid. **Titrate:** Increase by 5 mg/d q2-3d. **Usual:** 20-30 mg/d. **Max:** 60 mg/d.	B v
Chloral Hydrate CIV	**Cap:** 500 mg; **Sup:** 325 mg, 650 mg; **Syr:** 500 mg/5 ml	**Adults: Insomnia:** 500 mg-1 gm 15-30 min before retiring. **Sedative:** 250 mg tid. **Peds: Insomnia:** 50 mg/kg or 1.5 gm/m^2. **Max:** 1 gm. **Sedative:** 8 mg/kg or 250 mg/m^2 tid. **Max:** 500 mg tid.	C >
Eszopiclone CIV (Lunesta)	**Tab:** 1 mg, 2 mg, 3 mg	**Insomnia: Adults 18-65 yo: Initial:** 2 mg qhs. **Max:** 3 mg qhs. **≥65 yo: Difficulty Falling Asleep: Initial:** 1 mg qhs. **Max:** 2 mg qhs. **Difficulty Staying Asleep: Intial/Max:** 2 mg qhs.	C > **H**
Ramelteon (Rozerem)	**Tab:** 8 mg	**Adults:** 8 mg within 30 min of bedtime. Do not take w/ or after high fat meal.	C v **H**
Zaleplon CIV (Sonata)	**Cap:** 5 mg, 10 mg	**Insomnia: Adults:** 10 mg qhs. **Low-Wt Patients: Initial:** 5 mg qhs. **Max:** 20 mg qhs. **Debilitated Patients:** 5 mg qhs. **Max:** 10 mg qhs.	C v **H**
Zolpidem Tartrate CIV (Ambien CR)	**Tab, ER** 6.25 mg, 12.5 mg	**Insomnia: Adults: ≥18 yo:** 12.5 mg qhs. **Elderly/ Debilitated/Hepatic Insufficiency:** 6.25 mg qhs.	C v **H**
Zolpidem Tartrate CIV (Ambien)	**Tab:** 5 mg, 10 mg	**Insomnia: Adults: ≥18 yo:** 10 mg qhs. **Elderly/Debilitated/ Hepatic Insufficiency:** 5 mg qhs. May need to decrease dose w/ other CNS depressants.	B v **H**

Anticonvulsants

NAME	FORM/STRENGTH	DOSAGE	COMMENTS
BENZODIAZEPINES			
Clonazepam CIV (Klonopin, Klonopin Wafers)	**Tab:** 0.5 mg, 1 mg, 2 mg; **Tab,Dissolve:** (Wafer) 0.125 mg, 0.25 mg, 0.5 mg, 1 mg, 2 mg	**Seizure Disorder: Adults: Initial:** Up to 0.5 mg tid. **Titrate:** Increase by 0.5-1 mg q3d. **Max:** 20 mg/d. **Peds: Up to 10 yo or 30 kg: Initial:** 0.01-0.03 mg/kg/d (up to 0.05 mg/kg/d) given bid-tid. **Titrate:** Increase by 0.25-0.5 mg q3d. **Maint:** 0.1-0.2 mg/kg/d given tid.	D v
Diazepam CIV (Valium)	**Tab:** 2 mg, 5 mg, 10 mg	**Adults: PO:** 2-10 mg bid-qid. **Peds: ≥6 mths: Initial:** 1-2.5 mg tid-qid. **Titrate:** May increase gradually as needed & tolerated.	N >
Lorazepam CIV (Ativan Injection)	**Inj:** 2 mg/ml, 4 mg/ml	**Status Epilepticus: Adults: ≥18 yo:** 2 mg/min IV x 2 min, may repeat x 1 dose after 10-15 min. **Max:** 8 mg.	D v
CARBOXYLIC ACID DERIVATIVES			
Valproate Sodium (Depacon)	**Inj:** 100 mg/ml	**Complex Partial Seizure: Adults & Peds: ≥10 yo: IV: Initial:** 10-15 mg/kg/d. **Titrate:** Increase wkly by 5-10 mg/kg/d. **Max:** 60 mg/kg/d. **Simplex/Complex Absence Seizure: Adults: IV: Initial:** 15 mg/kg/d. **Titrate:** Increase wkly by 5-10 mg/kg/d. **Max:** 60 mg/kg/d.	D v Hepatic failure. Teratogenic. Pancreatitis. **H**

Valproic Acid (Depakene)	**Cap:** 250 mg; **Syr:** 250 mg/5 ml	**Complex Partial Seizure: Adults & Peds: ≥10 yo: Initial:** 10-15 mg/kg/d. **Titrate:** Increase wkly by 5-10 mg/kg/d. **Max:** 60 mg/kg/d. **Simplex/Complex Absence Seizure: Adults: Initial:** 15 mg/kg/d. **Titrate:** Increase wkly by 5-10 mg/kg/d. **Max:** 60 mg/kg/d.	D v Hepatic failure. Teratogenic. Pancreatitis. **H**
Valproic Acid (Stavzor)	**Cap,DR:** 125 mg, 250 mg, 500 mg	**Adults & Peds: ≥10 yo: Complex Partial Seizures: Initial:** 10-15 mg/kg/d. **Titrate:** Increase by 5-10 mg/kg/wk until optimal response (50-100 mcg/ml). **Max:** 60 mg/kg/d. **Conversion to Monotherapy:** Reduce concomitant antiepileptic drug (AED) dosage by 25% q2wks; withdrawal of AED highly variable, monitor closely for seizure frequency. **Simple/Complex Absence Seizures: Initial:** 15 mg/kg/d. **Titrate:** Increase at 1 wk interval by 5-10 mg/kg/d until optimal response (50-100 mcg/ml). **Max:** 60 mg/kg/d. If dose >250 mg/d, give in divided doses. **Elderly:** Reduce starting dose & increase slowly; monitor fluid, nutritional intake, and somnolence. Swallow whole.	D v **W** [101]

HYDANTOIN DERIVATIVES

Fosphenytoin Sodium (Cerebyx)	**Inj:** 50 mg/ml	**Adults: LD:** 10-20 mg PE/kg IV/IM (≤150 mg PE/min). **Maint:** 4-6 mg PE/kg/d. **Status Epilepticus: LD:** 15-20 mg PE/kg; administer as 100-150 mg PE/min.	D v **H R**

NAME	FORM/STRENGTH	DOSAGE	COMMENTS
Phenytoin (Dilantin)	**Cap, ER:** 30 mg, 100 mg; **Chewtab:** 50 mg; **Susp:** 125 mg/5 ml	**Tonic-Clonic & Complex Partial Seizures/Seizure Treatment or Prevention w/ Neurosurgery: Adults: Cap,ER: Initial:** 100 mg tid-qid. **Titrate:** Increase q7-10d. **Max:** 200 mg tid. May give ER qd if controlled on 300 mg/d. **LD:** 400 mg PO, then 300 mg q2h x 2 doses (total 1 gm). Start maint 24h later. **Chewtab: Initial:** 100 mg tid. **Titrate:** Increase q7-10d. **Usual:** 300-400 mg/d. **Max:** 600 mg/d. **Susp: Initial:** 125 mg tid. **Titrate:** Increase q7-10d. **Max:** 625 mg/d. **Peds: Initial:** 5 mg/kg/d given bid-tid. **Titrate:** Increase q7-10d. **Maint:** 4-8 mg/kg/d. **Max:** 300 mg/d. **>6 yo:** May require min adult dose (300 mg/d).	N v

SODIUM CHANNEL INACTIVATOR

NAME	FORM/STRENGTH	DOSAGE	COMMENTS
Lacosamide (Vimpat)	**Inj:** 10 mg/ml; **Tab:** 50 mg, 100 mg, 150 mg, 200 mg	**Partial Onset Seizures: Adults:** (PO/Inj) Initial: 50 mg bid (100 mg/d). **Titrate:** May increase at wkly intervals by 100 mg/d given as two divided doses. **Maint:** 200-400 mg/d based on response & tolerability. **Switching from Oral to IV Dosing:** Initial total daily IV dosage should be equivalent to total daily dosage & frequency of PO dosing & infused over 30-60 min. **Switching from IV to Oral Dosing:** Oral administration may be given at equivalent daily dosage and frequency of IV treatment.	C v **H R**

SULFONAMIDE

Zonisamide (Zonegran)	**Cap:** 25 mg, 100 mg	**Partial Seizures: Adults & Peds:** ≥**16 yo: Initial:** 100 mg qd. **Titrate:** Increase by 100 mg q2wks, given qd-bid. **Max:** 400 mg/d.	C v **H R**

TRIAZOLE DERIVATIVE

Rufinamide (Banzel)	**Tab:** 200 mg, 400 mg	**Adults: Initial:** 400-800 mg/d in two equally divided doses. **Titrate:** May increase by 400-800 mg/d q2d until max of 3200 mg/d, given in two equally divided doses, is reached. **Max:** 3200 mg/d. **Peds:** ≥**4 yo: Initial:** 10 mg/kg/d in two equally divided doses. **Titrate:** May increase by 10 mg/kg increments qod to target dose of 45 mg/kg/d or 3200 mg/d, whichever is less, given in two equally divided doses. **Max:** 45 mg/kg/d or 3200 mg/d. Take w/ food.	C v **H**

MISCELLANEOUS

Carbamazepine (Tegretol, Tegretol-XR)	**Chewtab:** 100 mg; **Susp:** 100 mg/5 ml; **Tab:** 200 mg; **Tab,ER:** (XR) 100 mg, 200 mg, 400 mg	**Partial/Tonic-Clonic/Mixed Seizures: Adults & Peds: >12 yo: Initial: Chewtab/Tab/Tab,ER:** 200 mg bid. **Susp:** 100 mg qid. **Titrate:** May increase wkly by 200 mg/d given tid-qid (Chewtab/Susp/Tab) or bid (Tab,ER). **Maint:** 800-1200 mg/d. **Max:** 1200 mg/d (>15 yo) or 1000 mg/d (12-15 yo). **6-12 yo: Chewtab/Tab/Tab,ER: Initial:** 100 mg bid. **Susp:** 50 mg qid. **Titrate:** May increase wkly by	D v **H W** [87]

Continued on Next Page

NAME	FORM/STRENGTH	DOSAGE	COMMENTS
Carbamazepine (Tegretol, Tegretol-XR) *Continued*		100 mg/d given tid-qid (Chewtab/Susp/Tab) or bid (Tab,ER). **Maint:** 400-800 mg/d. **Max:** 1000 mg/d. **6 mths-6 yo: Chewtab/Tab: Initial:** 10-20 mg/kg/d given bid-tid. **Susp:** 10-20 mg/kg/d given qid. **Titrate:** (Chewtab/Susp/Tab) May increase wkly tid-qid. **Max:** 35 mg/kg/d.	
Divalproex Sodium (Depakote ER)	**Tab, ER:** 250 mg, 500 mg	**Complex Partial Seizures: Adults & Peds: >10 yo: Initial:** 10-15 mg/kg qd. **Titrate:** Increase by 5-10 mg/kg/wk. **Usual:** <60 mg/kg/d. **Absence Seizures: Adults & Peds: >10 yo: Initial:** 15 mg/kg qd. **Titrate:** Increase by 5-10 mg/kg/wk. **Max:** 60 mg/kg/d.	D; v Hepatotoxic. Teratogenic. Pancreatitis.
Divalproex Sodium (Depakote)	**Cap, Delay:** (Sprinkle) 125 mg; **Tab, Delay:** 125 mg, 250 mg, 500 mg	**Complex Partial Seizures: Adults & Peds: >10 yo: Initial:** 10-15 mg/kg/d. **Titrate:** Increase by 5-10 mg/kg/wk. **Max:** 60 mg/kg/d. **Absence Seizures: Adults: Initial:** 15 mg/kg/d. **Titrate:** Increase by 5-10 mg/kg/wk. **Max:** 60 mg/kg/d.	D; v Hepatotoxic. Teratogenic. Pancreatitis.
Gabapentin (Neurontin)	**Cap:** 100 mg, 300 mg, 400 mg; **Sol:** 250 mg/5 ml; **Tab:** 600 mg, 800 mg	**Partial Seizures: Adults & Peds: ≥12 yo: Initial:** 300 mg tid. **Titrate:** Increase up to 1.8 gm/d. **Max:** 3.6 gm/d. **3-12 yo: Initial:** 10-15 mg/kg/d given tid. **Titrate:** Increase over 3d. **Usual: ≥5 yo:** 25-35 mg/kg/d given tid. **3-4 yo:** 40 mg/kg/d given tid. **Max:** 50 mg/kg/d.	C; > **R**
Lamotrigine (Lamictal, Lamictal CD, Lamictal ODT)	**Chewtab:** (CD) 2 mg, 5 mg, 25 mg; **Tab:** 25 mg, 100 mg, 150 mg, 200 mg; **Tab, Dissolve:**	**Lennox-Gastaut/Partial Seizures:** Special dosing requirements w/ VPA. **Adults & Peds: >12 yo: Concomitant EIAEDs w/ VPA:** 25 mg qod x 2 wks, then 25 mg qd x 2 wks. **Titrate:** Increase q1-2 wks by 25-50 mg/d. **Maint:**	C; v Serious rashes, Stevens-Johnson

	(ODT) 25 mg, 50 mg, 100 mg, 200 mg	100-400 mg/d, given qd or bid. **Concomitant EIAEDs w/o VPA:** 50 mg qd x 2 wks, then 50 mg bid x 2 wks. **Titrate:** Increase q1-2wks by 100 mg/d. **Maint:** 150-250 mg bid. **Conversion to Monotherapy from Single EIAED: ≥16 yo:** 50 mg qd x 2 wks, then 50 mg bid x 2 wks. **Titrate:** Increase q1-2wks by 100 mg/d. **Maint:** 250 mg bid. Withdraw EIAED over 4 wks. **Conversion to Monotherapy from VPA: ≥16 yo: Step 1:** Follow concomitant AEDs w/ VPA dosing regimen to achieve lamotrigine dose of 200 mg/d. Maintain previous VPA dose. **Step 2:** Maintain lamotrigine 200 mg/d. Decrease VPA to 500 mg/d by decrements of ≤500 mg/d per wk. Maintain VPA 500 mg/d x 1 wk. **Step 3:** Increase to lamotrigine 300 mg/d x 1 wk. Decrease VPA simultaneously to 250 mg/d x 1 wk. **Step 4:** D/C VPA. Increase lamotrigine 100 mg/d qwk to maint dose of 500 mg/d. **Peds: 2-12 yo: ≥6.7 kg: Concomitant EIAEDs w/o VPA:** 0.3 mg/kg bid x 2 wks, then 0.6 mg/kg bid x 2 wks. **Titrate:** Increase q1-2wks by 1.2 mg/kg/d. **Maint:** 2.5-7.5 mg/kg bid. **Max:** 400 mg/d. Round dose down to nearest whole tab.	syndrome reported. **H R**
Levetiracetam (Keppra XR)	**Tab,ER:** 500 mg, 750 mg	**Partial Onset Seizures: Adults & Peds: ≥16 yo: Initial:** 1000 mg qd. **Titrate:** Adjust dose in increments of 1000 mg q2wks. **Max:** 3000 mg. Swallow whole.	◙C ❀v **R**

NAME	FORM/STRENGTH	DOSAGE	COMMENTS
Levetiracetam (Keppra)	**Inj:** 500 mg/ml; **Sol:** 100 mg/ml; **Tab:** 250 mg, 500 mg, 750 mg, 1000 mg	**Adults & Peds: ≥16 yo: Partial Onset Seizures (IV/PO) or ≥16 yo (IV)/ ≥12 yo (PO): Juvenile Myoclonic Epilepsy: Initial:** 500 mg bid. **Titrate:** Increase q2wks by 1000 mg/d. **Recommended/Max:** 3 gm/d. **Replacement Therapy: IV:** Initial total daily dosage & frequency should equal total daily dosage & frequency of PO therapy. Dilute inj in 100 ml of compatible diluent & give as 15 min IV infusion. **Peds: Partial Onset Seizures (4-<16 yo) or Primary Generalized Tonic-Clonic Seizures (6-<16 yo): PO: Initial:** 10 mg/kg bid. **Titrate:** Increase q2wks by 20 mg/kg/d. **Recommended/Max:** 30 mg/kg bid.	◙C ✲> **R**
Oxcarbazepine (Trileptal)	**Susp:** 300 mg/5 ml; **Tab:** 150 mg, 300 mg, 600 mg	**Partial Seizures: Monotherapy: Adults: Initial:** 300 mg bid. **Titrate:** Increase by 300 mg/d q3d. **Maint:** 1200 mg/d. **4-16 yo: Initial:** 4-5 mg/kg bid. **Titrate:** Increase by 5 mg/kg/d q3d. **Maint (mg/d): 20 kg: Initial:** 600 mg. **Max:** 900 mg. **25-30 kg: Initial:** 900 mg. **Max:** 1200 mg. **35-40 kg: Initial:** 900 mg. **Max:** 1500 mg. **45 kg: Initial:** 1200 mg. **Max:** 1500 mg. **50-55 kg: Initial:** 1200 mg. **Max:** 1800 mg. **60-65 kg: Initial:** 1200 mg. **Max:** 2100 mg. **70 kg: Initial:** 1500 mg. **Max:** 2100 mg. **Adjunct Therapy: Adults: Initial:** 300 mg bid. **Titrate:** Increase wkly by max of 600 mg/d. **Maint:** 600 mg bid. **4-16 yo: Initial:** 4-5 mg/kg bid. **Max:** 600 mg/d. **Titrate:** Increase over 2 wks. **Maint (mg/d): 20-29 kg:** 900 mg. **29.1-39 kg:** 1200 mg. **>39 kg:** 1800 mg. **Conversion to Monotherapy:**	◙C ✲v **R**

		Adults: Initial: 300 mg bid while reducing other AEDs. **Titrate:** Increase wkly by 600 mg/d. **Maint:** 2400 mg/d. **4-16 yo: Initial:** 4-5 mg/kg bid while reducing other AEDs. **Titrate:** Increase wkly by max of 10 mg/kg/d to target dose. Withdraw other AEDs over 3-6 wks.	
Pregabalin CV (Lyrica)	**Cap:** 25 mg, 50 mg, 75 mg, 100 mg, 150 mg, 200 mg, 225 mg, 300 mg	**Partial Seizures: Adults: Initial:** 150 mg/d divided bid-tid. **Max:** 600 mg/d.	C v **R**
Primidone (Mysoline)	**Tab:** 50 mg, 250 mg	**Grand Mal/Psychomotor/Focal Seizures: Adults & Peds: ≥8 yo: Initial/Titrate: Days 1-3:** 100-125 mg qhs. **Days 4-6:** 100-125 mg bid. **Days 7-9:** 100-125 mg tid. **Day 10-Maint:** 250 mg tid. **Max:** 500 mg qid. **<8 yo: Initial/Titrate: Days 1-3:** 50 mg qhs. **Days 4-6:** 50 mg bid. **Days 7-9:** 100 mg bid. **Day 10-Maint:** 125-250 mg tid or 10-25 mg/kg/d in divided doses.	N >
Topiramate (Topamax, Topamax Sprinkle Capsules)	**Cap:** 15 mg, 25 mg; **Tab:** 25 mg, 50 mg, 100 mg, 200 mg	**Partial Onset/Tonic-Clonic Seizures: Monotherapy: Adults & Peds: ≥10 yo: Initial:** 25 mg qam & qpm x 1 wk. **Titrate:** Increase am & pm dose by 25 mg qwk until 200 mg qam & qpm. **Partial Onset/Tonic-Clonic/Lennox-Gastaut Seizures: Adjunctive Therapy: Adults & Peds: ≥17 yo: Initial:** 25-50 mg qd. **Titrate:** Increase qwk by 25-50 mg. **Usual:** 100-200 mg bid (partial seizures) or 200 mg bid	C > **R**

Continued on Next Page

NAME	FORM/STRENGTH	DOSAGE	COMMENTS
Topiramate (Topamax, Topamax Sprinkle Capsules) *Continued*		(tonic-clonic seizures). **Max:** 1600 mg/d. **Peds: 2-16 yo: Initial:** 1-3 mg/kg/d qpm x 1 wk. **Titrate:** Increase by 1-3 mg/kg/d q1-2wks. **Usual:** 5-9 mg/kg/d given as bid.	

Antidepressant Agents

DOPAMINE/NOREPINEPHRINE REUPTAKE INHIBITOR

NAME	FORM/STRENGTH	DOSAGE	COMMENTS
Bupropion HCl (Wellbutrin XL)	**Tab, ER:** 150 mg, 300 mg	**Adults: ≥18 yo: Initial:** 150 mg qam, may increase to 300 mg qam after 3d. **Usual:** 300 mg qam. **Max:** 450 mg qam. Swallow whole.	C v **H R W** 29
Bupropion Hydrobromide (Aplenzin)	**Tab,ER:** 174 mg, 348 mg, 522 mg	**Adults: ≥18 yo:** Give in morning. Swallow whole. **Initial:** 174 mg qd. **Titrate:** May increase to 348 mg qd on Day 4 if tolerated. **Max:** 522 mg/d given as single dose if no clinical improvement after several wks. **Switching from Wellbutrin, Wellbutrin SR, or Wellbutrin XL:** Give equivalent dose. 522 mg bupropion HBr = 450 mg bupropion HCl, 348 mg bupropion HBr = 300 mg bupropion HCl, 174 mg bupropion HBr = 150 mg bupropion HCl. **Mild-Moderate Hepatic Cirrhosis/Renal Impairment:** Reduce frequency and/or dose. **Severe Hepatic Cirrhosis: Max:** 174 mg qod.	C v **H R W** 29
Bupropion (Wellbutrin, Wellbutrin SR)	**Tab:** 75 mg, 100 mg; **Tab, ER:** 100 mg, 150 mg, 200 mg	**Adults: ≥18 yo: Tab: Initial:** 100 mg bid. **Maint:** 100 mg tid. **Max:** 450 mg/d. **Tab, ER: Initial:** 150 mg qam. **Maint:** 150 mg bid. **Max:** 200 mg bid.	C v **H R W** 29

MAOIS

Selegiline (Emsam)	**Patch:** 6 mg/24h, 9 mg/24h, 12 mg/24h	**Adults:** Apply to dry, intact skin on upper torso, upper thigh, or outer surface of upper arm once q24h. **Initial/Target Dose:** 6 mg/24h. **Titrate:** May increase in increments of 3 mg/24h at intervals no less than 2 wks. **Max:** 12 mg/24h. **Elderly:** 6 mg/24h. Increase dose cautiously & monitor closely.	C > **W** [29]

PARTIAL D2/5HT1A AGONIST/5HT2A ANTAGONIST

Aripiprazole (Abilify, Abilify Discmelt)	**Sol:** 1 mg/ml; **Tab:** 2 mg, 5 mg, 10 mg, 15 mg, 20 mg, 30 mg; **Tab, Dissolve:** (Discmelt) 10 mg, 15 mg	**Adults: Initial: PO:** 2-5 mg/d. **Titrate:** May adjust dose at increments of ≤5 mg/d at intervals ≥1 wk. **Range:** 2-15 mg/d. **Max:** 15 mg/d. Oral sol can be given on mg-per-mg basis up to 25 mg. Patients receiving 30 mg tabs should receive 25 mg of sol. Adjust dose w/ CYP3A4 inducers/inhibitors or CYP2D6 inhibitors.	C v **W** [29, 30]

SEROTONIN/NOREPINEPHRINE REUPTAKE INHIBITORS

Desvenlafaxine (Pristiq)	**Tab, ER:** 50 mg, 100 mg	**Adults: Initial:** 50 mg qd. **Range:** 50-400 mg/d. Do not divide, crush, chew or dissolve.	C v **H R W** [29]
Duloxetine (Cymbalta)	**Cap,Delay:** 20 mg, 30 mg, 60 mg	**Adults: Initial:** 40 mg/d (given as 20 mg bid) to 60 mg/d (given once daily or as 30 mg bid). Re-evaluate periodically. Do not chew or crush.	C v **H R W** [29]
Venlafaxine (Effexor XR)	**Cap, ER:** 37.5 mg, 75 mg, 150 mg	**Adults: ≥18 yo: Initial:** 75 mg/d. **Titrate:** Increase by 75 mg/d at intervals not less than 4d. **Max:** 225 mg/d.	C v **H R W** [29]

NAME	FORM/STRENGTH	DOSAGE	COMMENTS
Venlafaxine (Effexor)	**Tab:** 25 mg, 37.5 mg, 50 mg, 75 mg, 100 mg	**Adults: ≥18 yo: Tab: Initial:** 37.5 mg bid or 25 mg tid. **Titrate:** Increase by 75 mg/d q4d to 150-225 mg/d. **Max:** 375 mg/d.	C v **H R W** [29]
SSRIS & COMBINATIONS			
Citalopram (Celexa)	**Sol:** 10 mg/5 ml; **Tab:** 10 mg, 20 mg, 40 mg	**Adults: Initial:** 20 mg qd, in am or pm. **Titrate:** May increase by 20 mg at intervals ≥1 wk, to 40 mg/d. **Max:** 60 mg/d. **Elderly/Hepatic Impairment:** 20 mg qd. May titrate to 40 mg/d for nonresponding patients.	C v **H W** [29]
Escitalopram Oxalate (Lexapro)	**Sol:** 5 mg/5 ml; **Tab:** 5 mg, 10 mg, 20 mg	**Adults & Peds: 12-17 yo: Initial:** 10 mg qd, in am or pm. **Titrate:** May increase to 20 mg after at least 1 wk (adults) or 3 wks (peds). **Max:** 20 mg qd. **Elderly/Hepatic Impairment:** 10 mg qd. Re-evaluate periodically.	C v **H R W** [29]
Fluoxetine (Prozac Weekly)	**Cap, ER:** 90 mg	**Adults: Initial:** One 90 mg cap 7d after last daily dose of Prozac 20 mg. Must be stabilized on 20 mg/d prior to initiation.	C v **H W** [29]
Fluoxetine (Prozac)	**Cap:** 10 mg, 20 mg, 40 mg; **Sol:** 20 mg/5 ml; **Tab:** 10 mg	**Adults: Daily Dosing: Initial:** 20 mg qam. **Titrate:** Increase dose if no improvement after several wks. Doses >20 mg/d, give qam or bid (am & noon). **Max:** 80 mg/d. **Peds: ≥8 yo: Higher Wt Peds: Initial:** 10 or 20 mg/d. After 1 wk at 10 mg/d, may increase to 20 mg/d. **Lower Wt Peds: Initial:** 10 mg/d. **Titrate:** May increase to 20 mg/d after several wks if clinical improvement not observed.	C v **H W** [29]

Olanzapine/Fluoxetine HCl (Symbyax)	**Cap:** 3-25 mg, 6-25 mg, 6-50 mg, 12-25 mg, 12-50 mg	**Adults: ≥18 yo: Depressive Episodes Associated w/ Bipolar I Disorder/Treatment Resistant Depression: Initial:** 6-25 mg qd in evening. **Titrate:** Adjust dose based on efficacy and tolerability. **Max:** 18-75 mg/d. **Hypotension Risk/Slow Metabolizers: Initial:** 3-25 mg to 6-25 mg qd in evening. **Titrate:** Increase cautiously. Re-evaluate periodically.	C v **H W** [29, 30]
Paroxetine HCl (Paxil CR)	**Tab, CR:** 12.5 mg, 25 mg, 37.5 mg	**Adults: Initial:** 25 mg/d. **Titrate:** May increase wkly by 12.5 mg/d. **Max:** 62.5 mg/d.	D > **H R W** [29]
Paroxetine HCl (Paxil)	**Susp:** 10 mg/5 ml; **Tab:** 10 mg, 20 mg, 30 mg, 40 mg; **Tab, CR:** 12.5 mg, 25 mg, 37.5 mg	**Adults: Susp/Tab: Initial:** 20 mg qam. **Max:** 50 mg/d. **Tab,CR: Initial:** 25 mg/d. **Titrate:** May increase wkly by 12.5 mg/d. **Max:** 62.5 mg/d.	D > **H R W** [29]
Paroxetine Mesylate (Pexeva)	**Tab:** 10 mg, 20 mg, 30 mg, 40 mg	**Adults: Initial:** 20 mg/d. **Max:** 50 mg/d.	C > **H R W** [29]
Sertraline (Zoloft)	**Sol:** 20 mg/ml; **Tab:** 25 mg, 50 mg, 100 mg	**Adults: Initial:** 50 mg qd. **Titrate:** Adjust wkly. **Max:** 200 mg/d.	C > **H W** [29]

TETRACYCLICS

Mirtazapine (Remeron, Remeron SolTab)	**Tab, Dissolve:** (SolTab) 15 mg, 30 mg, 45 mg; **Tab:** 15 mg, 30 mg, 45 mg	**Adults: Initial:** 15 mg qhs. **Titrate:** Increase q1-2wks. **Maint:** 15-45 mg qd. **Max:** 45 mg qd.	C > **W** [29]

NAME	FORM/STRENGTH	DOSAGE	COMMENTS
TRICYCLIC ANTIDEPRESSANTS			
Amitriptyline	**Inj:** 10 mg/ml; **Tab:** 10 mg, 25 mg, 50 mg, 75 mg, 100 mg, 150 mg	**Adults: PO: Initial:** (Outpatient) 75 mg/d in divided doses or 50-100 mg qhs. (Inpatient) 100 mg/d. **Titrate:** (Outpatient) Increase by 25-50 mg qhs. (Inpatient) Increase to 200 mg/d. **Maint:** 50-100 mg qhs. **Max:** (Outpatient) 150 mg/d. (Inpatient) 300 mg/d. **Peds: ≥12 yo & Elderly:** 10 mg tid or 20 mg qhs. **Adults & Peds: ≥12 yo: IM: Initial:** 20-30 mg qid.	C v **W** 29
Desipramine (Norpramin)	**Tab:** 10 mg, 25 mg, 50 mg, 75 mg, 100 mg, 150 mg	**Adults: Usual:** 100-200 mg qd. **Max:** 300 mg/d. **Adolescents: Usual:** 25-100 mg qd. **Max:** 150 mg/d.	N > **W** 29
Doxepin (Sinequan)	(Generic) **Cap:** 10 mg, 25 mg, 50 mg, 75 mg, 100 mg, 150 mg; **Sol:** 10 mg/ml; (Sinequan) **Cap:** 10 mg, 25 mg, 50 mg, 75 mg	**Adults & Peds: ≥12 yo: Mild Illness: Usual:** 25-50 mg/d. **Mild-Moderate: Initial:** 75 mg/d. **Usual:** 75-150 mg/d. **Severely Ill:** Up to 300 mg/d.	N > **W** 29
Imipramine HCl (Tofranil)	**Tab:** 10 mg, 25 mg, 50 mg	**Adults: Initial:** (Inpatients) 100 mg/d; may increase to 200 mg/d x 2 wks, then 250-300 mg/d if needed. (Outpatients) 75 mg/d; may increase to 150 mg/d, then to 200 mg/d if needed. **Maint:** 50-150 mg/d. **Adolescents: Initial:** 30-40 mg qhs. **Max:** 100 mg/d.	N v **W** 29

Nortriptyline HCl (Pamelor)	**Cap:** 10 mg, 25 mg, 50 mg, 75 mg; **Sol:** 10 mg/5 ml	**Adults: Usual:** 25 mg tid-qid. **Max:** 150 mg/d. **Adolescents:** 30-50 mg/d.	◉N ✽> **W** [29]

MISCELLANEOUS

Trazodone	**Tab:** 50 mg, 100 mg, 150 mg, 300 mg	**Adults: ≥18 yo: Initial:** 150 mg/d in divided doses. **Titrate:** Increase by 50 mg/d q3-4d. **Max:** (Outpatients) 400 mg/d, (Inpatients) 600 mg/d.	◉C ✽> **W** [29]

Antiparkinson's Agents

ANTICHOLINERGIC AGENTS

Benztropine Mesylate	**Inj:** 1 mg/ml; **Tab:** 0.5 mg, 1 mg, 2 mg	**Adults: Initial:** 0.5-1 mg PO/IV/IM qhs. **Usual:** 1-2 mg/d. **Max:** 6 mg/d.	◉N ✽>
Trihexyphenidyl	**Eli:** 2 mg/5 ml; **Tab:** 2 mg, 5 mg	**Adults: Idiopathic:** 1 mg on Day 1. **Titrate:** Increase by 2 mg q3-5d. **Usual:** 6-10 mg/d. **Max:** 15 mg/d. **Drug-Induced: Initial:** 1 mg, increase until achieve control. **Usual:** 5-15 mg/d.	◉N ✽>

NAME	FORM/STRENGTH	DOSAGE	COMMENTS
CHOLINESTERASE INHIBITORS			
Rivastigmine Tartrate (Exelon)	**Cap:** 1.5 mg, 3 mg, 4.5 mg, 6 mg; **Sol:** 2 mg/ml; **Patch:** 4.6 mg/24h, 9.5 mg/24h	**Dementia Associated w/ Parkinson's Disease: Adults: PO: Initial:** 1.5 mg bid. **Titrate:** May increase by 1.5 mg q4wks. Take w/ food in am & pm. **Patch: Initial:** Apply 4.6 mg/24h patch qd to clean, dry, hairless intact skin. **Maint:** May increase dose after 4 wks. **Max:** 9.5 mg/24h if well tolerated. **Switching from PO: Total PO Daily Dose <6mg:** Switch to 4.6 mg/24h patch. **Total PO Daily Dose 6-12 mg:** Switch to 9.5 mg/24h patch. Apply 1st patch on day following last PO dose.	B v
COMT INHIBITOR			
Entacapone (Comtan)	**Tab:** 200 mg	**Adults:** 200 mg w/ each levodopa/carbidopa dose. **Max:** 1600 mg/d.	C >
DOPAMINE AGONISTS			
Bromocriptine Mesylate (Parlodel)	**Cap:** 5 mg; **Tab:** 2.5 mg	**Adults: Initial:** 1.25 mg bid. **Titrate:** Increase by 2.5 mg/d q2-4wks. **Max:** 100 mg/d.	B v
Pramipexole Dihydrochloride (Mirapex)	**Tab:** 0.125 mg, 0.25 mg, 0.5 mg, 0.75 mg, 1 mg, 1.5 mg	**Adults: Initial:** 0.125 mg tid. **Titrate:** Increase q5-7d (eg, Wk 2: 0.25 mg tid; Wk 3: 0.5 mg tid; Wk 4: 0.75 mg tid; Wk 5: 1 mg tid; Wk 6: 1.25 mg tid; Wk 7: 1.5 mg tid). **Maint:** 0.5-1.5 mg tid. **Max:** 1.5 mg tid.	C v **R**

Ropinirole HCl (Requip)	**Tab:** 0.25 mg, 0.5 mg, 1 mg, 2 mg, 3 mg, 4 mg, 5 mg	**Adults: Initial:** 0.25 mg tid. **Titrate/Maint:** Increase wkly by 0.25 mg tid x 4 wks. After wk 4, increase wkly by 1.5 mg/d up to 9 mg/d, then by 3 mg/d wkly to 24 mg/d. **Max:** 24 mg/d. **Withdrawal:** Decrease dose to bid x 4d, then qd x 3d.	C v
Ropinirole HCl (Requip XL)	**Tab,ER:** 2 mg, 4 mg, 8 mg, 12 mg	**Adults: Initial:** 2 mg qd x 1-2 wks. **Titrate:** May increase by 2 mg/d at ≥1 wk intervals, depending on response & tolerability. **Max:** 24 mg/d. Swallow whole. **Switching from Immediate-Release (IR) to XL:** Initial dose should match total daily dose of IR formulation. See PI for more info.	C v

DOPAMINE PRECURSOR/DOPA-DECARBOXYLASE INHIBITOR

Carbidopa/Levodopa (Sinemet, Sinemet CR)	**Tab:** 10-100 mg, 25-100 mg, 25-250 mg; **Tab, ER:** (CR) 25-100 mg, 50-200 mg.	**Adults: ≥18 yo: Tab: Initial:** 10-100 mg tab tid-qid or 25-100 mg tab tid. **Titrate:** May increase by 1 tab qd or qod until 8 tabs/d. **Maint:** 70-100 mg/d carbidopa required. **Max:** 200 mg/d carbidopa. **Tab, ER: No Prior Levodopa Use: Initial:** 50-200 mg tab bid at intervals ≥6 hrs. Do not chew or crush. **Titrate:** May increase/decrease dose or interval accordingly. Adjust dose q3d. **Usual:** 400-1600 mg/d levodopa, given in 4-8h intervals while awake. **Conversion to Tab, ER:** See PI.	C >

NAME	FORM/STRENGTH	DOSAGE	COMMENTS
DOPAMINE PRECURSOR/DOPA-DECARBOXYLASE INHIBITOR/COMT INHIBITOR			
Carbidopa/Entacapone/ Levodopa (Stalevo)	**Tab:** 12.5/50/200 mg, 18.75/75/200 mg, 25/100/200 mg, 31.25/125/200 mg, 37.5/150/200 mg, 50/200/200 mg	**Adults: Currently Taking Carbidopa/Levodopa & Entacapone:** May switch directly to corresponding strength of levodopa/carbidopa. **Currently Taking Carbidopa/ Levodopa but not Entacapone:** First titrate individually w/ carbidopa/levodopa product & entacapone product then transfer to corresponding dose. **Max:** 8 tabs/d (Stalevo 50/Stalevo 75/Stalevo 100/Stalevo 125/Stalevo 150) or 6 tabs/d (Stalevo 200).	C >
MAOIS			
Rasagiline (Azilect)	**Tab:** 0.5 mg, 1 mg	**Adults: Monotherapy:** 1 mg qd. **Adjunctive Therapy: Initial:** 0.5 mg qd. **Titrate:** May increase to 1 mg qd. Adjust dose of levodopa w/ concomitant use. **Concomitant Ciprofloxacin or Other CYP1A2 Inhibitors/Hepatic Impairment:** 0.5 mg qd.	C > H
Selegiline HCl (Eldepryl)	**Cap:** 5 mg	**Adults:** 5 mg bid, at breakfast & lunch. **Max:** 10 mg/d.	C v

Antipsychotic Agents

BENZISOXAZOLE DERIVATIVE

Paliperidone (Invega)	**Tab,ER:** 3 mg, 6 mg, 9 mg	**Acute/Maint Treatment of Schizophrenia: Adults:** 6 mg qd in am. **Range:** 3-12 mg/d. **Titrate:** May increase by 3 mg/d at intervals of >5 days. **Max:** 12 mg/d. Swallow whole.	C v **R W** 30
Risperidone (Risperdal, Risperdal M-Tab)	**Sol:** 1 mg/ml; **Tab:** 0.25 mg, 0.5 mg, 1 mg, 2 mg, 3 mg, 4 mg; **Tab,Dissolve:** 0.5 mg, 1 mg, 2 mg, 3 mg, 4 mg	**Schizophrenia: Adults: PO: Initial:** 1 mg bid. **Maint:** 2-8 mg/d given qd-bid. **Max:** 16 mg/d. **Elderly/Debilitated/ Hypotension/Severe Renal or Hepatic Impairment: Initial:** 0.5 mg bid. **Peds: 13-17 yo: PO: Initial:** 0.5 mg qd in morning or evening. **Titrate:** Adjust dose, if needed, in increments of 0.5 or 1 mg/d & at intervals not <24h as tolerated to a recommended dose of 3 mg/d. **Max:** 6 mg/d.	C v **H W** 30
Ziprasidone (Geodon, Geodon for Injection)	**Cap:** 20 mg, 40 mg, 60 mg, 80 mg; **Inj:** 20 mg/ml	**Schizophrenia: Adults: Initial: PO:** 20 mg bid w/ food. **Max:** 80 mg bid. **Acute Agitation: IM:** 10 mg q2h or 20 mg q4h up to 40 mg/d x 3d.	C v **W** 30

BUTYROPHENONES

Haloperidol (Haldol, Haldol Decanoate)	(Haldol) **Inj:** (Decanoate) 50 mg/ml, 100 mg/ml, (Lactate) 5 mg/ml; (Generic) **Cnt:** 2 mg/ml; **Inj:** (Decanoate)	**Adults: Usual: PO:** 0.5-5 mg bid-tid. **IM:** (Lactate) 2-5 mg q4-8h or q1h prn. **Max:** 100 mg/d. (Decanoate) Give q4wks. 10-20x daily PO dose up to 100 mg. Give remainder of dose 3-7d later if initial dose >100 mg. **Peds:**	C v **W** 30

Continued on Next Page

NAME	FORM/STRENGTH	DOSAGE	COMMENTS
Haloperidol (Haldol, Haldol Decanoate) *Continued*	50 mg/ml, 100 mg/ml, (Lactate) 5 mg/ml; **Tab:** 0.5 mg, 1 mg, 2 mg, 5 mg, 10 mg, 20 mg	**3-12 yo (15-40 kg): PO:** 0.05-0.15 mg/kg/d given bid-tid. **Max:** 6 mg/d.	
DIBENZAPINE DERIVATIVE			
Clozapine (Clozaril)	**Tab:** 12.5 mg, 25 mg, 100 mg	**Schizophrenia/Suicidal Behavior Risk Reduction: Adults: Initial:** 12.5 mg qd-bid. **Titrate:** Increase by 25-50 mg/d, up to 300-450 mg/d by end of 2nd wk, then increase wkly or bi-wkly by up to 100 mg. **Usual:** 100-900 mg/d given tid. **Max:** 900 mg/d. If at risk of suicidal behavior then treat for at least 2 yrs then assess; reassess thereafter at regular intervals. To d/c, gradually reduce dose over 1-2 wks.	◙B ❋v **W** 26, 30
Clozapine (Fazaclo)	**Tab, Dissolve:** 12.5 mg, 25 mg, 50 mg, 100 mg	**Schizophrenia: Adults: Initial:** 12.5 mg qd-bid. **Titrate:** Increase by 25-50 mg/d, up to 300-450 mg/d by end of 2 wks, then increase wkly or bi-wkly by up to 100 mg increments. **Ususal:** 100-900 mg/d given tid. **Max:** 900 mg/d. To d/c, gradually reduce dose over 1-2 wks.	◙B ❋v **W** 26,30
Olanzapine (Zyprexa, Zyprexa Zydis, Zyprexa IntraMuscular)	**Inj:** 10 mg; **Tab:** 2.5 mg, 5 mg, 7.5 mg, 10 mg, 15 mg, 20 mg; **Tab,Dissolve:** (Zydis) 5 mg, 10 mg, 15 mg, 20 mg	**Schizophrenia: Adults: PO: Initial/Usual:** 5-10 mg qd. **Titrate:** Adjust wkly by 5 mg/d. **Max:** 20 mg/d. **Agitation Associated w/ Schizophrenia: Inj: Initial:** 10 mg IM. **Range:** 2.5-10 mg IM. **Max:** 3 doses of 10 mg IM q2-4h. May initiate PO therapy when clinically appropriate.	◙C ❋v **W** 30

Quetiapine Fumarate (Seroquel XR)	**Tab,ER:** 50 mg, 150 mg, 200 mg, 300 mg, 400 mg	**Schizophrenia:** Give qd, preferably in evening. **Initial:** 300 mg/d. **Titrate:** To within range of 400-800 mg/d depending on response & tolerance. Dose increases may be made at intervals as short as 1 day and in increments up to 300 mg/d. Re-evaluate periodically. **Elderly/Hepatic Impairment: Initial:** 50 mg/d; may increase in increments of 50 mg/d depending on response and tolerance. **Reinitiation of Treatment: If off >1 wk:** Follow initial dosing schedule. **If <1 wk:** No dose escalation required, reinitiate maint dose. **Switching from Seroquel:** May switch to Seroquel XR at equivalent total daily dose given qd. Swallow whole.	C v **H W** [29, 30]
Quetiapine Fumarate (Seroquel)	**Tab:** 25 mg, 50 mg, 100 mg, 200 mg, 300 mg, 400 mg	**Schizophrenia: Adults: Tab: Initial:** 25 mg bid. **Titrate:** Increase by 25-50 mg bid-tid daily on Day 2 & Day 3, up to target dose of 300-400 mg/d by Day 4. May adjust by 25-50 mg bid at intervals of ≥2 days. **Hepatic Impairment: Initial:** 25 mg/d. **Titrate:** Increase by 25-50 mg/d to effective dose. **Elderly/Debilitated/Predisposition to Hypotension:** Consider slower rate of dose titration & lower target dose. **Max:** 800 mg/d.	C v **H W** [29, 30]

NAME	FORM/STRENGTH	DOSAGE	COMMENTS
PARTIAL D2/5HT1A AGONIST/5HT2A ANTAGONIST			
Aripiprazole (Abilify, Abilify Discmelt)	**Sol:** 1 mg/ml; **Tab:** 2 mg, 5 mg, 10 mg, 15 mg, 20 mg, 30 mg; **Tab,Dissolve:** (Discmelt) 10 mg, 15 mg; **Inj:** 7.5 mg/ml	**(PO) Schizophrenia: Adults: Initial/Target:** 10-15 mg qd. **Titrate:** Should not increase before 2 wks. **Maint:** Periodically reassess. **Max:** 30 mg/d. **Peds: 13-17 yo: Initial:** 2 mg/d. **Titrate:** 5 mg after 2d. May adjust dose in 5 mg/d increments. **Recommended:** 10 mg/d. **Max:** 30 mg/d. Oral sol can be given on a mg-per-mg basis up to 25 mg. Patients receiving 30 mg tabs should receive 25 mg of sol. **(Inj) Agitation Associated w/ Schizophrenia: Adults:** 9.75 mg IM; **Range:** 5.25-15 mg IM. **Max:** 30 mg/d; Initiate PO therapy ASAP. Adjust dose w/ CYP3A4 inducers/strong inhibitors or CYP2D6 inhibitors.	C v **W** [29, 30]
PHENOTHIAZINES			
Chlorpromazine	**Cap, ER:** 30 mg, 75 mg, 150 mg; **Inj:** 25 mg/ml; **Sup:** 25 mg, 100 mg; **Syr:** 10 mg/5 ml; **Tab:** 10 mg, 25 mg, 50 mg, 100 mg, 200 mg	**Adults: Inpatient: Acute State:** 25 mg IM, then 25-50 mg IM in 1h if needed. **Titrate:** Increase up to 400 mg q4-6h until controlled then switch to PO. **Max:** 1 gm/d PO. **Outpatient:** 10 mg PO tid-qid or 25 mg PO bid-tid. **Titrate:** After 1-2d, increase by 20-50 mg BIW.	N v

Fluphenazine	(HCl) **Cnt:** 5 mg/ml; **Inj:** 2.5 mg/ml; **Eli:** 2.5 mg/5 ml; **Tab:** 1 mg, 2.5 mg, 5 mg, 10 mg; (Decanoate) **Inj:** 25 mg/ml	**Adults: PO: Initial:** 2.5-10 mg/d given q6-8h. **Titrate:** Increase up to 40 mg/d. **Maint:** 1-5 mg qd. **Inj, HCl: Initial:** 1.25 mg IM q6-8h. **Max:** 10 mg/d. **Decanoate: Initial:** 12.5-25 mg IM/SC q4-6wks. **Max:** 100 mg/dose.	◙N ❁>
Perphenazine	**Tab:** 2 mg, 4 mg, 8 mg, 16 mg	**Adults: Outpatients: Initial:** 4-8 mg tid. **Maint:** Reduce to min effective dose. **Inpatients:** 8-16 mg bid-qid. **Max:** 64 mg/d. **Peds: ≥12 yo:** Use lower limits of adult dose.	◙N ❁>
Thioridazine	**Tab:** 10 mg, 15 mg, 25 mg, 50 mg, 100 mg, 150 mg, 200 mg	**Adults: Initial:** 50-100 mg tid. **Maint:** 200-800 mg/d given bid-qid. **Max:** 800 mg/d. **Peds: Initial:** 0.6 mg/kg/d in divided doses. **Max:** 3 mg/kg/d.	◙N ❁> QTc prolongation.
Trifluoperazine	**Tab:** 1 mg, 2 mg, 5 mg, 10 mg	**Psychotic Disorders: Adults: Initial:** 2-5 mg bid. **Usual:** 15-20 mg/d. **Max:** 40 mg/d or more if needed. **Peds: 6-12 yo: Initial:** 1 mg qd-bid. Increase gradually until symptoms controlled. **Usual:** 15 mg/d. **Non-Psychotic Anxiety: Adults:** 1-2 mg bid. **Max:** 6 mg/d or >12 wks.	◙N ❁v

THIOXANTHENE DERIVATIVES

Thiothixene (Navane)	**Cap:** 2 mg, 5 mg, 10 mg, 20 mg	**Adults & Peds: ≥12 yo: Mild Condition: Initial:** 2 mg tid. **Titrate:** May increase to 15 mg/d. **Severe Condition: Initial:** 5 mg bid. **Usual:** 20-30 mg/d. **Max:** 60 mg/d.	◙N ❁v **W** 30

Bipolar Agents

NAME	FORM/STRENGTH	DOSAGE	COMMENTS
Aripiprazole (Abilify, Abilify Discmelt)	**Sol:** 1 mg/ml; **Tab:** 2 mg, 5 mg, 10 mg, 15 mg, 20 mg, 30 mg; **Tab, Dissolve:** (Discmelt) 10 mg, 15 mg; **Inj:** 7.5 mg/ml	**(PO) Bipolar I Disorder: Acute Manic & Mixed Episodes: Adults: Initial:** 15 mg qd. **Titrate:** May increase to 30 mg/d based on response. **Max:** 30 mg/d. **Peds: 10-17 yo: Initial:** 2 mg/d. **Titrate:** May increase to 5 mg/d after 2 days, then to target of 10 mg/d after 2 additional days. May increase by 5 mg/d thereafter. **Max:** 30 mg/d. Oral sol can be given on mg-per-mg basis up to 25 mg. Patients receiving 30 mg tabs should receive 25 mg of sol. **(Inj) Agitation Associated w/ Manic or Mixed Episodes: Adults:** 9.75 mg IM; **Range:** 5.25-15 mg IM; **Max:** 30 mg/d; Initiate PO therapy ASAP. Adjust dose w/ CYP3A4 inducers/inhibitors or CYP2D6 inhibitors.	C v **W** [29, 30]
Carbamazepine (Equetro)	**Cap, ER:** 100 mg, 200 mg, 300 mg	**Bipolar I Disorder: Acute Manic & Mixed Episodes: Adults: Initial:** 400 mg/d, given in divided doses, bid. **Titrate:** 200 mg/d. **Max:** 1600 mg/d.	D v **W** [87]
Divalproex Sodium (Depakote ER)	**Tab, ER:** 250 mg, 500 mg	**Bipolar Disorder: Manic Episodes: Adults: Initial:** 25 mg/kg/d. **Titrate:** May increase rapidly to clinical effect. **Max:** 60 mg/kg/d.	D v Hepatotoxic. Teratogenic. Pancreatitis.
Divalproex Sodium (Depakote)	**Tab, Delay:** 125 mg, 250 mg, 500 mg	**Bipolar Disorder: Manic Episodes: Adults: Initial:** 750 mg qd in divided doses. **Titrate:** May increase rapidly to clinical effect. **Max:** 60 mg/kg/d.	D v Hepatotoxic. Teratogenic. Pancreatitis.

Lamotrigine (Lamictal, Lamictal CD, Lamictal ODT)	**Chewtab:** (CD) 2 mg, 5 mg, 25 mg; **Tab:** 25 mg, 100 mg, 150 mg, 200 mg; **Tab, Dissolve:** (ODT) 25 mg, 50 mg, 100 mg, 200 mg	**Bipolar I Disorder: Maintenance: Adults: Patients Not Taking Carbamazepine (CBZ), Other Enzyme-Inducing Drugs (EIDs) or VPA: Wks 1 & 2:** 25 mg/d. **Wks 3 & 4:** 50 mg/d. **Wk 5:** 100 mg/d. **Wks 6 & 7:** 200 mg/d. **Patients taking VPA: Wks 1 & 2:** 25 mg qod. **Wks 3 & 4:** 25 mg/d. **Wk 5:** 50 mg/d. **Wks 6 & 7:** 100 mg/d. **Patients Taking CBZ (or other EIDs) & Not Taking VPA: Wks 1 & 2:** 50 mg/d. **Wks 3 & 4:** 100 mg/d (divided doses). **Wk 5:** 200 mg/d (divided doses). **Wk 6:** 300 mg/d (divided doses). **Wk 7:** Up to 400 mg/d (divided doses). **After D/C of Psychotropic Dugs Excluding VPA, CBZ, or Other EIDs:** Maintain current dose. **After D/C of VPA & Current Lamotrigine Dose of 100 mg/d: Wk 1:** 150 mg/d. **Wk 2 & Onward:** 200 mg/d. **After D/C of CBZ or Other EIDs & Current Lamotrigine Dose of 400 mg/d: Wk 1:** 400 mg/d. **Wk 2:** 300 mg/d. **Wk 3 & Onward:** 200 mg/d.	◉C ❊v Serious rashes, Stevens-Johnson syndrome reported. **H R**
Lithium Carbonate	**Cap:** 150 mg, 300 mg, 600 mg; **Tab:** 300 mg	**Adults & Peds: ≥12 yo: Acute Mania:** 600 mg tid. Effective serum levels are 1-1.5 mEq/L; monitor levels twice wkly until stabilized. **Maint:** 300 mg tid-qid to maintain serum levels of 0.6-1.2 mEq/L; monitor levels q2mths.	◉D ❊v Lithium toxicity related to serum levels.
Lithium Carbonate (Lithobid)	**Tab, ER:** 300 mg	**Adults & Peds: ≥12 yo: Acute Mania: Initial:** 900 mg bid or 600 mg tid to achieve effective serum levels of 1-1.5 mEq/L; monitor levels twice wkly until stabilized. Maint: 900-1200 mg/d, given bid-tid to maintain serum levels of 0.6-1.2 mEq/L; monitor levels q2mths.	◉D ❊v Lithium toxicity related to serum levels.

NAME	FORM/STRENGTH	DOSAGE	COMMENTS
Olanzapine (Zyprexa, Zyprexa Zydis, Zyprexa IntraMuscular)	**Inj:** 10 mg; **Tab:** 2.5 mg, 5 mg, 7.5 mg, 10 mg, 15 mg, 20 mg; **Tab, Dissolve:** (Zydis) 5 mg, 10 mg, 15 mg, 20 mg	**Bipolar I Disorder: Acute Manic & Mixed Episodes: Adults: Monotherapy: PO: Initial:** 10-15 mg qd. **Combination Therapy w/ Lithium or Valproate: Initial:** 10 mg qd. **Range:** 5-20 mg/d. **Max:** 20 mg/d. **Titrate:** Adjust by 5 mg/d. **Max:** 20 mg/d. **Maintenance Monotherapy:** 5-20 mg/d. **Agitation Associated w/ Bipolar Mania: Inj: Initial:** 10 mg IM. **Range:** 2.5-10 mg IM. **Max:** 3 doses of 10 mg IM q2-4h. May initiate PO therapy when clinically appropriate.	C v **W** [30]
Quetiapine Fumarate (Seroquel XR)	**Tab,ER:** 50 mg, 150 mg, 200 mg, 300 mg, 400 mg	**Adults: Bipolar Depressive Episodes:** Give qd in evening. **Day 1:** 50 mg/d. **Day 2:** 100 mg/d. **Day 3:** 200 mg/d. **Day 4:** 300 mg/d. **Bipolar Mania: Monotherapy/Adjunct:** Give qd in evening. **Day 1:** 300 mg. **Day 2:** 600 mg. **Titrate:** May adjust dose between 400-800 mg beginning on Day 3 depending on response and tolerance. **Maint of Bipolar I Disorder:** 400-800 mg/d given bid. Re-evaluate periodically. **Elderly/Hepatic Impairment: Initial:** 50 mg/d; may increase in increments of 50 mg/d depending on response and tolerance. **Reinitiation of Treatment: If off >1 wk:** Follow initial dosing schedule. **If <1 wk:** No dose escalation required, reinitiate maint dose. **Switching from Seroquel:** May switch to Serquel XR at equivalent total daily dose given qd. Swallow whole.	C v **H W** [29, 30]

Quetiapine Fumarate (Seroquel)	**Tab:** 25 mg, 50 mg, 100 mg, 200 mg, 300 mg, 400 mg	**Adults: Bipolar I Disorder: Acute Manic Episodes: Monotherapy or Adjunct Therapy w/ Lithium or Divalproex: Initial:** 100 mg/d given bid on Day 1. **Titrate:** Increase to 400 mg/d given bid on Day 4 in increments of up to 100 mg/d given in bid divided doses. Adjust doses up to 800 mg/d by Day 6 in increments ≤200 mg/d. **Max:** 800 mg/d. **Bipolar I Disorder Maint:** 400-800 mg/d given bid. **Bipolar Depressive Episodes:** Give once daily hs. **Day 1:** 50 mg/d. **Day 2:** 100 mg/d. **Day 3:** 200 mg/d. **Day 4:** 300 mg/d. **Hepatic Impairment: Initial:** 25 mg/d. **Titrate:** Increase by 25-50 mg/d to effective dose. **Elderly/ Debilitated/Predisposition to Hypotension:** Consider slower rate of dose titration & lower target dose.	C v **H W** [29, 30]
Risperidone (Risperdal, Risperdal M-Tab)	**Sol:** 1 mg/ml; **Tab:** 0.25 mg, 0.5 mg, 1 mg, 2 mg, 3 mg, 4 mg; **Tab,Dissolve:** 0.5 mg, 1 mg, 2 mg, 3 mg, 4 mg	**Bipolar I Disorder: Acute Manic & Mixed Episodes: Adults: Monotherapy or Adjunct Therapy w/ Lithium or Valproate: Initial:** 2-3 mg qd. **Titrate:** Increase by 1 mg qd. **Max:** 6 mg/d. **Peds: 10-17 yo: Monotherapy: Initial:** 0.5 mg qd in morning or evening. **Titrate:** Adjust dose, if needed, in increments of 0.5 or 1 mg/d & at intervals not <24h as tolerated to recommended dose of 2.5 mg/d. **Max:** 6 mg/d.	C v **H R W** [30]

NAME	FORM/STRENGTH	DOSAGE	COMMENTS
Valproic Acid (Stavzor)	**Cap,DR:** 125 mg, 250 mg, 500 mg	**Manic Episodes w/Bipolar Disorder: Adults: Initial:** 750 mg qd in divided doses. **Titrate:** Increase rapidly to produce desired clinical effect or plasma level (50-125 mcg/ml). **Max:** 60 mg/kg/d. **Elderly:** Reduce starting dose & increase slowly; monitor fluid, nutritional intake, and somnolence. Swallow whole.	D v **W** 101
Ziprasidone (Geodon)	**Cap:** 20 mg, 40 mg, 60 mg, 80 mg	**Bipolar Disorder: Acute Manic & Mixed Episodes: Adults: Initial:** 40 mg bid w/ food. **Titrate:** Increase to 60-80 mg bid on 2nd day of treatment. **Maint:** 40-80 mg bid.	C v **W** 30

Migraine Therapy

5-HT$_1$ AGONISTS & COMBINATIONS

NAME	FORM/STRENGTH	DOSAGE	COMMENTS
Almotriptan Malate (Axert)	**Tab:** 6.25 mg, 12.5 mg	**Acute Therapy: Adults & Peds: 12-17 yo: Initial:** 6.25 mg or 12.5 mg; may repeat after 2h. **Max:** 2 doses/24h.	C > **H R**
Eletriptan HBr (Relpax)	**Tab:** 20 mg, 40 mg	**Acute Therapy: Adults: ≥18 yo: Initial:** 20 mg or 40 mg; may repeat after 2h. **Max:** 40 mg/dose or 80 mg/d.	C > **H**
Frovatriptan Succinate (Frova)	**Tab:** 2.5 mg	**Acute Therapy: Adults: ≥18 yo: Initial:** 2.5 mg; may repeat after 2h. **Max:** 7.5 mg/d.	C >
Naproxen Sodium/ Sumatriptan Succinate (Treximet)	**Tab:** 500/85 mg	**Adults: Initial:** 1 tab; may repeat after 2h. **Max:** 2 tabs/24h. Do not split, crush, or chew.	C v CI w/ hepatic impairment. **H R W** 100

Naratriptan HCl (Amerge)	**Tab:** 1 mg, 2.5 mg	**Acute Therapy: Adults: ≥18 yo: Initial:** 1 mg or 2.5 mg; may repeat once after 4h. **Max:** 5 mg/24h.	C > **H R**
Rizatriptan Benzoate (Maxalt, Maxalt-MLT)	**Tab:** 5 mg, 10 mg; **Tab, Dissolve (ODT):** (MLT) 5 mg, 10 mg	**Acute Therapy: Adults: ≥18 yo: Initial:** 5 or 10 mg; may repeat q2h. **Max:** 30 mg/24h. Place ODT on tongue.	C > Adjust dose w/ propranolol.
Sumatriptan Succinate (Imitrex)	**Inj:** 6 mg/0.5 ml; **Nasal Spr:** 5 mg/spr, 20 mg/spr; **Tab:** 25 mg, 50 mg, 100 mg	**Acute Therapy: Adults: ≥18 yo: Initial: Inj:** 6 mg SC; may repeat in 1h. **Tab:** 25-100 mg PO; may repeat in 2h. **Nasal Spr:** 5 mg, 10 mg, or 20 mg; may repeat in 2h. **Max:** 12 mg/24h SC; 200 mg/24h PO; 40 mg/24h nasal spr.	C > **H** (Tab)
Zolmitriptan (Zomig, Zomig Nasal Spray, Zomig-ZMT)	**Tab:** 2.5 mg, 5 mg; **Tab, Dissolve (ODT):** 2.5 mg, 5 mg; **Nasal Spr:** 5 mg/spr	**Acute Therapy: Adults: ≥18 yo: Initial: PO:** 2.5 mg or lower; may repeat after 2h. **Max:** 10 mg/24h. **Nasal Spr:** 1 spr; may repeat after 2h. **Max:** 2 spr/24h. Place ODT on tongue.	C >**H**

MISCELLANEOUS

Divalproex Sodium (Depakote ER)	**Tab, ER:** 250 mg, 500 mg	**Prophylaxis: Adults: Initial:** 500 mg qd x 1 wk. **Titrate:** May increase to 1000 mg/d.	D v Hepatotoxic. Teratogenic. Pancreatitis.
Divalproex Sodium (Depakote)	**Tab, Delay:** 125 mg, 250 mg, 500 mg	**Prophylaxis: Adults: ≥16 yo: Initial:** 250 mg bid. **Max:** 1000 mg/d.	D v Hepatotoxic. Teratogenic. Pancreatitis.

NAME	FORM/STRENGTH	DOSAGE	COMMENTS
Topiramate (Topamax, Topamax Sprinkle Capsules)	**Cap:** 15 mg, 25 mg; **Tab:** 25 mg, 50 mg, 100 mg, 200 mg	**Prophylaxis: Titrate: Adults: Wk 1:** 25 mg qpm. **Wk 2:** 25 mg bid. **Wk 3:** 25 mg qam & 50 mg qpm. **Wk 4:** 50 mg bid. **Usual:** 50 mg bid.	C > **R**
Valproic Acid (Stavzor)	**Cap,DR:** 125 mg, 250 mg, 500 mg	**Prophylaxis: Adults: Initial:** 250 mg bid. **Max:** 1000 mg/d. **Elderly:** Reduce starting dose & increase slowly; monitor fluid, nutritional intake, and somnolence. Swallow whole.	D v **W** [101]

Muscle Relaxants

NAME	FORM/STRENGTH	DOSAGE	COMMENTS
Baclofen (Kemstro)	**Tab:** (Generic) 10 mg, 20 mg; **Tab (ODT):** (Kemstro) 10 mg, 20 mg	**Adults & Peds: ≥12 yo: Initial:** 5 mg tid x 3d. **Titrate:** Increase q3d by 5 mg tid. **Usual:** 40-80 mg/d. **Max:** 80 mg/d (20 mg qid).	C > **R**
Carisoprodol (Soma)	**Tab:** 250 mg, 350 mg	**Adults/Peds: 16-65 yo:** 250-350 mg tid & hs.	C >
Cyclobenzaprine (Amrix)	**Cap, ER:** 15 mg, 30 mg	**Adults: Usual:** 15 mg qd. Titrate: May increase to 30 mg qd if needed. Use for longer than 2-3 wks not recommended.	B > **H**
Cyclobenzaprine (Flexeril)	**Tab:** 5 mg, 10 mg	**Adults & Peds: ≥15 yo: Usual:** 5 mg tid. **Titrate:** May increase to 10 mg tid. Do not exceed 2-3 wks of therapy.	B > **H**
Metaxalone (Skelaxin)	**Tab:** 800 mg	**Adults & Peds: >12 yo:** 800 mg tid-qid.	N v
Methocarbamol (Robaxin, Robaxin Injection, Robaxin-750)	**Inj:** 100 mg/ml; **Tab:** 500 mg, 750 mg	**Adults: Tab: Initial:** (500 mg tab) 1.5 gm qid x 2-3d. **Maint:** 1 gm qid. **Initial:** (750 mg tab) 1.5 gm qid x 2-3d. **Maint:** 750 mg q4h or 1.5 gm tid. **Max:** 6 gm/d x 2-3d; 8 gm/d if severe. **IM/IV: Moderate Symptoms:** 1 gm.	C v

Tizanidine HCl (Zanaflex)	**Cap:** 2 mg, 4 mg, 6 mg; **Tab:** 2 mg, 4 mg	**Adults: Initial:** 4 mg q6-8h. **Titrate:** Increase by 2-4 mg. **Usual:** 8 mg q6-8h. **Max:** 3 doses/24h or 36 mg/d.	C >

Obsessive-Compulsive Disorder

SSRIS & COMBINATIONS

Fluoxetine (Prozac)	**Cap:** 10 mg, 20 mg, 40 mg; **Sol:** 20 mg/5 ml; **Tab:** 10 mg	**Adults: Initial:** 20 mg qam. **Maint:** 20-60 mg/d given qd or bid, am & noon. **Max:** 80 mg/d. **Peds: ≥7 yo: Adolescents & Higher-Wt Peds: Initial:** 10 mg/d. **Titrate:** Increase to 20 mg/d after 2 wks. Consider additional dose increases after several more wks if clinical improvement not observed. **Usual:** 20-60 mg/d. **Lower-Wt Peds: Initial:** 10 mg/d. **Titrate:** Consider additional dose increases after several wks if clinical improvement not observed. **Usual:** 20-30 mg/d. **Max:** 60 mg/d.	C v **H W** [29]
Fluvoxamine Maleate (Luvox CR)	**Cap,ER:** 100 mg, 150 mg	**Adults: Initial:** 100 mg qhs. **Titrate:** May increase by 50 mg qwk. **Maint:** 100-300 mg/d. **Max:** 300 mg/d. **Elderly/Hepatic Impairment:** Titrate slowly following initial dose.	C v **W** [29]
Fluvoxamine	**Tab:** 25 mg, 50 mg, 100 mg	**Adults: Initial:** 50 mg qhs. **Titrate:** Increase by 50 mg q4-7d. **Maint:** 100-300 mg/d. **Max:** 300 mg/d. **8-17 yo: Initial:** 25 mg qhs. **Titrate:** Increase by 25 mg q4-7d. **Maint:** 50-200 mg/d. **Max: 8-11 yo:** 200 mg/d. **Adolescents:** 300 mg/d.	C v **H W** [29]

NAME	FORM/STRENGTH	DOSAGE	COMMENTS
Paroxetine HCl (Paxil)	**Susp:** 10 mg/5 ml; **Tab:** 10 mg, 20 mg, 30 mg, 40 mg	**Adults: Initial:** 20 mg qam. **Usual:** 40 mg/d. **Max:** 60 mg/d.	D > **H R W** [29]
Paroxetine Mesylate (Pexeva)	**Tab:** 10 mg, 20 mg, 30 mg, 40 mg	**Adults: Initial:** 40 mg/d. **Max:** 60 mg/d.	C > **H R W** [29]
Sertraline (Zoloft)	**Sol:** 20 mg/ml; **Tab:** 25 mg, 50 mg, 100 mg	**Initial: Adults & Peds: ≥13 yo:** 50 mg qd. **6-12 yo:** 25 mg qd. **Titrate:** Adjust wkly. **Max:** 200 mg/d.	C > **H W** [29]

TRICYCLIC ANTIDEPRESSANTS

NAME	FORM/STRENGTH	DOSAGE	COMMENTS
Clomipramine HCl (Anafranil)	**Cap:** 25 mg, 50 mg, 75 mg	**Adults: Initial:** 25 mg/d, increase to 100 mg/d within 1st 2 wks. **Titrate:** Increase over several wks. **Max:** 250 mg/d. May give qhs. **Peds: >10 yo: Initial:** 25 mg/d, increase to 3 mg/kg/d or 100 mg/d within 1st 2 wks. **Titrate:** Increase over several wks. **Max:** 3 mg/kg/d or 200 mg/d. May give qhs.	C v **W** [29]

Miscellaneous

NAME	FORM/STRENGTH	DOSAGE	COMMENTS
Pramipexole Dihydrochloride (Mirapex)	**Tab:** 0.125 mg, 0.25 mg, 0.5 mg, 0.75 mg, 1 mg, 1.5 mg	**Moderate-to-Severe Primary Restless Legs Syndrome: Adults: Initial:** 0.125 mg qd, 2-3 h before bedtime. **Titrate:** May double dose q4-7d up to 0.5 mg/d.	C v **R**

Risperidone (Risperdal, Risperdal M-Tab)	**Sol:** 1 mg/ml; **Tab:** 0.25 mg, 0.5 mg, 1 mg, 2 mg, 3 mg, 4 mg; **Tab,Dissolve:** 0.5 mg, 1 mg, 2 mg, 3 mg, 4 mg	**Irritability Associated w/ Autistic Disorder: Peds: 5-16 yo: (Sol,Tab) Initial: <20 kg:** 0.25 mg/d; **≥20 kg:** 0.5 mg/d. **Titrate:** After at least 4d: **<20 kg:** Increase by 0.5 mg/d; **≥20 kg:** 1 mg/d. **Maint:** For minimum of 14d. **Inadequate Response:** Increase at ≥2-wk intervals: **<20kg:** Increase by 0.25 mg/d; **≥20 kg:** Increase by 0.5 mg/d. Caution in patients <15 kg. **Max: <20 kg:** 1 mg/d; **≥20 kg:** 2.5 mg/d; **>45 kg:** 3 mg/d.	◉C ❁v **H R W** 30
Ropinirole HCl (Requip)	**Tab:** 0.25 mg, 0.5 mg, 1 mg, 2 mg, 3 mg, 4 mg, 5 mg	**Moderate-to-Severe Primary Restless Legs Syndrome: Adults: Initial:** 0.25 mg qd, 1-3h before bedtime. **Titrate:** 0.5 mg qd on Days 3-7, then 1 mg qd during Wk 2, then increase by 0.5 mg wkly. **Max:** 4 mg/d.	◉C ❁v
Sodium Oxybate CIII (Xyrem)	**Sol:** 500 mg/ml	**Excessive Daytime Sleepiness/Cataplexy Associated w/ Narcolepsy: Adults & Peds: ≥13 yo: Initial:** 2.25 gm qhs, then 2.25 gm 2.5-4 h later. **Titrate:** Increase by 0.75 gm/dose q1-2wks. **Range:** 6-9 gm/night. **Max:** 9 gm/night. Take 1st dose at bedtime while in bed & 2nd dose while sitting in bed. Dilute each dose w/ 2 oz water.	◉B ❁> **H W** 54

PULMONARY/RESPIRATORY

Asthma/COPD Preparations

NAME	FORM/STRENGTH	DOSAGE	COMMENTS
ANTICHOLINERGICS			
Ipratropium Bromide (Atrovent HFA)	**MDI:** 0.017 mg/inh	**COPD: Adults: Initial:** 2 inh qid. **Max:** 12 inh/24h.	B >
Tiotropium Bromide (Spiriva)	**Cap,Inh:** 18 mcg	**COPD: Adults:** Inhale contents of 1 cap qd w/ HandiHaler device.	C >
BRONCHODILATOR (BETA AGONISTS/ANTICHOLINERGICS)			
Albuterol Sulfate/ Ipratropium Bromide (Combivent)	**MDI:** 0.09-0.018 mg/inh	**COPD: Adults:** 2 inh qid. **Max:** 12 inh/24h.	C v
BRONCHODILATOR COMBINATIONS			
Albuterol Sulfate/ Ipratropium Bromide (Duoneb)	**Sol,Neb:** 3-0.5 mg/3 ml	**Adults:** 3 ml qid via nebulizer. May give 2 additional doses/d if needed.	C (albuterol) B (ipratropium) v
Fluticasone Propionate/ Salmeterol Xinafoate (Advair HFA)	**MDI:** (45/21) 0.045 mg-0.021 mg/inh, (115/21) 0.115 mg-0.021 mg/inh, (230/21) 0.230 mg-0.021 mg/inh	**Asthma: Adults & Peds: ≥12 yo:** 2 inh q12h. **Without Prior Inhaled Corticosteroid (CS): Initial:** 2 inh of 45/21 bid or 1 inh of 115/21 bid. **Max:** 2 inh of 230-21 bid. **Current Inhaled CS: Beclomethasone:** ≤160 mcg/d, use 2 inh of 45/21 bid; 320 mcg/d, use 2 inh of 115/21 bid; 640 mcg/d,	C > Asthma-related deaths reported.

		use 2 inh of 230/21 bid. **Budesonide:** ≤400 mcg/d, use 2 inh of 45/21 bid; 800-1200 mcg/d, use 2 inh of 115/21 bid; 1600 mcg/d, use 2 inh of 230/21 bid. **Flunisolide:** ≤1000 mcg/d, use 2 inh of 45/21 bid; 1250-2000 mcg/d, use 2 inh of 115/21 bid. **Flunisolide HFA:** ≤320 mcg/d, use 2 inh of 45/21 bid; 640 mcg/d, use 2 inh of 115/21 bid. **Fluticasone Aerosol:** ≤176 mcg/d, use 2 inh of 45/21 bid; 440 mcg/d, use 2 inh of 115/21 bid; 660-880 mcg/d, use 2 inh of 230/21 bid. **Fluticasone Pow:** ≤200 mcg/d, use 2 inh of 45/21 bid; 500 mcg/d, use 2 inh of 115/21 bid; 1000 mcg/d, use 2 inh of 230/21 bid. **Mometasone Pow:** 220 mcg/d, use 2 inh of 45/21 bid; 440 mcg/d, use 2 inh of 115/21 bid; 880 mcg/d, use 2 inh of 230/21 bid. **Triamcinolone:** ≤1000 mcg/d, use 2 inh of 45/21 bid; 1100-1600 mcg/d, use 2 inh of 115/21 bid. If no response within 2 wks, increase to higher strength.	
Fluticasone Propionate/ Salmeterol Xinafoate (Advair)	**MDI:** (Diskus) 100-50 mcg/inh, 250-50 mcg/inh, 500-50 mcg/inh	**Asthma: Adults & Peds: ≥12 yo:** 1 inh q12h. **Without Prior Inhaled Corticosteroid (CS) Therapy/Inadequate Control on Current Inhaled CS: Initial:** 100/50 or 250/50 bid. **Max:** 500/50 bid. If no response within 2 wks, may increase to higher strength. **Symptomatic on Inhaled CS: 4-11 yo:** (100/50 only) 1 inh q12h. **COPD: Adults:** (250/50 only) 1 inh q12h. Rinse mouth after use.	◙C ❊> Asthma-related deaths reported.

NAME	FORM/STRENGTH	DOSAGE	COMMENTS
Formoterol Fumarate dihydrate/Budesonide (Symbicort)	**MDI:** (Budesonide-Formoterol) 80/4.5 mcg/inh, 160/4.5 mcg/inh	**Asthma: Adults & Peds: ≥12 yo: Initial:** Individualize dose. 2 inh bid of 80/4.5 or 160/4.5. **Maint:** 2 inh bid of 80/4.5 or 160/4.5. **No Current Inhaled Corticosteroid:** 2 inh bid of 80/4.5 or 160/4.5 depending on asthma severity. **Max:** 160/4.5 bid. Patients not responding to starting dose after 1-2 wks of therapy w/ 80/4.5, may replace w/ 160/4.5 for better asthma control. **COPD: Adults:** 2 inh bid of 160/4.5. If asthma or shortness of breath occurs in period between doses, use short-acting $beta_2$-agonist for immediate relief. Rinse mouth after use.	C > Asthma-related deaths reported.

BRONCHODILATORS (BETA AGONISTS)

NAME	FORM/STRENGTH	DOSAGE	COMMENTS
Albuterol Sulfate (AccuNeb)	**Sol, Neb:** 0.63 mg/3 ml, 1.25 mg/3 ml	**Bronchospasm/Asthma: Peds: 6-12 yo w/ Severe Asthma or >40 kg or 11-12 yo: Initial:** 1.25 mg tid-qid. **2-12 yo:** 0.63 mg or 1.25 mg tid-qid via nebulizer.	C v
Albuterol Sulfate (ProAir HFA)	**MDI:** 0.09 mg/inh	**Adults & Peds: ≥4 yo:** 2 inh q4-6h or 1 inh q4h. **Exercise-Induced Bronchospasm:** 2 inh 15 min before activity.	C v
Albuterol Sulfate (Proventil HFA)	**MDI:** 0.09 mg/inh	**Adults & Peds: ≥4 yo: Bronchospasm:** 2 inh q4-6h or 1 inh q4h. **Exercise-Induced Bronchospasm:** 2 inh 15-30 min before exercise.	C v
Albuterol Sulfate (Ventolin HFA)	**MDI:** 0.09 mg/inh	**Adults & Peds: ≥4 yo: Bronchospasm:** 2 inh q4-6h or 1 inh q4h. **Exercise-Induced Bronchospasm:** 2 inh 15-30 min before exercise.	C v

Albuterol Sulfate (VoSpire ER)	**Tab,ER:** 4 mg, 8 mg	**Bronchospasm: Adults/Peds: >12 yo: Usual:** 4-8 mg q12h. **Low Body Weight: Initial:** 4 mg q12h. **Titrate:** May increase to 8 mg q12h. **Max:** 32 mg/d in divided doses. **6-12 yo: Usual:** 4 mg q12h. **Max:** 24 mg/d in divided doses. Swallow whole w/ liquids.	C v
Formoterol Fumarate (Foradil)	**MDI:** 12 mcg/inh	**Adults & Peds: ≥5 yo: Asthma/COPD:** 12 mcg q12h. **Max:** 24 mcg/d. **Exercise-Induced Bronchospasm:** 12 mcg 15 min prior to exercise. Do not give added dose if on q12h schedule. Give only by inhalation w/ Aerolizer inhaler.	C > Asthma-related deaths reported.
Levalbuterol HCl (Xopenex HFA)	**HFA MDI:** 45 mcg/inh	**Adults & Peds: ≥4 yo: Bronchospasm:** 2 inh (90 mcg) q4-6h or 1 inh (45 mcg) q4h may be sufficient.	C v
Levalbuterol HCl (Xopenex)	**Sol,Neb:** 0.31 mg/3 ml, 0.63 mg/3 ml, 1.25 mg/3 ml	**Adults & Peds: ≥12 yo: Bronchospasm: Initial:** 0.63 mg tid q6-8h. **Severe Asthma:** 1.25 mg tid q6-8h. **6-11 yo:** 0.31 mg tid. **Max:** 0.63 mg tid. Administer via neb.	C v
Metaproterenol Sulfate (Alupent)	(Alupent) **MDI:** 0.65 mg/inh; (Generic) **Sol,Neb:** 0.4%, 0.6%; **Syr:** 10 mg/5 ml; **Tab:** 10 mg, 20 mg	**Bronchospasm: Adults & Peds: ≥12 yo: MDI:** 2-3 inh q3-4h. **Max:** 12 inh/d. **Sol,Neb 0.4%, 0.6%:** 2.5 ml by IPPB tid-qid, up to q4h prn. **Syr/Tab: >9 yo or >60 lbs:** 20 mg tid-qid. **6-9 yo or <60 lbs:** 10 mg tid-qid.	C >
Pirbuterol Acetate (Maxair, Maxair Autohaler)	**Autohaler:** 0.2 mg/inh **MDI:** 0.2 mg/inh	**Adults & Peds: ≥12 yo:** 1-2 inh q4-6h. **Max:** 12 inh/d.	C >

NAME	FORM/STRENGTH	DOSAGE	COMMENTS
Salmeterol Xinafoate (Serevent)	**Diskus:** 50 mcg	**Adults & Peds: ≥4 yo: Asthma/COPD:** 1 inh q12h. **Exercise-Induced Bronchospasm Prevention:** 1 inh 30 min before exercise (do not give preventive doses if already on bid dose).	C v Asthma-related deaths reported.
INHALED CORTICOSTEROIDS			
Beclomethasone Dipropionate (Qvar)	**MDI:** 40 mcg/inh, 80 mcg/inh	**Adults & Adolescents: Previous Bronchodilator Only:** 40-80 mcg bid. **Max:** 320 mcg bid. **Previous Inhaled Corticosteroid Therapy:** 40-160 mcg bid. **Max:** 320 mcg bid. **5-11 yo: Previous Bronchodilator Only or Inhaled Corticosteroid:** 40 mcg bid. **Max:** 80 mcg bid. **Adults & Peds: ≥5 yo: Maint w/ Oral Corticosteroids:** May attempt gradual reduction of oral dose after 1 wk on inhaled therapy.	C v
Budesonide (Pulmicort Flexhaler, Pulmicort Respules)	**Sus,Inh:** (Respules) 0.25 mg/2 ml; 0.5 mg/2 ml; **Pow,Inh:** (Flexhaler) 90 mcg/dose, 180 mcg/dose	**Adults & Peds: ≥6 yo: Flexhaler:** Individualize dose. **Initial:** 180-360 mcg bid. **Max:** 720 mcg (adults) or 360 mcg (peds) bid. **Respules: 1-8 yo: Previous Bronchodilator Only: Initial:** 0.5 mg qd or 0.25 mg bid. Administer via jet neb. **Max:** 0.5 mg/d. **Previous Inhaled Corticosteroid:** 0.5 mg qd or 0.25 mg bid. **Max:** 1 mg/d. **Previous Oral Corticosteroid:** 1 mg qd or 0.5 mg bid. **Max:** 1 mg/d. Gradually reduce PO corticosteroid after 1 wk of budesonide.	B > (Respules) B v (Flexhaler)

Ciclesonide (Alvesco)	**MDI:** 80 mcg/inh, 160 mcg/inh	**Adults: Previous Bronchodilator Only: Initial:** 80 mcg bid. **Max:** 160 mcg bid. **Previous Inhaled Corticosteroids: Initial:** 80 mcg bid. **Max:** 320 mcg bid. **Previous Oral Corticosteroids: Initial:** 320 mcg bid. **Max:** 320 mcg bid.	C ❋>
Flunisolide (Aerobid, Aerobid-M)	**MDI:** 0.25 mg/inh	**Adults & Peds: ≥6 yo: Initial:** 2 inh bid. **Max: Adults:** 4 inh bid.	C ❋>
Fluticasone Propionate (Flovent HFA)	**MDI:** 44 mcg/inh, 110 mcg/inh, 220 mcg/inh	**Adults & Peds: ≥12 yo: Previous Bronchodilator Only: Initial:** 88 mcg bid. **Max:** 440 mcg bid. **Previous Inhaled Corticosteroids: Initial:** 88-220 mcg bid. **Max:** 440 mcg bid. **Previous Oral Corticosteroids: Initial:** 440 mcg bid. **Max:** 880 mcg bid. **4-11 yo: Initial/Max:** 88 mcg bid. Reduce PO prednisone no faster than 2.5 mg/d wkly; begin at least 1 wk after start fluticasone.	C ❋>
Mometasone Furoate (Asmanex)	**MDI:** 110 mcg/inh, 220 mcg/inh	**Adults & Peds: ≥12 yo: Previous Therapy w/ Bronchodilators Alone or Inhaled Corticosteroids (CS): Initial:** 220 mcg qpm. **Max:** 440 mcg qpm or 220 mcg bid. **Previous Therapy w/ Oral CS: Initial:** 440 mcg bid. **Max:** 880 mcg/d. **Peds: 4-11 yo:** 110 mcg qpm regardless of prior therapy. Titrate to lowest effective dose once asthma stability achieved.	C ❋>
Triamcinolone Acetonide (Azmacort)	**MDI:** 100 mcg/inh	**Adults & Peds: >12 yo:** 2 inh tid-qid or 4 inh bid. **Severe Asthma: Initial:** 12-16 inh/d. **Max:** 16 inh/d. **6-12 yo:** 1-2 inh tid-qid or 2-4 inh bid. **Max:** 12 inh/d.	C ❋>

NAME	FORM/STRENGTH	DOSAGE	COMMENTS
LEUKOTRIENE MODIFIERS			
Montelukast Sodium (Singulair)	**Chewtab:** 4 mg, 5 mg; **Granules:** 4 mg/pkt; **Tab:** 10 mg	**Asthma: Adults & Peds: ≥15 yo:** 10 mg qpm. **6-14 yo:** 5 mg qpm. **2-5 yo: Chewtab/Granules:** 4 mg qpm. **12-23 mths: Granules:** 4 mg qpm. **Exercise-Induced Bronchoconstriction: Adults & Peds: ≥15 yo:** 10 mg 2 hrs before exercise. Do not take additional dose within 24 hrs of previous dose.	B >
Zafirlukast (Accolate)	**Tab:** 10 mg, 20 mg	**Asthma: Adults & Peds: ≥12 yo:** 20 mg bid. **5-11 yo:** 10 mg bid. Administer 1h ac or 2h pc.	B v
MAST CELL STABILIZERS			
Cromolyn Sodium (Intal)	(Generic) **MDI:** 0.8 mg/inh; **Sol,Neb:** 10 mg/ml; (Intal) **MDI:** 0.8 mg/inh	**Asthma: MDI: Adults & Peds: ≥5 yo: Usual/Max:** 2 inh qid. **Sol: ≥2 yo:** 20 mg qid via neb. **Acute Bronchospasm Prevention: MDI: ≥5 yo: Usual:** 2 inh 10-60 min before precipitant exposure. **Sol: ≥2 yo:** 20 mg via neb shortly before precipitant exposure.	B > **H R**
XANTHINE DERIVATIVES			
Theophylline (Theo-24)	**Cap,ER:** 100 mg, 200 mg, 300 mg, 400 mg	**Adults & Peds: ≥12 yo & >45 kg: Initial:** 300-400 mg/d. **Titrate:** Increase to 400-600 mg/d after 3d if tolerated, then to >600 mg/d if needed & tolerated after 3 more days. **Elderly/CHF: Max:** 400 mg/d. **Fast Metabolizers:** May give in divided doses q12h. **≥12 yo & <45 kg: Initial:**	C > **H R**

12-14 mg/kg/d (Max: 300 mg/d). After 3d, may increase to 16 mg/kg/d (Max: 400 mg/d). After 3 more days, may increase to 20 mg/kg/d (Max: 600 mg/d) if tolerated & needed.

Miscellaneous

BRONCHODILATORS (ALPHA/BETA AGONISTS)

Epinephrine (EpiPen, EpiPen Jr.)	**Inj:** (EpiPen) 1 mg/ml (1:1000), (EpiPen Jr) 0.5 mg/ml (1:2000)	**Allergic Reactions/Anaphylaxis:** Inject IM into thigh. **Adults:** 0.3 mg. **Peds:** 0.15 mg or 0.3 mg (0.01 mg/kg). May repeat if severe.	C >
Epinephrine (Twinject)	**Inj:** 1 mg/ml (1:1000)	**Allergic Reactions/Anaphylaxis: Adults/Peds:** Inject IM or SC into thigh. **15-30 kg:** (Twinject 0.15 mg) 0.15 mg. **≥30 kg:** (Twinject 0.3 mg) 0.3 mg. May repeat if needed.	C >

MUCOLYTIC

Acetylcysteine	**Sol:** 10%, 20%	**Adults & Peds: Mucolytic: Nebulization (face mask, mouth piece, tracheostomy):** 1-10 ml of 20% or 2-10 ml of 10% q2-6h. **Usual:** 3-5 ml of 20% or 6-10 ml of 10% 3-4x/d. **Closed Tent or Croupette:** Up to 300 ml of 10% or 20%. **Direct Instillation:** 1-2 ml of 10% or 20% q1-4h. **Percutaneous Intratracheal Catheter:** 1-2 ml of 20% or 2-4 ml of 10% q1-4h. **Diagnostic Bronchograms:** Give before procedure. 2-3 doses of 1-2 ml of 20% or 2-4 ml of 10%.	B >

UROLOGY

Benign Prostatic Hypertrophy

ALPHA$_1$ RECEPTOR BLOCKERS

NAME	FORM/STRENGTH	DOSAGE	COMMENTS
Doxazosin Mesylate (Cardura XL)	**Tab,ER:** 4 mg, 8 mg	**Adults: Initial:** 4 mg qd w/ breakfast. **Titrate:** May increase to 8 mg after 3-4 wks. **Max:** 8 mg. Swallow whole.	C v
Doxazosin Mesylate (Cardura)	**Tab:** 1 mg, 2 mg, 4 mg, 8 mg	**Adults: Initial:** 1 mg qd (am or pm). **Titrate:** May double dose q1-2wks. **Max:** 8 mg/d.	C >
Silodosin (Rapaflo)	**Cap:** 4 mg, 8 mg	**Adults:** 8 mg qd. Take w/ meal. **CrCl 30-50 ml/min:** 4 mg qd.	B v CI w/ severe hepatic impairment. **H R**
Tamsulosin HCl (Flomax)	**Cap:** 0.4 mg	**Adults:** 0.4 mg qd, 1/2h after same meal qd. If fail to respond after 2-4 wks, may increase to 0.8 mg qd. If therapy interrupted for several days, restart w/ 0.4 mg qd.	B v
Terazosin HCl (Hytrin)	**Cap:** 1 mg, 2 mg, 5 mg, 10 mg	**Adults: Initial:** 1 mg qhs. **Titrate:** Increase stepwise to 10 mg qd. **Max:** 20 mg.	C >

ALPHA-REDUCTASE INHIBITORS

NAME	FORM/STRENGTH	DOSAGE	COMMENTS
Dutasteride (Avodart)	**Cap:** 0.5 mg	**Adults: Monotherapy:** 0.5 mg qd. **Combination w/ Tamsulosin:** 0.5 mg qd & tamsulosin 0.4 mg qd. Swallow whole.	X v

Finasteride (Proscar)	**Tab:** 5 mg	**Adults:** 5 mg qd.	X v

Erectile Dysfunction

PHOSPHODIESTERASE TYPE 5 INHIBITOR

Sildenafil Citrate (Viagra)	**Tab:** 25 mg, 50 mg, 100 mg	**Adults: Usual:** 50 mg 1h (range 0.5-4h) before sexual activity up to once daily. **Titrate:** May decrease to 25 mg qd or increase to 100 mg qd. **Max:** 100 mg qd. **Elderly/ Concomitant CYP3A4 Inhibitors: Initial:** 25 mg qd. **Concomitant Ritonavir: Max:** 25 mg q48h. **Concomitant α-blocker:** Avoid doses >25 mg of sildenafil within 4h of α-blocker.	B v CI w/ nitrates. **H R**
Tadalafil (Cialis)	**Tab:** 5 mg, 10 mg, 20 mg	**Adults: PRN Use:** Take prior to sexual activity. **Initial:** 10 mg. **Range:** 5-20 mg. **With Potent CYP3A4 Inhibitors: Max:** 10 mg/72h. **Once-Daily Use: Initial:** 2.5 mg qd without regard to timing of sexual activity. **Titrate:** May increase to 5 mg qd based on efficacy and tolerability. **With Potent CYP3A4 Inhibitors: Max:** 2.5 mg.	B v CI w/ nitrates. **H R**

NAME	FORM/STRENGTH	DOSAGE	COMMENTS
Vardenafil HCl (Levitra)	**Tab:** 2.5 mg, 5 mg, 10 mg, 20 mg	**Adults: Initial:** 10 mg 60 min prior to sexual activity at frequency of up to once daily. **Titrate:** May decrease to 5 mg or increase to max of 20 mg based on response. **Elderly: ≥65 yo: Initial:** 5 mg. **Concomitant Ritonavir: Max:** 2.5 mg/72h. **Concomitant Indinavir/Saquinavir/ Atazanavir/Ketoconazole 400 mg daily/Itraconazole 400 mg daily: Max:** 2.5 mg/24h. **Concomitant Ketoconazole 200 mg daily/Itraconazole 200 mg daily/ Erythromycin: Max:** 5 mg/24h.	◉B ✽> CI w/ nitrates or nitric oxide donors. **H**

Urinary Retention

PARASYMPATHETIC STIMULANTS

NAME	FORM/STRENGTH	DOSAGE	COMMENTS
Bethanechol Chloride (Urecholine)	**Tab:** 5 mg, 10 mg, 25 mg, 50 mg	**Adults: Initial:** 5-10 mg. **Titrate:** May repeat q1h until satisfactory response or 50 mg given. **Usual:** 10-50 mg tid-qid. **Max:** 200 mg/d.	◉C ✽v

Urinary Tract Antispasmodics

PARASYMPATHOLYTICS

NAME	FORM/STRENGTH	DOSAGE	COMMENTS
Darifenacin (Enablex)	**Tab,ER:** 7.5 mg, 15 mg	**OAB: Adults: Initial:** 7.5 mg qd w/ liquid. **Titrate:** May increase up to 15 mg qd after 2 wks. **Concomitant CYP3A4 Inhibitors:** Do not exceed 7.5 mg/d. Avoid use with severe hepatic impairment.	◉C ✽> **H**

Fesoterodine Fumarate (Toviaz)	**Tab,ER:** 4 mg, 8 mg	**OAB: Adults: Usual:** 4 mg qd. **Titrate:** May increase to 8 mg based on response and tolerability. **Potent CYP3A4 Inhibitors:** Should not exceed 4 mg. Swallow whole.	C v **R**
Hyoscyamine Sulfate	**Tab,Disintegrating:** 0.125 mg	**Adults & Peds: ≥12 yo:** 0.125-0.25 mg q4h or prn. **Max:** 1.5 mg/24h. **2 to <12 yo:** 0.0625-0.125 mg q4h or prn. **Max:** 0.75 mg/24h.	C >
Hyoscyamine Sulfate (Cystospaz)	**Tab:** 0.15 mg	**Adults:** 0.15-0.3 mg up to qid prn.	C >
Hyoscyamine Sulfate (Levbid, Levsin, Levsinex)	(Levbid) **Tab,ER:** 0.375 mg; (Levsin) **Drops:** 0.125 mg/ml; **Eli:** 0.125 mg/5 ml; **Inj:** 0.5 mg/ml; **Tab:** 0.125 mg; **Tab,SL:** 0.125 mg; (Levsinex) **Cap,ER:** 0.375 mg	**Adults & Peds: ≥12 yo: Drops/Eli/Tab/Tab,SL:** 0.125-0.25 mg q4h or prn. **Max:** 1.5 mg/24h. **Cap, Tab,ER:** 0.375-0.75 mg q12h; or 1 cap q8h. **Max:** 1.5 mg/24h. **2 to <12 yo: Tab/Tab,SL:** 0.0625-0.125 mg q4h or prn. **Max:** 0.75 mg/24h. **Eli:** Give q4h or prn. **10 kg:** 1.25 ml. **20 kg:** 2.5 ml. **40 kg:** 3.75 ml. **50 kg:** 5 ml. **Max:** 30 ml/24h. **Drops:** 0.25-1 ml q4h or prn. **Max:** 6 ml/24h. **<2 yo: Drops:** Give q4h or prn. **3.4 kg:** 4 gtts. **Max:** 24 gtts/24h. **5 kg:** 5 gtts. **Max:** 30 gtts/24h. **7 kg:** 6 gtts. **Max:** 36 gtts/24h. **10 kg:** 8 gtts. **Max:** 48 gtts/24h.	C >
Oxybutynin Chloride (Ditropan, Ditropan XL)	**Syr:** 5 mg/5 ml; **Tab:** 5 mg; **Tab,ER:** 5 mg, 10 mg, 15 mg	**OAB: Adults: Tab/Syr:** 5 mg bid-tid. **Max:** 5 mg qid. **Frail Elderly:** 2.5 mg bid-tid. **Tab,ER: Initial:** 5 or 10 mg qd. **Titrate:** May increase wkly by 5 mg. **Max:** 30 mg/d. **Peds: >5 yo: Tab/Syr:** 5 mg bid. **Max:** 5 mg tid. **Detrusor Overactivity: Peds: ≥6 yo: Tab,ER: Initial:** 5 mg qd. **Titrate:** May increase wkly by 5 mg. **Max:** 20 mg/d.	B >

NAME	FORM/STRENGTH	DOSAGE	COMMENTS
Oxybutynin Chloride (Gelnique)	**Gel:** 10%	**OAB: Adults:** Apply qd to dry, intact skin on abdomen, upper arms/shoulders, or thighs. Rotate sites.	B >
Oxybutynin (Oxytrol)	**Patch:** 3.9 mg/d	**OAB: Adults:** Apply to dry, intact skin on abdomen, hip, or buttock twice weekly (q3-4d). Rotate sites.	B >
Solifenacin Succinate (VESIcare)	**Tab:** 5 mg, 10 mg	**OAB: Adults: Usual:** 5 mg qd. **Max:** 10 mg qd. **Potent CYP3A4 Inhibitors: Max:** 5 mg qd. Avoid use with severe hepatic impairment.	C v **H R**
Tolterodine Tartrate (Detrol, Detrol LA)	**Cap,ER:** 2 mg, 4 mg; **Tab:** 1 mg, 2 mg	**OAB: Adults: Cap,ER: Usual:** 4 mg qd. May decrease to 2 mg qd depending on response & tolerability. **Tab: Initial:** 2 mg bid. **Maint:** 1-2 mg bid.	C v **H R**
Trospium Chloride (Sanctura, Sanctura XR)	**Cap,ER:** 60 mg; **Tab:** 20 mg	**OAB: Adults:** (Tab) 20 mg bid. (Cap,ER) 60 mg qd in am. Take at least 1h before meals or on empty stomach. **Elderly ≥75 yo:** (Tab) May titrate to 20 mg qd based on tolerability.	C > **R**

ANTIHISTAMINES

DRUG	RX/OTC	FORM/STRENGTH	DOSAGE	COMMENTS
Azelastine (Astelin)	RX	**Spr:** 137 mcg/spray	**Seasonal Allergic Rhinitis: Adults & Peds: ≥12 yo:** 2 sprays per nostril bid. **5-11 yo:** 1 spray per nostril bid. **Vasomotor Rhinitis: Adults & Peds: ≥12 yo:** 2 sprays per nostril bid.	◙C ✿>
Brompheniramine Maleate (Lodrane 24)	RX	**Cap,ER:** 12 mg	**Adults & Peds: ≥12 yo:** 12-24 mg qd. **6-12 yo:**12 mg qd.	◙C ✿v
Carbinoxamine Maleate (Palgic)	RX	**Sol:** 4 mg/5 ml; **Tab:** 4 mg	**Adults & Peds: ≥6 yo: Usual:** 4 mg prn. **Max:** 24 mg/day given q6-8h; **1-6 yo: Usual:** 2 mg prn. May increase to 0.2-0.4 mg/kg/day given q6-8h.	◙C ✿v
Cetirizine HCl (Zyrtec)	RX	**Chewtab:** 5mg, 10 mg; **Syr:** 1 mg/ml; **Tab:** 5 mg, 10 mg	**Seasonal or Perennial Allergic Rhinitis/ Urticaria: Adults & Peds ≥6 yo:** 5-10 mg qd. **Syr: 2-5 yo:** 2.5 ml (2.5 mg) qd. **Max:** 5 mg/d. **Perennial Allergic Rhinitis/Urticaria: 6 mo-23 mo:** 2.5 ml (2.5 mg) qd. **12 mo-23 mo:** May increase to max 5 mg/d.	◙B ✿v **H R**
Chlorpheniramine Maleate (Chlor-Trimeton)	OTC	**Syr:** 2 mg/5 ml; **Tab:** 4 mg; **Tab,ER:** 8 mg, 12 mg	**Adults & Peds ≥12 yo: Syr/Tab:** 4 mg q4-6h. **Tab,ER:** 8 mg q8-12h or 12 mg q12h. **Max:** 24 mg/d. **6-11 yo: Syr/Tab:** 2 mg q4-6h. **Max:** 12 mg/d.	◙N ✿>

(Tavist)	1.34 mg); RX (Tab 2.68 mg, Syr 0.5 mg/ 5 ml)	(Generic) **Syr:** 0.5 mg/ 5 ml; **Tab:** 1.34 mg, 2.68 mg	2.68 mg qd. **Max:** 8.04 mg/d. **Syr:** 1-2 mg bid. **Max:** 6 mg/d. **6-12 yo: Syr:** 0.5-1 mg bid. **Max:** 3 mg/d.	B v
Cyproheptadine HCl	RX	**Syr:** 2 mg/5 ml; **Tab:** 4 mg	**Adults: Initial:** 4 mg tid. **Usual:** 4-20 mg/d. **Max:** 0.5 mg/kg/d. **7-14 yo:** 4 mg bid-tid. **Max:** 16 mg/d. **2-6 yo:** 2 mg bid-tid. **Max:** 12 mg/d.	B v
Desloratadine (Clarinex, Clarinex Reditabs, Clarinex Syrup)	RX	**ODT:** (Reditab) 2.5 mg, 5 mg; **Syr:** 0.5 mg/ml; **Tab:** 5 mg	**Perennial Allergic Rhinitis/Urticaria: Adults & Peds: Tabs: ≥12 yo:** 5 mg qd. **6-11 yo:** 2.5 mg qd. **Syr: ≥12 yo:** 10 ml (5 mg) qd. **6-11 yo:** 5 ml (2.5 mg) qd. **12 mths - 5 yo:** 2.5 ml (1.25 mg) qd. **6-11 mths:** 2 ml (1 mg) qd. **Seasonal Allergic Rhinitis: Adults & Peds: Tabs: ≥12 yrs:** 5 mg qd. **6-11 yo:** 2.5 mg qd. **Syr: ≥12 yo:** 10 ml (5 mg) qd. **6-11 yo:** 5 ml (2.5 mg) qd. **2-5 yo:** 2.5 ml (1.25 mg) qd.	C v **H R**
Diphenhydramine HCl (Benadryl)	OTC (PO), RX (Inj), OTC/RX (50 mg cap)	**Cap:** 25 mg, 50 mg; **Chewtab:** 12.5 mg; **Inj:** 50 mg/ml; **Syr:** 12.5 mg/5 ml; **Tab:** 25 mg, 50 mg	**Adults: PO:** 25-50 mg q4-6h. **Max:** 300 mg/d **Inj:** 10-50 mg IV or up to 100 mg deep IM. **Max:** 400 mg/d. **6-11 yo: PO:** 12.5-25 mg q4-6h. **Max:** 150 mg/d. **Peds: Inj:** 5 mg/kg/d or 150 $mg/m^2/d$ IV/IM in 4 divided doses. **Max:** 300 mg/d.	B v

NAME	RX/OTC	FORM/STRENGTH	DOSAGE	COMMENTS
Fexofenadine HCl (Allegra)	RX	**Susp:** 30 mg/5 ml; **Tab:** 30 mg, 60 mg 180 mg **Tab,Dissolve:** 30 mg	**Seasonal Allergic Rhinitis: Tab: Adults & Peds: >12 yo:** 60 mg bid or 180 mg qd. **6-11 yo:** 30 mg bid. **Susp: Peds: 2-11 yo:** 30 mg bid. **Chronic Idiopathic Urticaria: Tab: Adults & Peds: >12 yo:** 60 mg bid. **6-11 yo:** 30 mg bid. **Susp: Peds: 2-11 yo:** 30 mg (5 ml) bid. **6 mths to <2 yo:** 15 mg (2.5 ml) bid.	◙C ❉> **R**
Hydroxyzine HCl (Atarax)	RX	(Atarax) **Syr:** 10 mg/ 5 ml; (Generic) **Syr:** 10 mg/5 ml; **Tab:** 10 mg, 25 mg, 50 mg	**Adults:** 25 mg tid-qid. **≥6 yo:** 50-100 mg/d in divided doses. **<6 yo:** 50 mg/d in divided doses.	◙N ❉v
Hydroxyzine Pamoate (Vistaril)	RX	(Vistaril) **Cap:** 25 mg 50 mg; (Generic) **Cap:** 25 mg, 50 mg, 100 mg	**Adults:** 25 mg tid-qid. **Ped: ≥6 yo:** 50-100 mg/d in divided doses. **<6 yo:** 50 mg/d in divided doses.	◙N ❉v
Levocetirizine Dihydrochloride (Xyzal)	RX	**Sol:** 2.5 mg/5 ml **Tab:** 5 mg	**Seasonal or Perennial Allergic Rhinitis/ Urticaria: Adults & Peds: ≥12 yo:** 5 mg qd in evening. **6-11 yo:** 2.5 mg qd in evening.	◙B ❉v **R**
Loratadine (Alavert, Claritin, Claritin Reditabs)	OTC	**ODT:** (Reditab) 10 mg; **Syr:** 1 mg/ml; **Tab:** 10 mg	**Adults & Peds: ≥6 yo: ODT/Syr/Tab:** 10 mg qd. **2-5 yo: Syr:** 5 mg qd. **Max:** 10 mg/d.	◙B ❉> **H R**

(Phenergan)		25 mg/ml,50 mg/ml; **Sup:** 12.5 mg, 25 mg, 50 mg; **Syr:** 6.25 mg/5 ml; **Tab:** 12.5 mg, 25 mg, 50 mg; (Phenergan) **Inj:** 25 mg/ml, 50 mg/ml; **Sup:** 12.5 mg, 25 mg, 50 mg; **Tab:** 12.5 mg, 25 mg, 50 mg	**Peds: ≥2 yo:** 25 mg or 0.5 mg/lb PO/PR qhs or & qhs; 25 mg IM/IV and repeat in 2h if needed. 6.25-12.5 mg tid; up to 12.5 mg IM/IV.	

COUGH & COLD COMBINATIONS

DRUG	RX/OTC	ANTIHISTAMINE	DECONGESTANT	COUGH SUPPRESSANT	OTHER CONTENT	DOSE
Actifed Cold & Sinus Caplets	OTC	Chlorpheniramine Maleate, 2 mg	Pseudoephedrine HCl, 30 mg		Acetaminophen, 500 mg	≥12 yo: 2 q6h. Max: 8/24h.
Advil Cold & Sinus	OTC		Pseudoephedrine HCl, 30 mg		Ibuprofen, 200 mg	≥12 yo: 1-2 q4-6h. Max: 6/24h.
Aleve Cold & Sinus	OTC		Pseudoephedrine HCl, 120 mg		Naproxen Sodium, 220 mg	≥12 yo: 1 q12h. Max: 2/24h.
Allegra-D 12 Hour Extended-Release Tablets	RX	Fexofenadine HCl, 60 mg	Pseudoephedrine HCl, 120 mg			≥12 yo: 1 tab bid.
Allegra-D 24 Hour Extended-Release Tablets	RX	Fexofenadine HCl, 180 mg	Pseudoephedrine HCl, 240 mg			≥12 yo: 1 tab qd.
Clarinex-D 12 Hour Extended-Release Tablets	RX	Desloratadine, 2.5 mg	Pseudoephedrine Sulfate, 120 mg			≥12 yo: 1 tab bid.
Clarinex-D 24 Hour Extended-Release Tablets	RX	Desloratadine, 5 mg	Pseudoephedrine Sulfate, 240 mg			≥12 yo: 1 tab qd.
Claritin-D 12 Hour	OTC	Loratadine, 5 mg	Pseudoephedrine Sulfate,			≥12 yo: 1 tab

Tablet			240 mg			
Contac Severe Cold & Flu Maximum Strength Caplet	OTC	Chlorpheniramine Maleate, 2 mg	Pseudoephedrine HCl, 30 mg	Dextromethorphan HBr, 15 mg	Acetaminophen, 500 mg	≥12 yo: 2 q6h.
Coricidin HBP Cough/Cold Tablet	OTC	Chlorpheniramine Maleate, 4 mg		Dextromethorphan HBr, 30 mg		≥12 yo: 1 tab q6h. Max: 4/24h.
DayQuil Cold/Flu	OTC		Phenylephrine HCl, 5 mg/15 ml	Dextromethorphan HBr, 10 mg/15 ml	Acetaminophen, 325 mg/15 ml	≥12 yo: 2 tbsp q4h. 6 to <12 yo: 1 tbsp q4h. Max: 5 doses (child) or 6 doses (adult)/ 24h.
Delsym Suspension	OTC			Dextromethorphan Polistirex, 30 mg/5 ml		≥12 yo: 2 tsp q12h. Max: 4 tsp/ 24h. 6 to <12 yo: 1 tsp q12h. Max: 2 tsp/24h. 2 to <6 yo: 1/2 tsp q12h. Max: 1 tsp/24h.
Dimetapp Cold & Allergy Elixir	OTC	Brompheniramine Maleate, 1 mg/5 ml	Phenylephrine HCl, 2.5 mg/5 ml			≥12 yo: 4 tsp q4h. 6 to <12 yo: 2 tsp q4h. Max: 6 doses/24h.

DRUG	RX/OTC	ANTIHISTAMINE	DECONGESTANT	COUGH SUPPRESSANT	OTHER CONTENT	DOSE
Drixoral Cold & Allergy Tablet	OTC	Dexbrompheniramine Maleate, 6 mg	Pseudoephedrine Sulfate, 120 mg			≥12 yo: 1 tab q12h.
Entex PSE Tablet	RX		Pseudoephedrine HCl, 120 mg		Guaifenesin, 400 mg	≥12 yo: 1 tab q12h. 6 to <12 yo: 1/2 tab q12h.
Hycodan Syrup	CIII			Hydrocodone Bitartrate, 5 mg/5 ml	Homatropine MBr, 1.5 mg/5 ml	>12 yo: 1 tsp q4-6h. Max: 6 tsp/24h. 6-12 yo: 1/2 tsp q4-6h. Max: 3 tsp/24h
Mucinex	OTC				Guaifenesin 600 mg	≥12 yo: 1-2 tabs q12h. Max: 4/24h
Mucinex DM	OTC			Dextromethorphan HBr, 30 mg	Guaifenesin, 600 mg	≥12 yo: 1-2 tabs q12h. Max: 4/24h
NyQuil Cold/Flu	OTC	Doxylamine 6.25 mg/15 ml		Dextromethorphan HBr, 15 mg/15 ml	Acetaminophen 500 mg/15 ml	≥12 yo: 2 tbsp q6h. Max: 4 doses/24h
Phenergan w/ Codeine	CV	Promethazine 6.25 mg/5 ml		Codeine 10 mg/5 ml		≥16 yo: 1 tsp q4-6h. Max: 30 ml/24h

				Codeine 10 mg/5 ml	Guaifenesin 100 mg/5 ml	≥12 yo: 1-2 tsp q4h. 6 to <12 yo: 1 tsp q4h. 2 to <6 yo: 1-1.5 mg/kg/d of codeine in 4 divided doses.
Robitussin CF	OTC		Phenylephrine HCl, 5 mg/5 ml	Dextromethorphan HBr, 10 mg/5 ml	Guaifenesin, 100 mg/5 ml	≥12 yo: 2 tsp q4h. 6 to <12 yo: 1 tsp q4h. 2 to <6 yo: 1/2 tsp q4h.
Robitussin DM Syrup	OTC			Dextromethorphan HBr, 10 mg/5 ml	Guaifenesin, 100 mg/5 ml	≥12 yo: 2 tsp q4h. 6 to <12 yo: 1 tsp q4h. 2 to <6 yo: 1/2 tsp q4h.
Robitussin PE Syrup	OTC		Phenylephrine HCl, 5 mg/5 ml		Guaifenesin, 100 mg/5 ml	≥12 yo: 2 tsp q4h. 6 to <12 yo: 1 tsp q4h. 2 to <6 yo: 1/2 tsp q4h.
Ryna-12X Suspension	RX	Pyrilamine Tannate, 30 mg	Phenylephrine Tannate, 5 mg		Guaifenesin, 100 mg/5ml	≥6 yo: 1-2 tsp q12h. 2 to <6 yo: 1/2-1 tsp q12h.
Sudafed Cold & Cough	OTC		Pseudoephedrine HCl, 30 mg	Dextromethorphan HBr, 10 mg	Guaifenesin, 100 mg Acetaminophen, 250 mg	≥12 yo: 2 caps q4h. Max: 8/24h

DRUG	RX/OTC	ANTIHISTAMINE	DECONGESTANT	COUGH SUPPRESSANT	OTHER CONTENT	DOSE
Theraflu Cold & Sore Throat Hot Liquid	OTC	Pheniramine Maleate, 20 mg	Phenylephrine HCl, 10 mg		Acetaminophen, 325 mg	≥12 yo: 1 pkt q4h. Max: 6 pkts/24h
Triaminic Day Time Cold & Cough Liquid	OTC		Phenylephrine HCl, 2.5 mg/5 ml	Dextromethorphan HBr, 5 mg/5 ml		6 to <12 yo: 2 tsp q4h. 2 to <6 yo: 1 tsp q4h. Max: 6 doses/24h.
Triaminic Softchews Cough & Runny Nose	OTC	Chlorpheniramine Maleate, 1 mg		Dextromethorphan HBr, 5 mg		6 to <12 yo: 2 tabs q4-6h. Max: 6 doses/24h.
Triaminic Flu, Cough & Fever Liquid	OTC	Chlorpheniramine Maleate, 1 mg/5 ml		Dextromethorphan HBr, 7.5 mg/5 ml	Acetaminophen, 160 mg/5 ml	6 to <12 yo: 2 tsp q6h. Max: 4 doses/24h.
Triaminic Night Time Cough & Cold Liquid	OTC	Diphenhydramine HCl, 6.25 mg/5 ml	Phenylephrine HCl, 2.5 mg/5 ml			6-12 yo: 2 tsp q4h. Max 6 doses/24h.
Triaminic Softchews Cough & Sore Throat	OTC			Dextromethorphan HBr, 5 mg	Acetaminophen, 160 mg	6 to <12 yo: 2 tabs q4h. 2 to <6 yo: 1 tab q4h. Max: 5 doses/24h.

Suspension		30 mg	5 mg	Tannate, 30 mg		≥6 yo: 1-2 tsp q12h. 2 to <6 yo: 1/2-1 tsp q12h.
Tussionex Pennkinetic Suspension	CIII	Chlorpheniramine Polistirex, 8 mg/5 ml			Hydrocodone Polistirex, 10 mg/5 ml	>12 yo: 1 tsp q12h. 6-12 yo: 1/2 tsp q12h.
Tylenol Cold Day Caplet	OTC		Pseudoephedrine HCl, 30 mg	Dextromethorphan HBr, 15 mg	Acetaminophen, 325 mg	≥12 yo: 2 q6h. Max: 8/24h.
Zyrtec-D 12 Hour Tablet	RX	Cetirizine HCl, 5 mg	Pseudoephedrine HCl, 120 mg			≥12 yo: 1 tab bid.

IMMUNIZATIONS

RECOMMENDED IMMUNIZATION SCHEDULE FOR PERSONS AGED 0–6 YEARS • UNITED STATES, 2009

Vaccine ▼ Age ▶	Birth	1 month	2 months	4 months	6 months	12 months	15 months	18 months	19–23 months	2–3 years	4–6 years
Hepatitis B[1]	HepB	HepB		*see footnote 1*	HepB						
Rotavirus[2]			RV	RV	*RV*[2]						
Diphtheria, Tetanus, Pertussis[3]			DTaP	DTaP	DTaP	*see footnote 3*	DTaP				DTaP
Haemophilus influenzae type b[4]			Hib	Hib	*Hib*[4]	Hib					
Pneumococcal[5]			PCV	PCV	PCV	PCV				PPSV	
Inactivated Poliovirus			IPV	IPV	IPV						IPV
Influenza[6]					Influenza (Yearly)						
Measles, Mumps, Rubella[7]						MMR		*see footnote 7*			MMR
Varicella[8]						Varicella		*see footnote 8*			Varicella
Hepatitis A[9]						HepA (2 doses)				HepA Series	
Meningococcal[10]										MCV	

This schedule indicates the recommended ages for routine administration of currently licensed vaccines, as of December 1, 2008, for children aged 0 through 6 years. Any dose not administered at the recommended age should be administered at a subsequent visit, when indicated and feasible. Licensed combination vaccines may be used whenever any component of the combination is indicated and other components are not contraindicated and if approved by the Food and Drug Administration for that dose of the series. Providers should consult the relevant Advisory Committee on Immunization Practices statement for detailed recommendations, including high-risk conditions: *http://www.cdc.gov/vaccines/pubs/acip-list.htm*. Clinically significant adverse events that follow immunization should be reported to the Vaccine Adverse Event Reporting System (VAERS). Guidance about how to obtain and complete a VAERS form is available at *http://www.vaers.hhs.gov* or by telephone, 800-822-7967.

1. **Hepatitis B vaccine (HepB).** *(Minimum age: birth)*
   At birth:
   - Administer monovalent HepB to all newborns before hospital discharge.
   - If mother is hepatitis B surface antigen (HBsAg)-positive, administer HepB and 0.5 mL of hepatitis B immune globulin (HBIG) within 12 hours of birth.
   - If mother's HBsAg status is unknown, administer HepB within 12 hours of birth. Determine mother's HBsAg status as soon as possible and, if HBsAg-positive, administer HBIG (no later than age 1 week).

   After the birth dose:
   - The HepB series should be completed with either monovalent HepB or a combination vaccine containing HepB. The second dose should be administered at age 1 or 2 months. The final dose should be administered no earlier than age 24 weeks.
   - Infants born to HBsAg-positive mothers should be tested for HBsAg and antibody to HBsAg (anti-HBs) after completion of at least 3 doses of the HepB series, at age 9 through 18 months (generally at the next well-child visit).

   4-month dose:
   - Administration of 4 doses of HepB to infants is permissible when combination vaccines containing HepB are administered after the birth dose.
2. **Rotavirus vaccine (RV).** *(Minimum age: 6 weeks)*
   - Administer the first dose at age 6 through 14 weeks (maximum age: 14 weeks 6 days). Vaccination should not be initiated for infants aged 15 weeks or older (i.e., 15 weeks 0 days or older).
   - Administer the final dose in the series by age 8 months 0 days.
   - If Rotarix® is administered at ages 2 and 4 months, a dose at 6 months is not indicated.

3. **Diphtheria and tetanus toxoids and acellular pertussis vaccine (DTaP).** *(Minimum age: 6 weeks)*
   - The fourth dose may be administered as early as age 12 months, provided at least 6 months have elapsed since the third dose.
   - Administer the final dose in the series at age 4 through 6 years.
4. ***Haemophilus influenzae* type B conjugate vaccine (Hib).** *(Minimum age: 6 weeks)*
   - If PRP-OMP (PedvaxHIB® or Comvax® [HepB-Hib]) is administered at ages 2 and 4 months, a dose at age 6 months is not indicated.
   - TriHiBit® (DTaP/Hib) should not be used for doses at ages 2, 4, or 6 months but can be used as the final dose in children aged 12 months or older.
5. **Pneumococcal vaccine.** *(Minimum age: 6 weeks for pneumococcal conjugate vaccine [PCV]; 2 years for pneumococcal polysaccharide vaccine [PPSV])*
   - PCV is recommended for all children aged younger than 5 years. Administer 1 dose of PCV to all healthy children aged 24 through 59 months who are not completely vaccinated for their age.
   - Administer PPSV to children aged 2 years or older with certain underlying medical conditions (see *MMWR* 2000;49[No. RR-9]), including a cochlear implant.
6. **Influenza vaccine.** *(Minimum age: 6 months for trivalent inactivated influenza vaccine [TIV]; 2 years for live, attenuated influenza vaccine [LAIV])*
   - Administer annually to children aged 6 months through 18 years.
   - For healthy nonpregnant persons (i.e., those who do not have underlying medical conditions that predispose them to influenza complications) aged 2 through 49 years, either LAIV or TIV may be used.
   - Children receiving TIV should receive 0.25 mL if aged 6 through 35 months or 0.5 mL if aged 3 years or older.
   - Administer 2 doses (separated by at least 4 weeks) to children aged younger than 9 years who are receiving influenza vaccine for the first time or who were vaccinated for the first time during the previous influenza season but only received 1 dose.
7. **Measles, mumps, and rubella vaccine (MMR).** *(Minimum age: 12 months)*
   - Administer the second dose at age 4 through 6 years. However, the second dose may be administered before age 4, provided at least 28 days have elapsed since the first dose.
8. **Varicella vaccine.** *(Minimum age: 12 months)*
   - Administer the second dose at age 4 through 6 years. However, the second dose may be administered before age 4, provided at least

- For children aged 12 months through 12 years, the minimum interval between doses is 3 months. However, if the second dose was administered at least 28 days after the first dose, it can be accepted as valid.

9. **Hepatitis A vaccine (HepA).** *(Minimum age: 12 months)*
   - Administer to all children aged 1 year (i.e., aged 12 through 23 months). Administer 2 doses at least 6 months apart.
   - Children not fully vaccinated by age 2 years can be vaccinated at subsequent visits.
   - HepA also is recommended for children older than 1 year who live in areas where vaccination programs target older children or who are at increased risk of infection. See *MMWR* 2006;55(No. RR-7).
10. **Meningococcal vaccine.** *(Minimum age: 2 years for meningococcal conjugate vaccine [MCV] and for meningococcal polysaccharide vaccine [MPSV])*
    - Administer MCV to children aged 2 through 10 years with terminal complement component deficiency, anatomic or functional asplenia, and certain other high-risk groups. See *MMWR* 2005;54(No. RR-7).
    - Persons who received MPSV 3 or more years previously and who remain at increased risk for meningococcal disease should be revaccinated with MCV.

RECOMMENDED IMMUNIZATION SCHEDULE FOR PERSONS AGED 7–18 YEARS • UNITED STATES, 2009

Vaccine ▼ Age ▶	7–10 years	11–12 years	13–18 years
Tetanus, Diphtheria, Pertussis[1]	*see footnote 1*	Tdap	Tdap
Human Papillomavirus[2]	*see footnote 2*	HPV (3 doses)	HPV Series
Meningococcal[3]	MCV	MCV	MCV
Influenza[4]		Influenza (Yearly)	
Pneumococcal[5]		PPSV	
Hepatitis A[6]		HepA Series	
Hepatitis B[7]		HepB Series	
Inactivated Poliovirus[8]		IPV Series	
Measles, Mumps, Rubella[9]		MMR Series	
Varicella[10]		Varicella Series	

Range of recommended ages — Catch-up immunization — Certain high-risk groups

7 through 18 years. Any dose not administered at the recommended age should be administered at a subsequent visit, when indicated and feasible. Licensed combination vaccines may be used whenever any component of the combination is indicated and other components are not contraindicated and if approved by the Food and Drug Administration for that dose of the series. Providers should consult the relevant Advisory Committee on Immunization Practices statement for detailed recommendations, including high-risk conditions: *http://www.cdc.gov/vaccines/pubs/acip-list.htm*. Clinically significant adverse events that follow immunization should be reported to the Vaccine Adverse Event Reporting System (VAERS). Guidance about how to obtain and complete a VAERS form is available at *http://www.vaers.hhs.gov* or by telephone, 800-822-7967.

1. **Tetanus and diphtheria toxoids and acellular pertussis vaccine(Tdap).** *(Minimum age: 10 years for BOOSTRIX® and 11 years for ADACEL®)*
   - Administer at age 11 or 12 years for those who have completed the recommended childhood DTP/DTaP vaccination series and have not received a tetanus and diphtheria toxoid (Td) booster dose.
   - Persons aged 13 through 18 years who have not received Tdap should receive a dose.
   - A 5-year interval from the last Td dose is encouraged when Tdap is used as a booster dose; however, a shorter interval may be used if pertussis immunity is needed.
2. **Human papillomavirus vaccine (HPV).** *(Minimum age: 9 years)*
   - Administer the first dose to females at age 11 or 12 years.
   - Administer the second dose 2 months after the first dose and the third dose 6 months after the first dose (at least 24 weeks after the first dose).
   - Administer the series to females at age 13 through 18 years if not previously vaccinated.
3. **Meningococcal conjugate vaccine (MCV).**
   - Administer at age 11 or 12 years, or at age 13 through 18 years if not previously vaccinated.
   - Administer to previously unvaccinated college freshmen living in a dormitory.
   - MCV is recommended for children aged 2 through 10 years with terminal complement component deficiency, anatomic or functional asplenia, and certain other groups at high risk. See *MMWR* 2005;54(No. RR-7).
   - Persons who received MPSV 5 or more years previously and remain at increased risk for meningococcal disease should be revaccinated with MCV.
4. **Influenza vaccine.**
   - Administer annually to children aged 6 months through 18 years.
   - For healthy nonpregnant persons (i.e., those who do not have underlying medical conditions that predispose them to influenza

complications) aged 2 through 49 years, either LAIV or TIV may be used.
- Administer 2 doses (separated by at least 4 weeks) to children aged younger than 9 years who are receiving influenza vaccine for the first time or who were vaccinated for the first time during the previous influenza season but only received 1 dose.

5. **Pneumococcal polysaccharide vaccine (PPSV).**
   - Administer to children with certain underlying medical conditions (see *MMWR* 1997;46[No. RR-8]), including a cochlear implant. A single revaccination should be administered to children with functional or anatomic asplenia or other immunocompromising condition after 5 years.
6. **Hepatitis A vaccine (HepA).**
   - Administer 2 doses at least 6 months apart.
   - HepA is recommended for children older than 1 year who live in areas where vaccination programs target older children or who are at increased risk of infection. See *MMWR* 2006;55(No. RR-7).
7. **Hepatitis B vaccine (HepB).**
   - Administer the 3-dose series to those not previously vaccinated.
   - A 2-dose series (separated by at least 4 months) of adult formulation Recombivax HB® is licensed for children aged 11 through 15 years.
8. **Inactivated poliovirus vaccine (IPV).**
   - For children who received an all-IPV or all-oral poliovirus (OPV) series, a fourth dose is not necessary if the third dose was administered at age 4 years or older.
   - If both OPV and IPV were administered as part of a series, a total of 4 doses should be administered, regardless of the child's current age.
9. **Measles, mumps, and rubella vaccine (MMR).**
   - If not previously vaccinated, administer 2 doses or the second dose for those who have received only 1 dose, with at least 28 days between doses.
10. **Varicella vaccine.**
    - For persons aged 7 through 18 years without evidence of immunity (see *MMWR* 2007;56[No. RR-4]), administer 2 doses if not previously vaccinated or the second dose if they have received only 1 dose.
    - For persons aged 7 through 12 years, the minimum interval between doses is 3 months. However, if the second dose was administered at least 28 days after the first dose, it can be accepted as valid.
    - For persons aged 13 years and older, the minimum interval between doses is 28 days.

CATCH-UP IMMUNIZATION SCHEDULE FOR PERSONS AGED 4 MONTHS–18 YEARS WHO START LATE OR WHO ARE MORE THAN 1 MONTH BEHIND • UNITED STATES, 2009

CATCH-UP SCHEDULE FOR PERSONS AGED 4 MONTHS THROUGH 6 YEARS					
Vaccine	Minimum Age for Dose 1	Minimum Interval Between Doses			
		Dose 1 to Dose 2	Dose 2 to Dose 3	Dose 3 to Dose 4	Dose 4 to Dose 5
Hepatitis B[1]	Birth	4 weeks	8 weeks (and at least 16 weeks after first dose)		
Rotavirus[2]	6 wks	4 weeks	4 weeks[2]		
Diphtheria, Tetanus, Pertussis[3]	6 wks	4 weeks	4 weeks	6 months	6 months[3]
Haemophilus influenzae type b[4]	6 wks	**4 weeks** if first dose administered at younger than age 12 months **8 weeks (as final dose)** if first dose administered at age 12-14 months **No further doses needed** if first dose administered at age 15 months or older	**4 weeks[4]** if current age is younger than 12 months **8 weeks (as final dose)[4]** if current age is 12 months or older and second dose administered at younger than age 15 months **No further doses needed** if previous dose administered at age 15 months or older	**8 weeks (as final dose)** This dose only necessary for children aged 12 months through 59 months who received 3 doses before age 12 months	
Pneumococcal[5]	6 wks	**4 weeks** if first dose administered at younger than age 12 months **8 weeks** (as final dose for healthy children) if first dose administered at age 12 months or older or current age 24 through 59 months **No further doses needed** for healthy children if first dose administered at age 24 months or older	**4 weeks** if current age is younger than 12 months **8 weeks** (as final dose for healthy children) if current age is 12 months or older **No further doses needed** for healthy children if previous dose administered at age 24 months or older	**8 weeks** (as final dose) This dose only necessary for children aged 12 months through 59 months who received 3 doses before age 12 months or for high-risk children who received 3 doses at any age	
Inactivated Poliovirus[6]	6 wks	4 weeks	4 weeks	4 weeks[6]	
Measles, Mumps, Rubella[7]	12 mos	4 weeks			
Varicella[8]	12 mos	3 months			
Hepatitis A[9]	12 mos	6 months			

CATCH-UP SCHEDULE FOR PERSONS AGED 7 THROUGH 18 YEARS					
Tetanus, Diphtheria/ Tetanus, Diphtheria, Pertussis[10]	7 yrs[10]	4 weeks	**4 weeks** if first dose administered at younger than age 12 months **6 months** if first dose administered at age 12 months or older	**6 months** if first dose administered at younger than age 12 months	
Human Papillomavirus[11]	9 yrs	Routine dosing intervals are recommended[11]			
Hepatitis A[9]	12 mos	6 months			
Hepatitis B[1]	Birth	4 weeks	**8 weeks** (and at least 16 weeks after first dose)		
Inactivated Poliovirus[6]	6 wks	4 weeks	4 weeks	4 weeks[6]	
Measles, Mumps, Rubella[7]	12 mos	4 weeks			
Varicella[8]	12 mos	**3 months** if the person is younger than age 13 years **4 weeks** if the person is aged 13 years or older			

1. **Hepatitis B vaccine (HepB).**
   - Administer the 3-dose series to those not previously vaccinated.
   - A 2-dose series (separated by at least 4 months) of adult formulation Recombivax HB® is licensed for children aged 11 through 15 years.
2. **Rotavirus vaccine (RV).**
   - The maximum age for the first dose is 14 weeks 6 days. Vaccination should not be initiated for infants aged 15 weeks or older (i.e., 15 weeks 0 days or older).
   - Administer the final dose in the series by age 8 months 0 days.
   - If Rotarix® was administered for the first and second doses, a third dose is not indicated.
3. **Diphtheria and tetanus toxoids and acellular pertussis vaccine (DTaP).**
   - The fifth dose is not necessary if the fourth dose was administered at age 4 years or older.
4. ***Haemophilus influenzae* type B conjugate vaccine (Hib).**
   - Hib vaccine is not generally recommended for persons aged 5 years or older. No efficacy data are available on which to base a recommendation concerning use of Hib vaccine for older children and adults. However, studies suggest good immunogenicity in persons who have sickle cell disease, leukemia, or HIV infection, or who have had a splenectomy; administering 1 dose of Hib vaccine to these

- If the first 2 doses were PRP-OMP (PedvaxHIB® or Comvax®), and administered at age 11 months or younger, the third (and final) dose should be administered at age 12 through 15 months and at least 8 weeks after the second dose.
- If the first dose was administered at age 7 through 11 months, administer 2 doses separated by 4 weeks and a final dose at age 12 through 15 months.

5. **Pneumococcal vaccine.**
   - Administer 1 dose of pneumococcal conjugate vaccine (PCV) to all healthy children aged 24 through 59 months who have not received at least 1 dose of PCV on or after age 12 months.
   - For children aged 24 through 59 months with underlying medical conditions, administer 1 dose of PCV if 3 doses were received previously or administer 2 doses of PCV at least 8 weeks apart if fewer than 3 doses were received previously.
   - Administer pneumococcal polysaccharide vaccine (PPSV) to children aged 2 years or older with certain underlying medical conditions (see *MMWR* 2000;49[No. RR-9]), including a cochlear implant, at least 8 weeks after the last dose of PCV.
6. **Inactivated poliovirus vaccine (IPV).**
   - For children who received an all-IPV or all-oral poliovirus (OPV) series, a fourth dose is not necessary if the third dose was administered at age 4 years or older.
   - If both OPV and IPV were administered as part of a series, a total of 4 doses should be administered, regardless of the child's current age.
7. **Measles, mumps, and rubella vaccine (MMR).**
   - Administer the second dose at age 4 through 6 years. However, the second dose may be administered before age 4, provided at least 28 days have elapsed since the first dose.
   - If not previously vaccinated, administer 2 doses with at least 28 days between doses.
8. **Varicella vaccine.**
   - Administer the second dose at age 4 through 6 years. However, the second dose may be administered before age 4, provided at least 3 months have elapsed since the first dose.
   - For persons aged 12 months through 12 years, the minimum interval between doses is 3 months. However, if the second dose was administered at least 28 days after the first dose, it can be accepted as valid.
   - For persons aged 13 years and older, the minimum interval between doses is 28 days.
9. **Hepatitis A vaccine (HepA).**
   - HepA is recommended for children older than 1 year who live in areas where vaccination programs target older children or who are at increased risk of infection. See *MMWR* 2006;55(No. RR-7).
10. **Tetanus and diphtheria toxoids vaccine (Td) and tetanus and diphtheriatoxoids and acellular pertussis vaccine (Tdap).**

- Doses of DTaP are counted as part of the Td/Tdap series
- Tdap should be substituted for a single dose of Td in the catch-up series or as a booster for children aged 10 through 18 years; use Td for other doses.

11. Human papillomavirus vaccine (HPV).

- Administer the series to females at age 13 through 18 years if not previously vaccinated.
- Use recommended routine dosing intervals for series catch-up (i.e., the second and third doses should be administered at 2 and 6 months after the first dose). However, the minimum interval between the first and second doses is 4 weeks. The minimum interval between the second and third doses is 12 weeks, and the third dose should be given at least 24 weeks after the first dose.

RECOMMENDED ADULT IMMUNIZATION SCHEDULE

FIGURE 1. RECOMMENDED ADULT IMMUNIZATION SCHEDULE, BY VACCINE AND AGE GROUP UNITED STATES, 2009

VACCINE ▼ AGE GROUP ▶	19–26 years	27–49 years	50–59 years	60–64 years	≥65 years
Tetanus, diphtheria, pertussis (Td/Tdap)[1,*]	Substitute 1-time dose of Tdap for Td booster; then boost with Td every 10 yr				Td booster every 10 yrs
Human papillomavirus (HPV)[2,*]	3 doses (females)				
Varicella[3,*]	2 doses				
Zoster[4]				1 dose	
Measles, mumps, rubella (MMR)[5,*]	1 or 2 doses		1 dose		
Influenza[6,*]	1 dose annually				
Pneumococcal (polysaccharide)[7,8]	1 or 2 doses				1 dose
Hepatitis A[9,*]	2 doses				
Hepatitis B[10,*]	3 doses				
Meningococcal[11,*]	1 or more doses				

*Covered by the Vaccine Injury Compensation Program.

- For all persons in this category who meet the age requirements and who lack evidence of immunity (e.g., lack documentation of vaccination or have no evidence of prior infection)
- Recommended if some other risk factor is present (e.g., on the basis of medical, occupational, lifestyle, or other indications)
- No recommendation

FIGURE 2. VACCINES THAT MIGHT BE INDICATED FOR ADULTS BASED ON MEDICAL AND OTHER INDICATIONS UNITED STATES, 2009

INDICATION ▶ VACCINE ▼	Pregnancy	Immuno-compromising conditions (excluding human immunodeficiency virus [HIV])[13]	HIV infection[3,12,13] CD4+ T lymphocyte count <200 cells/µL	HIV infection[3,12,13] CD4+ T lymphocyte count ≥200 cells/µL	Diabetes, heart disease, chronic lung disease, chronic alcoholism	Asplenia[12] (including elective splenectomy and terminal complement component deficiencies)	Chronic liver disease	Kidney failure, end-stage renal disease, receipt of hemodialysis	Health-care personnel
Tetanus, diphtheria, pertussis (Td/Tdap)[1,*]	Td	Substitute 1-time dose of Tdap for Td booster; then boost with Td every 10 yrs							
Human papillomavirus (HPV)[2,*]		3 doses for females through age 26 yrs							
Varicella[3,*]	Contraindicated			2 doses					
Zoster[4]	Contraindicated				1 dose				
Measles, mumps, rubella (MMR)[5,*]	Contraindicated			1 or 2 doses					
Influenza[6,*]	1 dose TIV annually								1 dose TIV or LAIV annually
Pneumococcal (polysaccharide)[7,8]	1 or 2 doses								
Hepatitis A[9,*]	2 doses								
Hepatitis B[10,*]	3 doses								
Meningococcal[11,*]	1 or more doses								

*Covered by the Vaccine Injury Compensation Program.

For all persons in this category who meet the age requirements and who lack evidence of immunity (e.g., lack documentation of vaccination or have

Recommended if some other risk factor is present (e.g., on the basis of medical, occupational, lifestyle, or other indications)

No recommendation

1. Tetanus, diphtheria, and acellular pertussis (Td/Tdap) vaccination

Tdap should replace a single dose of Td for adults aged 19 through 64 years who have not received a dose of Tdap previously.

Adults with uncertain or incomplete history of primary vaccination series with tetanus and diphtheria toxoid–containing vaccines should begin or complete a primary vaccination series. A primary series for adults is 3 doses of tetanus and diphtheria toxoid–containing vaccines; administer the first 2 doses at least 4 weeks apart and the third dose 6–12 months after the second. However, Tdap can substitute for any one of the doses of Td in the 3-dose primary series. The booster dose of tetanus and diphtheria toxoid–containing vaccine should be administered to adults who have completed a primary series and if the last vaccination was received 10 or more years previously. Tdap or Td vaccine may be used, as indicated.

If a woman is pregnant and received the last Td vaccination 10 or more years previously, administer Td during the second or third trimester. If the woman received the last Td vaccination less than 10 years previously, administer Tdap during the immediate postpartum period. A dose of Tdap is recommended for postpartum women, close contacts of infants aged less than 12 months, and all health-care personnel with direct patient contact if they have not previously received Tdap. An interval as short as 2 years from the last Td is suggested; shorter intervals can be used. Td may be deferred during pregnancy and Tdap substituted in the immediate postpartum period, or Tdap may be administered instead of Td to a pregnant woman after an informed discussion with the woman.

Consult the ACIP statement for recommendations for administering Td as prophylaxis in wound management.

2. Human papillomavirus (HPV) vaccination

HPV vaccination is recommended for all females aged 11 through 26 years (and may begin at age 9 years) who have not completed the vaccine series. History of genital warts, abnormal Papanicolaou test, or positive HPV DNA test is not evidence of prior infection with all vaccine HPV types; HPV vaccination is recommended for persons with such histories.

Ideally, vaccine should be administered before potential exposure to HPV through sexual activity; however, females who are sexually active should still be vaccinated consistent with age-based recommendations. Sexually active females who have not been infected with any of the four HPV vaccine types receive the full benefit of the vaccination. Vaccination is less beneficial for females who have already been infected with one or more of the HPV vaccine types.

A complete series consists of 3 doses. The second dose should be administered 2 months after the first dose; the third dose should be administered 6 months after the first dose.

HPV vaccination is not specifically recommended for females with the medical indications described in Figure 2, "Vaccines that might be indicated for adults based on medical and other indications." Because HPV vaccine is not a live-virus vaccine, it may be administered to persons with the medical indications described in Figure 2. However, the immune response and vaccine efficacy might be less for persons with the medical indications described in Figure 2 than in persons who do not have the medical indications described or who are immunocompetent. Health-care personnel are not at increased risk because of occupational exposure, and should be vaccinated consistent with age-based recommendations.

3. Varicella vaccination

All adults without evidence of immunity to varicella should receive 2 doses of single-antigen varicella vaccine if not previously vaccinated or the second dose if they have received only one dose, unless they have a medical contraindication. Special consideration should be given to those who 1) have close contact with persons at high risk for severe disease (e.g., health-care personnel and family contacts of persons with immunocompromising conditions) or 2) are at high risk for exposure or transmission (e.g., teachers; child care employees; residents and staff members of institutional settings, including correctional institutions; college students; military personnel; adolescents and adults living in households with children; nonpregnant women of childbearing age; and international travelers).

Evidence of immunity to varicella in adults includes any of the following: 1) documentation of 2 doses of varicella vaccine at least 4 weeks apart; 2) U.S.-born before 1980 (although for health-care personnel and pregnant women, birth before 1980 should not be considered evidence of immunity); 3) history of varicella based on diagnosis or verification of varicella by a health-care provider (for a patient reporting a history of or presenting with an atypical case, a mild case, or both, health-care providers should seek either an epidemiologic link to a typical varicella case or to a laboratory-confirmed case or evidence of laboratory confirmation, if it was performed at the time of acute disease); 4) history of herpes zoster based on health-care provider diagnosis or verification of herpes zoster by a health-care provider; or 5) laboratory evidence of immunity or laboratory confirmation of disease.

Pregnant women should be assessed for evidence of varicella immunity. Women who do not have evidence of immunity should receive the first dose of varicella vaccine upon completion or termination of pregnancy and before discharge from the health-care facility. The second dose should be administered 4–8 weeks after the first dose.

4. Herpes zoster vaccination

A single dose of zoster vaccine is recommended for adults aged 60 years and older regardless of whether they report a prior episode of herpes zoster. Persons with chronic medical conditions may be vaccinated unless their condition constitutes a contraindication.

5. Measles, mumps, rubella (MMR) vaccination

Measles component: Adults born before 1957 generally are considered immune to measles. Adults born during or after 1957 should receive 1 or more doses of MMR unless they have a medical contraindication, documentation of 1 or more doses, history of measles based on health-care provider diagnosis, or laboratory evidence of immunity.

A second dose of MMR is recommended for adults who 1) have been recently exposed to measles or are in an outbreak setting; 2) have been vaccinated previously with killed measles vaccine; 3) have been vaccinated with an unknown type of measles vaccine during 1963–1967; 4) are students in postsecondary educational institutions; 5) work in a health-care facility; or 6) plan to travel internationally.

Mumps component: Adults born before 1957 generally are considered immune to mumps. Adults born during or after 1957 should receive 1 dose of MMR unless they have a medical contraindication, history of mumps based on health-care provider diagnosis, or laboratory evidence of immunity.

A second dose of MMR is recommended for adults who 1) live in a community experiencing a mumps outbreak and are in an affected age group; 2) are students in postsecondary educational institutions; 3) work in a health-care facility; or 4) plan to travel internationally. For unvaccinated health-care personnel born before 1957 who do not have other evidence of mumps immunity, administering 1 dose on a routine basis should be considered and administering a second dose during an outbreak should be strongly considered.

Rubella component: 1 dose of MMR vaccine is recommended for women whose rubella vaccination history is unreliable or who lack laboratory evidence of immunity. For women of childbearing age, regardless of birth year, rubella immunity should be determined and women should be counseled regarding congenital rubella syndrome. Women who do not have evidence of immunity should receive MMR vaccine upon completion or termination of pregnancy and before discharge from the health-care facility.

6. Influenza vaccination

Medical indications: Chronic disorders of the cardiovascular or pulmonary systems, including asthma; chronic metabolic diseases, including diabetes mellitus, renal or hepatic dysfunction, hemoglobinopathies, or immunocompromising conditions (including immunocompromising conditions caused by medications or human immunodeficiency virus [HIV]); any condition that compromises respiratory function or the handling of respiratory secretions or that can increase the risk of aspiration (e.g., cognitive dysfunction, spinal cord injury, or seizure disorder or other neuromuscular disorder); and pregnancy during the influenza season. No data exist on the risk for severe or complicated influenza disease among persons with asplenia; however, influenza is a risk factor for secondary bacterial infections that can cause severe disease among persons with asplenia.

Occupational indications: All health-care personnel, including those employed by long-term care and assisted-living facilities, and caregivers of children less than 5 years old.

Other indications: Residents of nursing homes and other long-term care and assisted-living facilities; persons likely to transmit influenza to persons at high risk (e.g., in-home household contacts and caregivers of children aged less than 5 years old, persons 65 years old and older and persons of all ages with high-risk condition[s]); and anyone who would like to decrease their risk of getting influenza. Healthy, nonpregnant adults aged less than 50 years without high-risk medical conditions who are not contacts of severely immunocompromised persons in special care units can receive either intranasally administered live, attenuated influenza vaccine (FluMist®) or inactivated vaccine. Other persons should receive the inactivated vaccine.

7. Pneumococcal polysaccharide (PPSV) vaccination

Medical indications: Chronic lung disease (including asthma); chronic cardiovascular diseases; diabetes mellitus; chronic liver diseases, cirrhosis; chronic alcoholism, chronic renal failure or nephrotic syndrome; functional or anatomic asplenia (e.g., sickle cell disease or splenectomy [if elective splenectomy is planned, vaccinate at least 2 weeks before surgery]); immunocompromising conditions; and cochlear implants and cerebrospinal fluid leaks. Vaccinate as close to HIV diagnosis as possible.

Other indications: Residents of nursing homes or other long-term care facilities and persons who smoke cigarettes. Routine use of PPSV is not recommended for Alaska Native or American Indian persons younger than 65 years unless they have underlying medical conditions that are PPSV indications. However, public health authorities may consider recommending PPSV for Alaska Natives and American Indians aged 50 through 64 years who are living in areas in which the risk of invasive pneumococcal disease is increased.

8. Revaccination with PPSV

One-time revaccination after 5 years is recommended for persons with chronic renal failure or nephrotic syndrome; functional or anatomic asplenia (e.g., sickle cell disease or splenectomy); and for persons with immunocompromising conditions. For persons aged 65 years and older, one-time revaccination if they were vaccinated 5 or more years previously and were aged less than 65 years at the time of primary vaccination.

9. Hepatitis A vaccination

Medical indications: Persons with chronic liver disease and persons who receive clotting factor concentrates.

Behavioral indications: Men who have sex with men and persons who use illegal drugs.

Occupational indications: Persons working with hepatitis A virus (HAV)–infected primates or with HAV in a research laboratory setting.

Other indications: Persons traveling to or working in countries that have high or intermediate endemicity of hepatitis A (a list of countries is available at http://wwwn.cdc.gov/travel/contentdiseases.aspx) and any person seeking protection from HAV infection.

Single-antigen vaccine formulations should be administered in a 2-dose schedule at either 0 and 6–12 months (Havrix®), or 0 and 6–18 months (Vaqta®). If the combined hepatitis A and hepatitis B vaccine (Twinrix®) is used, administer 3 doses at 0, 1, and 6 months; alternatively, a 4-dose schedule, administered on days 0, 7, and 21 to 30 followed by a booster dose at month 12 may be used.

10. Hepatitis B vaccination

Medical indications: Persons with end-stage renal disease, including patients receiving hemodialysis; persons with HIV infection; and persons with chronic liver disease.

Occupational indications: Health-care personnel and public-safety workers who are exposed to blood or other potentially infectious body fluids.

Behavioral indications: Sexually active persons who are not in a long-term, mutually monogamous relationship (e.g., persons with more than 1 sex partner during the previous 6 months); persons seeking evaluation or treatment for a sexually transmitted disease (STD); current or recent injection-drug users; and men who have sex with men.

Other indications: Household contacts and sex partners of persons with chronic hepatitis B virus (HBV) infection; clients and staff members of institutions for persons with developmental disabilities; international travelers to countries with high or intermediate prevalence of chronic HBV infection (a list of countries is available at http://wwwn.cdc.gov/travel/contentdiseases.aspx); and any adult seeking protection from HBV infection.

Hepatitis B vaccination is recommended for all adults in the following settings: STD treatment facilities; HIV testing and treatment facilities; facilities providing drug-abuse treatment and prevention services; health-care settings targeting services to injection-drug users or men who have sex with men; correctional facilities; end-stage renal disease programs and facilities for chronic hemodialysis patients; and institutions and nonresidential daycare facilities for persons with developmental disabilities.

If the combined hepatitis A and hepatitis B vaccine (Twinrix®) is used, administer 3 doses at 0, 1, and 6 months; alternatively, a 4-dose schedule, administered on days 0, 7, and 21 to 30 followed by a booster dose at month 12 may be used.

Special formulation indications: For adult patients receiving hemodialysis or with other immunocompromising conditions, 1 dose of 40 µg/mL (Recombivax HB®) administered on a 3-dose schedule or 2 doses of 20 µg/mL (Engerix-B®) administered simultaneously on a 4-dose schedule at 0,1, 2 and 6 months.

11. Meningococcal vaccination

Medical indications: Adults with anatomic or functional asplenia, or terminal complement component deficiencies.

Other indications: First-year college students living in dormitories; microbiologists routinely exposed to isolates of *Neisseria meningitidis*; military recruits; and persons who travel to or live in countries in which meningococcal disease is hyperendemic or epidemic (e.g., the "meningitis belt" of sub-Saharan Africa during the dry season [December–June]), particularly if their contact with local populations will be prolonged. Vaccination is required by the government of Saudi Arabia for all travelers to Mecca during the annual Hajj.

Meningococcal conjugate vaccine (MCV) is preferred for adults with any of the preceding indications who are aged 55 years or younger, although meningococcal polysaccharide vaccine (MPSV) is an acceptable alternative. Revaccination with MCV after 5 years might be indicated for adults previously vaccinated with MPSV who remain at increased risk for infection (e.g., persons residing in areas in which disease is epidemic).

12. Selected conditions for which *Haemophilus influenzae* type B (Hib) vaccine may be used

Hib vaccine generally is not recommended for persons aged 5 years and older. No efficacy data are available on which to base a recommendation concerning use of Hib vaccine for older children and adults. However, studies suggest good immunogenicity in patients who have sickle cell disease, leukemia, or HIV infection or who have had a splenectomy; administering 1 dose of vaccine to these patients is not contraindicated.

13. Immunocompromising conditions

Inactivated vaccines generally are acceptable (e.g., pneumococcal, meningococcal, and influenza [trivalent inactivated influenza vaccine]) and live vaccines generally are avoided in persons with immune deficiencies or immunocompromising conditions. Information on specific conditions is available at *http://www.cdc.gov/vaccines/pubs/acip-list.htm.*

ORAL CONTRACEPTIVES

DRUG	ESTROGEN	PROGESTIN	STRENGTH (ESTROGEN-PROGESTIN)
MONOPHASIC			
Alesse, Aviane, Lessina	Ethinyl Estradiol	Levonorgestrel	20 mcg-0.1 mg
Apri, Desogen, Ortho-Cept	Ethinyl Estradiol	Desogestrel	30 mcg-0.15 mg
Brevicon, Necon 0.5/35, Nortrel 0.5/35	Ethinyl Estradiol	Norethindrone	35 mcg-0.5 mg
Demulen 1/35, Zovia 1/35E	Ethinyl Estradiol	Ethynodiol Diacetate	35 mcg-1 mg
Demulen 1/50, Zovia 1/50E	Ethinyl Estradiol	Ethynodiol Diacetate	50 mcg-1 mg
Levora, Nordette, Portia	Ethinyl Estradiol	Levonorgestrel	30 mcg-0.15 mg
Loestrin 1/20, Loestrin Fe 1/20 Microgestin Fe 1/20, Junel 1/20	Ethinyl Estradiol	Norethindrone Acetate	20 mcg-1 mg
Loestrin 21 1.5/30, Loestrin Fe 1.5/30, Microgestin 1.5/30, Junel 1.5/30	Ethinyl Estradiol	Norethindrone Acetate	30 mcg-1.5 mg
Lo/Ovral, Low-Ogestrol, Cryselle	Ethinyl Estradiol	Norgestrel	30 mcg-0.3 mg
Necon 1/35, Norinyl 1/35, Ortho-Novum 1/35, Norcept-E 1/35, Nortrel 1/35, Norethin 1/35E	Ethinyl Estradiol	Norethindrone	35 mcg-1 mg

Necon 1/50, Norinyl 1/50, Norethin 1/50M	Mestranol	Norethindrone	50 mcg-1 mg
Ortho-Cyclen, Previfem, Sprintec, Mononessa	Ethinyl Estradiol	Norgestimate	35 mcg-0.25 mg
Balziva, Ovcon 35	Ethinyl Estradiol	Norethindrone	35 mcg-0.4 mg
Ovcon 50	Ethinyl Estradiol	Norethindrone	50 mcg-1 mg
Ogestrel-28	Ethinyl Estradiol	Norgestrel	50 mcg-0.5 mg
Seasonale	Ethinyl Estradiol	Levonorgestrel	30 mcg-0.15 mg
Yasmin	Ethinyl Estradiol	Drospirenone	30 mcg-3 mg
YAZ	Ethinyl Estradiol	Drospirenone	20 mcg-3 mg
BIPHASIC			
Aranelle, Gencept 10/11, Necon 10/11, Ortho-Novum 10/11	Ethinyl Estradiol	Norethindrone	**Phase 1:** 35 mcg-0.5 mg **Phase 2:** 35 mcg-1 mg
Mircette, Kariva	Ethinyl Estradiol	Desogestrel	**Phase 1:** 20 mcg-0.15 mg **Phase 2:** 10 mcg-NONE
TRIPHASIC			
Cyclessa, Velivet	Ethinyl Estradiol	Desogestrel	**Phase 1:** 25 mcg-0.1 mg **Phase 2:** 25 mcg-0.125 mg **Phase 3:** 25 mcg-0.15 mg
Estrostep	Ethinyl Estradiol	Norethindrone	**Phase 1:** 20 mcg-1 mg **Phase 2:** 30 mcg-1 mg **Phase 3:** 35 mcg-1 mg

DRUG	ESTROGEN	PROGESTIN	STRENGTH (ESTROGEN-PROGESTIN)
Ortho-Novum 7/7/7, Necon 7/7/7, Nortrel 7/7/7	Ethinyl Estradiol	Norethindrone	**Phase 1:** 35 mcg-0.5 mg **Phase 2:** 35 mcg-0.75 mg **Phase 3:** 35 mcg-1 mg
Ortho Tri-Cyclen Tri-Sprintec, Tri-Previfem	Ethinyl Estradiol	Norgestimate	**Phase 1:** 35 mcg-0.18 mg **Phase 2:** 35 mcg-0.215 mg **Phase 3:** 35 mcg-0.25 mg
Ortho Tri-Cyclen Lo	Ethinyl Estradiol	Norgestimate	**Phase 1:** 25 mcg-0.18 mg **Phase 2:** 25 mcg-0.215 mg **Phase 3:** 25 mcg-0.25 mg
Expresse, Triphasil, Trivora	Ethinyl Estradiol	Levonorgestrel	**Phase 1:** 30 mcg-0.05 mg **Phase 2:** 40 mcg-0.075 mg **Phase 3:** 30 mcg-0.125 mg
Tri-Norinyl	Ethinyl Estradiol	Norethindrone	**Phase 1:** 35 mcg-0.5 mg **Phase 2:** 35 mcg-1 mg **Phase 3:** 35 mcg-0.5 mg
PROGESTIN ONLY			
Ortho-Micronor, Nor-Q.D, Camila, Errin		Norethindrone	0.35 mg
EMERGENCY			
Plan B		Levonorgestrel	0.75 mg

SYSTEMIC CORTICOSTEROIDS

CORTICOSTEROID	EQUIVALENT POTENCY	MINERALOCORTICOID POTENCY	FORM/STRENGTH	DOSAGE RANGE
Betamethasone (Celestone)	0.6 mg	0	**Syr:** 0.6 mg/5 ml	**Initial:** 0.6-7.2 mg/d PO.
Betamethasone Sodium Phosphate & Betamethasone Acetate (Celestone Soluspan)	0.6 mg	0	**Inj:** 3 mg-3 mg/ml	**Initial:** 0.25-9 mg/d IM.
Cortisone Acetate	25 mg	2	**Tab:** 25 mg	**Initial:** 25-300 mg/d PO.
Dexamethasone (Decadron)	0.5 mg	0	**Sol:** 0.5 mg/5 ml **Tab:** 0.5 mg, 0.75 mg, 1 mg, 1.5 mg, 2 mg, 4 mg, 6 mg	**Initial:** 0.75-9 mg/d PO.
Dexamethasone Sodium Phosphate (Decadron Phosphate)	0.5 mg	0	**Inj:** 4 mg/ml	**Initial:** 0.5-9 mg/d IM/IV.
Hydrocortisone (Cortef)	20 mg	2	**Tab:** 5 mg, 10 mg, 20 mg	**Initial:** 20-240 mg/d PO.
Hydrocortisone Cypionate (Cortef)	20 mg	2	**Susp:** 10 mg/5 ml	**Initial:** 20-240 mg/d PO.
Hydrocortisone Sodium Succinate (Solu-Cortef)	20 mg	2	**Inj:** 100 mg, 250 mg, 500 mg, 1000 mg	**Initial:** 100-500 mg IM/IV.

CORTICOSTEROID	EQUIVALENT POTENCY	MINERALOCORTICOID POTENCY	FORM/STRENGTH	DOSAGE RANGE
Methylprednisolone (Medrol)	4 mg	0	**Tab:** 2 mg, 4 mg, 8 mg, 16 mg, 24 mg, 32 mg	**Initial:** 4-48 mg/d PO.
Methylprednisolone Acetate (Depo-Medrol)	4 mg	0	**Inj:** 20 mg/ml, 40 mg/ml, 80 mg/ml	**Initial:** 40-120 mg/wk IM.
Methylprednisolone Sodium Succinate (Solu-Medrol)	4 mg	0	**Inj:** 40 mg, 125 mg, 500 mg, 1 gm, 2 gm	**Initial:** 10-40 mg IV.
Prednisolone (Prelone)	5 mg	1	**Syr:** 5 mg/5 ml, 15 mg/5 ml	**Initial:** 5-60 mg/d PO.
Prednisolone Sodium Phosphate (Pediapred)	5 mg	1	**Sol:** 5 mg/5 ml	**Initial:** 5-60 mg/d PO.
Prednisone (Deltasone)	5 mg	1	**Sol:** 5 mg/ml, 5 mg/5 ml; **Tab:** 1 mg, 2.5 mg, 5 mg, 10 mg, 20 mg, 50 mg	**Initial:** 5-60 mg/d PO.
Triamcinolone (Aristocort)	4 mg	0	**Tab:** 4 mg	**Initial:** 4-60 mg/d PO.
Triamcinolone Acetonide (Kenalog-10)	4 mg	0	**Inj:** 10 mg/ml	**Intra-articular/ Intrabursal:** 2.5-20 mg/d.

Triamcinolone Acetonide (Kenalog-40)	4 mg	0	**Inj:** 40 mg/ml	**Initial:** 2.5-60 mg/d IM or intra-articular.
Triamcinolone Hexacetonide (Aristospan Intra-lesional, Aristospan Intra-articular)	4 mg	0	**Inj:** 5 mg/ml (intralesional), 20 mg/ml (intra-articular)	**Intra-articular:** 2-48 mg. **Intra-lesional:** Up to 0.5 mg/in^2 of area affected.

TOPICAL CORTICOSTEROIDS—RELATIVE POTENCY AND DOSAGE

DRUG	DOSAGE FORM (S)	STRENGTH (%)	POTENCY	FREQUENCY
Alclometasone Dipropionate (Aclovate)	Cre, Oint	0.05	Low	bid/tid
Amcinonide (Cyclocort)	Cre, Lot, Oint	0.1	High	bid/tid
Augmented Betamethasone Dipropionate Diprolene, Diprolene AF)	Oint	0.05	Very High	qd/bid
	Cre, Lot	0.05	High	qd/bid
Betamethasone Dipropionate (Diprosone, Alphatrex)	Cre, Lot, Oint	0.05	High	qd/bid
Betamethasone Valerate (Beta-Val, Betaderm)	Cre, Lot, Oint	0.1	Medium	qd/tid
Betamethasone Valerate (Luxiq)	Foam	0.12	Medium	bid
Clobetasol Propionate (Clobevate, Clobex, Cormax, Olux, Olux-E, Temovate)	Cre, Foam, Gel Lot, Oint, Sol	0.05	Very High	bid
	Shampoo (Clobex)	0.05	Very High	qd
Clocortolone Pivalate (Cloderm)	Cre	0.1	Low	tid
Desonide (DesOwen, Tridesilon)	Cre, Lot, Oint	0.05	Low	bid/tid
Desoximetasone (Topicort)	Cre	0.05	Medium	bid
	Gel	0.05	High	bid
	Cre, Oint	0.25	High	bid
Diflorasone Diacetate (Florone, Florone E)	Cre, Oint (Florone)	0.05	High	qd/qid
	Cre, Oint (Psorcon)	0.05	Very High	qd/tid

Fluocinolone Acetonide (Capex, Derma-Smoothe/FS, Synalar)	Cre, Oint	0.025	Medium	bid/qid
	Oil	0.01	Medium	qd/tid
	Shampoo (Capex)	0.01	Medium	qd
	Sol	0.01	Medium	bid/qid
Fluocinonide (Lidex, Lidex-E, Vanos)	Cre, Gel, Oint, Sol	0.05	High	bid/qid
	Cre	0.1	High	qd/bid
Flurandrenolide (Cordran, Cordran SP)	Cre, Lot	0.05	Medium	bid/qid
	Tape	4 mcg/cm^2	Medium	qd/bid
Fluticasone Propionate (Cutivate)	Cre	0.05	Medium	qd/bid
	Oint	0.005	Medium	bid
Halcinonide (Halog)	Cre, Oint, Sol	0.1	High	qd/tid
Halobetasol Propionate (Ultravate)	Cre, Oint	0.05	Very High	qd/bid
Hydrocortisone (Ala-Scalp HP, Ala-Cort, Cortaid, Texacort, Cetacort)	Cre, Oint	0.5	Low	tid/qid
	Cre, Lot, Oint, Sol	1	Low	tid/qid
	Lot	2	Low	tid/qid
	Cre, Lot, Oint, Sol	2.5	Low	bid/qid
Hydrocortisone Butyrate (Locoid)	Cre, Oint, Sol	0.1	Medium	bid/tid
Hydrocortisone Probutate (Pandel)	Cre	0.1	Medium	qd/bid
Hydrocortisone Valerate (Westcort)	Cre, Oint	0.2	Medium	bid/tid
Mometasone Furoate (Elocon)	Cre, Lot, Oint	0.1	Medium	qd
Prednicarbate (Dermatop E)	Cre, Oint	0.1	Medium	bid

Triamcinolone Acetonide (Kenalog, Triacet)	Cre, Lot	0.025	Medium	bid/qid
	Cre, Lot, Oint	0.1	Medium	bid/tid
	Cre	0.5	High	bid/tid
	Spr	0.147 mg/gm	Medium	tid/qid

INDEX

D

F

G

H

S

U

V